AMERICAN JOURNAL of PUBLIC HEALTH
APRIL 2025
Issue 4

AJPH

A PUBLICATION OF THE
AMERICAN PUBLIC HEALTH ASSOCIATION

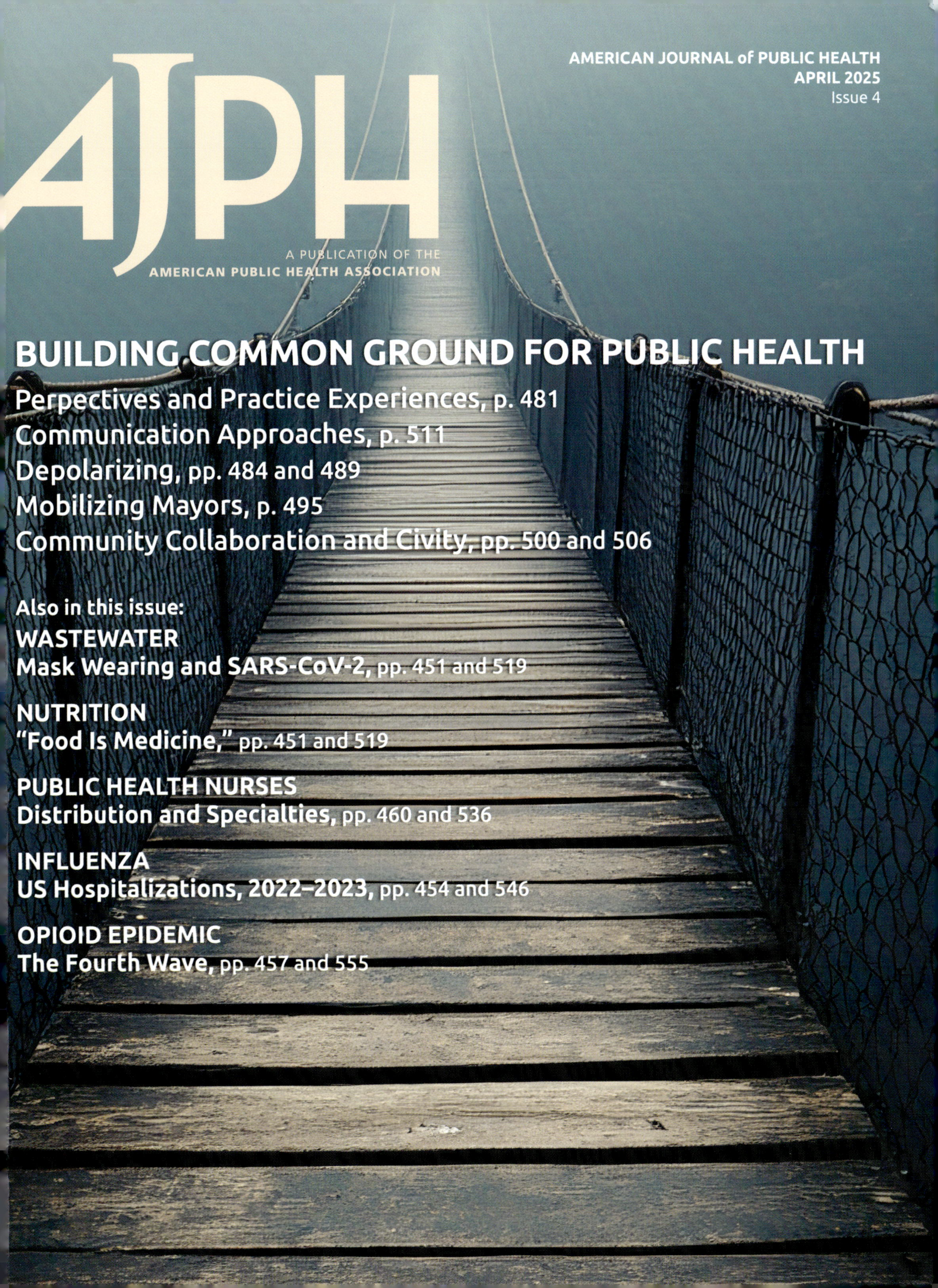

BUILDING COMMON GROUND FOR PUBLIC HEALTH

Perpectives and Practice Experiences, p. 481
Communication Approaches, p. 511
Depolarizing, pp. 484 and 489
Mobilizing Mayors, p. 495
Community Collaboration and Civity, pp. 500 and 506

Also in this issue:

WASTEWATER
Mask Wearing and SARS-CoV-2, pp. 451 and 519

NUTRITION
"Food Is Medicine," pp. 451 and 519

PUBLIC HEALTH NURSES
Distribution and Specialties, pp. 460 and 536

INFLUENZA
US Hospitalizations, 2022–2023, pp. 454 and 546

OPIOID EPIDEMIC
The Fourth Wave, pp. 457 and 555

APHA
AMERICAN PUBLIC HEALTH ASSOCIATION
For science. For action. For health.

AJPH®, published monthly, is the official Journal of the American Public Health Association®, 800 I St NW, Washington, DC 20001-3710; (202) 777- APHA; TDD (202) 777-2500. APHA is a nongovernmental professional society founded in 1872, representing all disciplines and specialties in public health.

The *American Journal of Public Health*® (*AJPH*) (print ISSN: 0090-0036; electronic ISSN: 1541- 0048), first published in 1911, is the official journal of the American Public Health Association® (APHA). The oldest and largest organization of public health professionals in the world, APHA represents approximately 30 000 members from more than 50 occupations of public health.

Submissions: Visit www.editorialmanager.com/ajph or ajph.edmgr.com for online manuscript preparation and submission guidelines. Contributions of original unpublished research, social science analyses, scholarly essays, critical commentaries, departments, and letters to the editor are welcome. Questions? Write ajph.submissions@apha.org or call APHA at (202) 777-2469.

Print plus online subscriptions: Institutional price (print copy with online access for a single institution and all authorized users, regardless of geographic location) varies by size of organization and ranges from $993–$1445 for US organizations, and $1073–$1526 for international organizations (air delivery); multiple campuses not permitted without special arrangement. Details of the tiered pricing system at https://subscriptionoffice.com/pages/apha-landing-page. To order, write apha.subscriptions@apha.org.

Online-only subscriptions: Institutional price for one institution and its authorized users (regardless of geographic location) is $878–$1307. To order, write apha.subscriptions@apha.org. For academic consortia or multisite corporate subscriptions, contact apha.subscriptions@apha.org.

Print-only subscriptions: Institutional price is US $701, $782 international.

Back print issues: A limited number of print issues are for sale. Single copies are US $65, $75 international (air delivery). Shipping included; prepay only. To order, write apha.subscriptions@apha.org.

Reprints: For prices and ordering information on 50 or more reprints, check the Reprints section at www.ajph.org. To order smaller quantities of reprints (rush delivery), use the "Purchase Article" link on the article site itself.

Electronic access: Online articles more than 10 years old are available free for personal use at www.ajph.org. Recent articles are available through pay-per-view: single PDF article for $24, single issue access for 24 hours for $33, or entire site access for 24 hours for $38.

Postal information: Periodicals postage paid at Washington, DC, and additional mailing offices. Postmaster: Send address changes to American Journal of Public Health, 800 I St NW, Washington, DC 20001-3710.

Address changes: Send to AJPH, Membership Department (members) or AJPH Subscriptions (subscribers), APHA, 800 I St NW, Washington, DC 20001-3710. Or write to membership.mail@apha.org (members) or apha.subscriptions@apha.org (subscribers).

Advertising: For pricing and other information, see www.ajph.org. Please write to brian.selzer@apha.org or call (202) 777-2470 for other advertising opportunities. Ask about special exhibit packages and sponsorships. Acceptance of advertising by the *Journal* does not imply endorsement of products.

Indexes: Publications that index or abstract articles from *AJPH* include the following: Ageline, Assia (Applied Social Science Index and Abstracts), Biological Abstracts, Chemical Abstracts, CINAHL, Criminal Justice Abstracts, EMBASE, EMCare, Environmental Abstracts, e-psyche, ERIC, ETOH (Alcohol and Alcohol Problems Science Database), Excerpta Medica, Food Science and Technology, General Science Index, Grateful Med, Hospital Literature Index, Human Resources Abstracts, International Pharmaceutical Abstracts (IPA), Medline, Physical Education Index, Pollution Abstracts, Psychological Abstracts, PsychINFO, Safety Science Abstracts, Sage Family Studies Abstracts, Sage Human Resources Abstracts, Science Citation Index, SCOPUS, SIIC Data Bases, Social Work Research and Abstracts, and Statistical Reference Index (SRI)/LexisNexis.

AJPH

A PUBLICATION OF THE
AMERICAN PUBLIC HEALTH ASSOCIATION

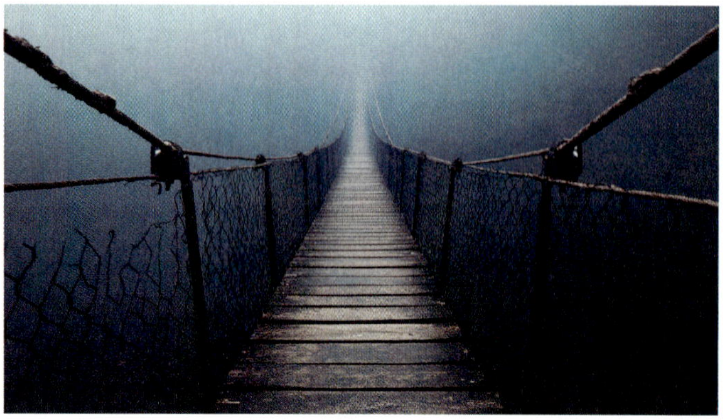

COVER: *AJPH* has stressed for many years that we need to communicate health information to all audiences. In public health we must deliver evidence-based information while going beyond simple fact corrections. Simultaneously focusing on our shared identities, common goals, and mutual empathy is a long-term solution to help create a dialogue and bridge divides.

Cover concept and selection by Aleisha Kropf. Image by vetrana / Adobe Stock, printed with permission.

APHA
AMERICAN PUBLIC HEALTH ASSOCIATION
For science. For action. For health.

Promoting public health research, policy, practice, and education is the *AJPH* mission. As we widen our scope to embrace global issues, we also sharpen our focus to support the needs of public health practitioners. We invite contributions of original unpublished research, opinion and commentary, and letters to the editor.

The *Journal* is printed on acid-free recycled paper.

AJPH April 2025, Vol. 115, No. 4

OPEN ACCESS ONLINE ONLY PODCAST DATA SUPPLEMENT AVAILABLE

EDITOR'S CHOICE

446 The State of the Public Health Union 2025
A. Morabia

BOOKS & MEDIA

448 The Challenger Disaster: NASA, Public Health, and the Precautionary Principle
N. Pearce

OPINIONS, IDEAS, & PRACTICE

EDITORIALS

451 Benefits of Masks as a School-Based Prevention Intervention Outweigh the Risks
C.A. Teasdale and S.A. Fleary

454 Using Surveillance Data to Estimate Infectious Disease Burden: Opportunities and Challenges
H. Hochheiser and P. Kumar

457 The Evolving Overdose Crisis: United States Needs Robust Policy Change to Address the Fourth Wave
S.V. Aronowitz and M.K. Reed

460 Considering the Complexity of Professional Identity for Public Health Nurse Workforce Enumeration
S.M. Kneipp

463 Can "Food Is Medicine" Interventions Be Positioned to Combat the Historical Effects of Racism in Black Communities Deprived of Food Resources?
C.R. Singleton

PERSPECTIVES

466 How US Grassroots Organizations Confront the Global Anti-LGBTQ+ Crisis and Support LGBTQ+ Asylum Seekers
C. Nnaji, A. Green, and N.J. Weeks

NOTES FROM THE FIELD

469 Better Together: Implementation of a Public Health Learning Community During the COVID-19 Pandemic
K.M. Brown, B. Courtot, Z. Porter, and S. Hinojosa

473 Outreach to Adolescents in Crisis on Social Media, YouthLine's Safe Social Spaces, 2019 to 2024
C. Leets, A. Nielsen, M. Buchanan, A. Zirikly, M. Dredze, L. Miller, H.C. Wilcox, and C. Gallo

477 A Novel Reentry Hotline Led by Community Health Workers to Address the Health Needs of People Returning From Incarceration: Transitions Clinic Network, California, June 2020–June 2023
B. Divakaran, A. Steiner, S. Lin, S. Fennix, and S. Shavit

COMMON GROUND

481 Building Common Ground for Public Health: Perspectives and Practice Experiences
W.J. Kassler, H. Rodenberg, and S.C. Fiala

484 Depolarization Through Public-Sector Leadership Development: Emerging Leaders and Fellows Programs, United States, 2015–2024
M.F. McDonald

489 Depolarizing Health Policy Through Intergenerational Conversations
B. Jain, J.C. Lin, and J.M. Adams

492 Toward Common Ground: Rethinking Both Public Health and Religion, Together
G. Gunderson, J.R. Cochrane, and T. Cutts

495 Mobilizing Mayors Across the Political Spectrum to Promote Population Health: The Move With the Mayor Initiative
E. Waugh, J. Childress, M. Snyder, C. Muryn, and J. Clymer

500 Exploring Democratic Deliberation in Public Health: Bridging Division and Enhancing Community Engagement
M. Bosché, R. Krust, A. Fung, and A.S. Pawar

506 A "Civity" Approach Helps Build the Civic Muscle That Underlies Healthy Communities
P.J. Strand and M.R. Kopell

RESEARCH & ANALYSIS

COMMON GROUND

511 Public Health Communication Approaches for Building Common Ground
W-Y.S. Chou, I.A. Iles, A. Gaysynsky, and W.M.P. Klein

CLIMATE CHANGE

519 Observed Mask Wearing and Presence of SARS-CoV-2 in School Wastewater, San Diego County, CA, 2022
R. Fielding-Miller, T. Gaines, A. Hassani, T. Le, V. Omaleki, M. Flores, A. Majnoonian, F.C. Wijaya, R. Knight, S. Karthikeyan, and R.S. Garfein

PERSPECTIVES FROM THE SOCIAL SCIENCES

528 Amplifying Lived Expertise on "Food Is Medicine" in the Mississippi Delta's Legacy of Racism
V. Nicholson-Robinson, D.M. Krobath, S. Dixit-Joshi, C. Hawkins, J. Miller, D.J. Schultz, and C. Economos

POLICY

536 Distribution and Specialties of Broadly Versus Narrowly Defined Public Health Nurses Working in Government Settings in the United States, 2022
B. Bekemeier, P.M. Kett, G. Whitman, K. Chadwick, and J.K. Edmonds

METHODS

546 State-Level Influenza Hospitalization Burden in the United States, 2022–2023
A. Couture, A.D. Iuliano, H.H. Chang, R. Threlkel, M. Gilmer, A. O'Halloran, D. Ujamaa, M. Biggerstaff, and C. Reed

HEALTH MONITORING

555 The Fourth Wave of the Opioid Epidemic: Increasing Combination of Fentanyl With Stimulants
K. Diekhans, J. Yu, S. Pearring, R. Almeida, and L.N. Rodda

566 State Child Abuse and Mandated Reporting Policies for Prenatal Substance Use and Congenital Syphilis Case Rates: United States, 2018–2022
A.E. Austin, K. O'Callaghan, J. Rushmore, R. Cramer, R. McDonald, and E.R. Learner

575 Syndromic Surveillance and Case Identification for Varicella Among Recent Immigrants: New York City, 2023
M. S. Askari, R. J. Arciuolo, O. Matalka, K. A. Graham, B. M. Isaac, R. Lall, A. Jean, and J. B. Rosen

OPEN-THEMED RESEARCH

579 Population-Level Risks for HIV Mortality During the COVID-19 Pandemic in the United States by Demographic Characteristics and Medicaid Access, 2020–2021
D. Purcell, W. A. Duffus, M. Standifer, R. Mayberry, and S. S. Hutchins

588 OSHA Injury Data: An Opportunity for Improving Work Injury Prevention
D. Michaels and G. R. Wagner

596 Navigating Dual-Harm: Integrating Self- and Other-Harm Into Public Health Inquiry
D. A. Díaz-Faes, S. Rajan, and C. C. Branas

605 Outcomes of Home Isolation Care Among COVID-19 Patients During the 2021 Epidemic Crisis in the Bangkok Metropolitan Region, Thailand
T. Lertwanichwattana, S. Srivanichakorn, S. Noknoy, S. S. N. Ratchaseema, N. Phanuphak, K. Wongthavarawat, A. Siriussawakul, V. Srinonprasert, P. Leelahavarong, P. Chevaisrakul, P. Lumjiaktase, A. Kumpitak, N. Phromsri, Y. Sirisinsuk, P. Kietdumrongwong, A. Aramrattana, and R. Rangsin

UPMC | HILLMAN CANCER CENTER

Associate Director for Community Outreach and Engagement
UPMC Hillman Cancer Center, Pittsburgh, PA

UPMC Hillman Cancer Center (UPMC Hillman) seeks a dynamic **Professor** level faculty leader with demonstrated experience in community-engaged outreach, research and/or practice to support bidirectional engagement with community members, community organizations, and other stakeholders. The **Associate Director for Community Outreach and Engagement (AD for COE)** will work closely with the Director, Deputy Director, and other Associate Directors to coordinate a community outreach and engagement agenda for UPMC Hillman.

Pittsburgh is routinely ranked as one of the top-most livable and affordable U.S. cities. Located in the city of Pittsburgh's Shadyside neighborhood, UPMC Hillman is an NCI-designated comprehensive matrix cancer center focused on state-of-the-art cancer research, training the next generation of cancer researchers, and community outreach. In 2020, UPMC Hillman celebrated its 34th anniversary and the renewal of its 5-year NCI Cancer Center Support Grant (CCSG) that resulted in Hillman Research Administration scoring in the 'Exceptional' range and qualifying UPMC Hillman for a 2-year merit extension. UPMC Hillman serves 29 western PA counties serving nearly 5 million individuals and provides unique opportunities to collaborate with clinical and translational research programs involved in cancer patient care, including the University of Pittsburgh, Magee-Women's Research Institute and UPMC Children's Hospital of Pittsburgh. UPMC Hillman has over 330 members, 7 scientific programs, 10 CCSG-supported shared resources, $110 million of peer-reviewed cancer-relevant funding with over $60 million from NCI, and an institutional funding base greater than $150 million.

The AD for COE reports directly to UPMC Hillman Cancer Center Director and is a member of UPMC Hillman's Senior Leadership Team. The AD for COE will play a critical role in leading community outreach and engagement as well as screening and prevention studies to quantify and intervene to overcome barriers to screening and early detection of cancer in under-represented minority and rural members of UPMC Hillman catchment area. These appointments are associated with an expectation of promoting external NCI peer reviewed funding, leading the designated programs specifically set forth in the NCI P30 CCSG RFA and stimulating collaborations and our UPMC Hillman network.

Current CCSG COE Specific Aims:
Aim 1: Identify and monitor the cancer burdens of UPMC Hillman catchment area through multiple data sources and stakeholder input.
Aim 2: Implement evidence-based interventions to address the cancer burden within the catchment area and beyond, through strategic community outreach, education, and engagement.
Aim 3: Promote, inform, enhance and disseminate UPMC Hillman research in order to address identified catchment area burdens, ensure representation in clinical trials, synergize policy and advance science.

Major AD for COE tasks includes:

- Designated Leader for COE at UPMC Hillman.
- Member of the Senior Leadership Team (reporting directly to the UPMC Hillman Director)
- Formalize, expand, and lead the Office of Community Outreach.
- Support the enrollment and retention of clinical trial participants representative of the catchment area.
- Work with clinicians and researchers across UPMC Hillman to grow cancer health equity research and service activities throughout the catchment area.

Successful candidates must have a MD, PhD, or equivalent, an exceptional scientific research record encompassing translational or population-based research using state-of-the-art approaches evidenced by scholarly productivity (e.g., grans, publications), a productive academic record of cancer-related research relevant to community outreach and/or engagement. Minimum of 8+ years' experience in a Cancer Center or university setting. Prior leadership experience related to strategic planning, program implementation and/or evaluation is preferred with excellent written and oral communication, computer, people management, and interpersonal skills.

Interested applicants should submit a CV and 1-page personal statement highlighting your qualifications and experience, UPMC Hillman Interim Director, Kathryn Schmitz, PhD, MPH (care of hollidaysm3@upmc.edu).

The State of the Public Health Union 2025

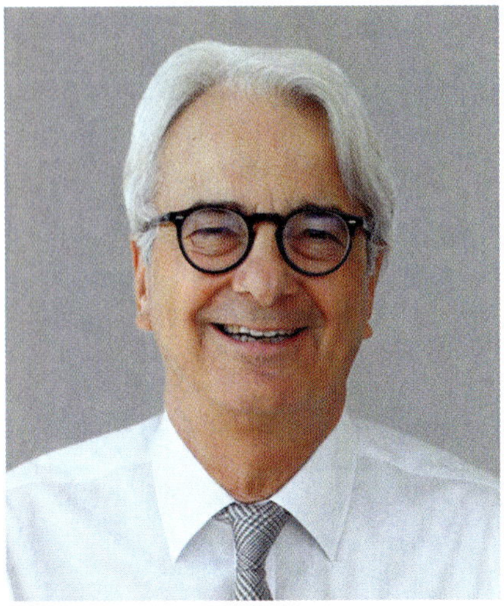

Alfredo Morabia, MD, PhD
Editor-in-Chief, *AJPH*

AJPH April 2025, Vol. 115, No. 4

It is an honor to address you on the State of the Public Health Union, especially as I prepare to step down as editor-in-chief of *AJPH* after 10 years of service. This role has provided a unique perspective on the pivotal events of the past decade, including the COVID-19 pandemic.

My central message is this: public health has never been stronger. Paradoxically, this strength has provoked unprecedented attacks that pose significant challenges.

Many may find this optimistic view surprising, given the persistent criticisms often amplified in the media. However, these criticisms stem from a vocal minority, which has influenced the narrative and, perhaps, key federal agencies. Yet, the data show no widespread distrust of public health among people in the United States, even amid today's political shifts.

Public health's accomplishments—particularly during COVID-19—are extraordinary. Consider vaccine uptake (bit.ly/3Ki0FKe): despite initial skepticism, by 2022, 93% of US adults aged 65 years and older were fully vaccinated, with even the lowest state coverage at 83%. Among adults aged 18 years and older, the national average was 74%. Such logistical and operational success highlights public health's resilience and effectiveness. No one would have predicted such success based on past attempts to mass vaccinate the US population or the usual coverage of the flu vaccine. Similarly, childhood vaccination rates remain high, with 93% of kindergarteners receiving required immunizations in 2022 (https://bit.ly/4hx6guj). These figures reflect enduring public trust.

However, history reminds us that pandemics often trigger fatigue. After the plague pandemics, cholera outbreaks, and even COVID-19, populations tired of prevention measures such as quarantines and isolation. This fatigue is normal and does not inherently threaten public health. What does threaten it are political attacks and disinformation. For example, states that downplayed vaccines saw higher COVID-19 mortality among younger adults (https://bit.ly/40F1Fj3). Alarmingly, childhood vaccination rates have declined in some states, such as Alabama, where rates for children aged 35 months fell from 82.5% in 2017 to 65.5% in 2021 (https://pubmed.ncbi.nlm.nih.gov/38341291).

Why does public health undergo a political backlash from far-right ideologues?

Continued on page 447...

HISTORY CORNER

13 YEARS AGO

The Common Ground Preparedness Framework

In 2006, 6 sites representing state or local public health agencies began a collaboration. "Common Ground: Transforming Public Health Information Systems," . . . Initial meetings revealed many potential business processes of varying scope and overlapping boundaries. It became apparent that some common framework was needed for organizing the processes. Participants considered their public health experience along with several frameworks, including the disaster management cycle, a preparedness framework from the CDC (prevent, detect and report, investigate, control, recover, and improve), the National Response Plan, and the Incident Command System (ICS). The participants drafted, circulated, and refined a progression of at least 8 frameworks, ultimately agreeing on 3 phases of emergency response and several business process groups, each containing specific processes. Advisors from the CDC, ASTHO, NACCHO, and a peer review group from the leadership of 10 state and local public health departments recognized the framework's potential. At their prompting, the Common Ground collaborators developed the comprehensive framework, and at their final meeting, they achieved consensus. . . . The CGPF identifies the business processes required to address an incident that threatens to overwhelm the routine capabilities of a public health system. The processes are grouped into

Because it is inherently inclusive. Public health serves everyone, regardless of documentation, religion, race, or orientation—a value incompatible with exclusionary ideologies. Racism and xenophobia undermine public health, whereas inclusivity strengthens it.

We must distinguish declining trust in political institutions from trust in public health itself. The backlash against public health is politically driven, not rooted in widespread public opinion. If unchecked, it could cause harm.

The pandemic taught us another critical lesson: public health cannot be improvised (https://bit.ly/40Tjb4e). Public health is different from clinical medicine. It requires trained experts capable of solving population-level problems; everyone in public health has to be a population thinker. The training must include public health department professionals, pharmacists, nurses, lab technicians, epidemiologists and statisticians, economists, engineers, doctors, nutritionists, dentists, informaticians, and more. Therefore, protecting public health education is crucial, as is ensuring that leaders and their teams in health institutions possess this expertise.

Democracy is also essential for public health because a public health system relies on both top-down expertise and bottom-up community participation. The transformative movement toward community engagement over the past decade demonstrates this. Programs like CEAL (Community Engagement Alliance Against COVID-19 Disparities; https://ajph.aphapublications.org/toc/ajph/114/S1) and RADx-UP (Rapid Acceleration of Diagnostics for Underserved Populations; https://ajph.aphapublications.org/toc/ajph/112/S9) show how engaging communities protects minoritized populations and counters disinformation.

Community engagement is the foundation of a resilient, inclusive public health system. It strengthens democracy and ensures that, as the theme of this address states, "Threats to democracy are threats to public health." The threats did not begin in 2025, but they are exacerbated by the current presidential administration's decision to eliminate all programs aimed at reducing inequities having structural roots and its attempts to carry out mass deportations of people who already suffered terribly to come to the United States and make a living for their families.

The movement toward a community-centered public health system is here to stay—and it is the future. AJPH

DOI: https://doi.org/10.2105/AJPH.2025.308048

HISTORY CORNER

6 categories: prepare, monitor, investigate, intervene, manage, and recover.

From *AJPH*, April 2012, p. 633

22 YEARS AGO

The Movement for Universal Health Insurance: Finding Common Ground

In 2003, almost no one overtly opposes the idea of universal health insurance, but virtually everyone disagrees with everyone else on how universal health insurance should be constructed.

The American public is now faced with a bewildering array of proposals—employer mandates, individual mandates, voluntary subsidies to employers or to individuals, tax credit plans, Medicaid expansion, Medicare expansion, and publicly administered plans, each with its academic and political supporters. The proposal that continues the pre-1971 idea of a public insurance program supported by social security or taxes is the "single-payer" plan, which I shall call the "public solution." My point of view is that the public solution is the best way to implement universal health insurance, but achieving universal health insurance will be easier if advocates of the public solution and well-intentioned supporters of solutions that contain some private or quasi-private elements seek common ground. How might supporters of the public solution and honest advocates of the private solution find common ground? To start with, they can search for agreement on a vision for a new health care system.

From *AJPH*, January 2003, pp. 112–113

The Challenger Disaster: NASA, Public Health, and the Precautionary Principle

Neil Pearce, PhD

ABOUT THE AUTHOR

Neil Pearce is with the Department of Medical Statistics, London School of Hygiene and Tropical Medicine, London, United Kingdom.

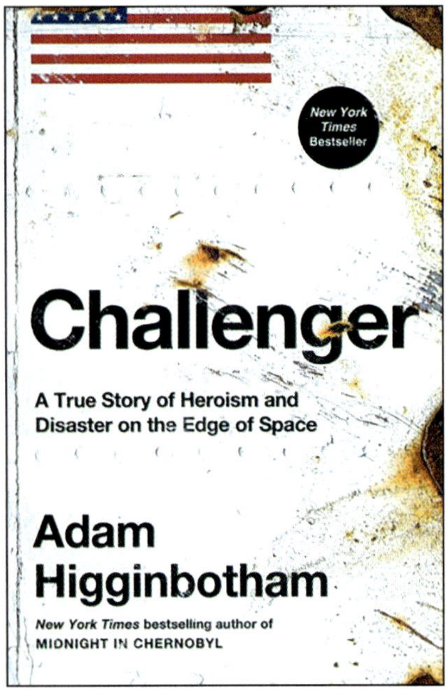

Challenger: A True Story of Heroism and Disaster on the Edge of Space
By Adam Higginbotham
Avid Reader Press/Simon & Schuster, New York, 2024
Hard cover
576 pages
ISBN13: 9781982176617

I can remember exactly where I was when I heard about the Challenger disaster. I was in my office at the University of North Carolina at Chapel Hill, where I was doing a postdoctoral fellowship. It was the height of the Reagan years, full of confidence and hubris. It all came crashing down on the morning of January 28, 1986 when, 73 seconds into its flight, the space shuttle Challenger exploded. The launch had more interest than usual because of Christa McAuliffe, a teacher, who was to become the first civilian in space. She would teach lessons to the world from space, and Reagan would highlight the flight in his State of the Union address that evening.

Concerns about the safety of the shuttle had been known for many years, and that engineers for the key contractor (Morton Thiokol) had recommended against launch, but had been overruled by NASA and by their own bosses. The proximate cause of the disaster had been the decision to go ahead with the launch despite strong evidence that the O-ring joints in the booster rockets would not function properly in cold temperatures. These problems hit the headlines when Richard Feynman, at the subsequent inquiry, showed that they lost their flexibility when dropped into a glass of ice water. Larry Mulloy, manager at the Marshall Space Flight Center, had received a recommendation from engineers not to go ahead in temperatures of less than 53°F; it was 29°F at the time of the launch.

Public health addresses these issues with the precautionary principle,[1] which argues that action should be taken to prevent harm even if some cause-and-effect relationships are not fully established scientifically. At a time when the precautionary principle, and public health in general, is under threat, the Challenger disaster provides a striking lesson in what can happen when corners are cut. In these turbulent times, the principle needs to remain central to our vision and practice. Adam Higginbotham's book *Challenger: A True Story of Heroism and Disaster on the Edge of Space* is not only a fantastic read, but provides striking and clearcut examples as to why the principle should be central to our work.

Of course, there is more to the Challenger story. Harm was not only done because of lack of evidence, but also because evidence was ignored. As with many tragedies, the story of the Challenger is full of "what ifs?" The proximate cause was the decision to go ahead with the launch in extreme cold conditions, against the objections of the Morton Thiokol engineers. But the story of the disaster stretches back right to the start of the space shuttle program.

Every step of the space shuttle story involved compromises, and cost-cutting, each of which slightly increased the risk of disaster. These included the initial decision to use booster rockets rather than a booster vehicle, to use solid booster rockets (they are cheaper than liquid boosters, but once they start, they can't be stopped), to manufacture the boosters in Utah (meaning they had to be shipped in segments and joined using the O-rings), and to have no escape mechanism for crew in the first few minutes of flight. Overlaying all of this was years of evidence, from previous flights, that the O-rings had often been badly damaged during launch, and that their performance was much worse in cold conditions. At a higher level was cost-cutting in the program, the possible loss of the contract by Morton Thiokol, pressure to launch from the politicians and the press, and the huge publicity about Christa McAuliffe's participation. All of this was exaggerated by several postponements, and the fact that a launch had been called off a few days earlier because of an erroneous weather forecast. Mulloy asked, "My God, Thiokol, when do you expect me to launch—next April?"

So the Challenger disaster was an accident waiting to happen. You can only be lucky for so long.

Higginbotham has written an utterly brilliant account of the Challenger disaster, following on from his equally brilliant account of Chernobyl.[2] The outcome is known from the beginning, but this does not make it any less gripping. It is interesting to speculate what the book tells us more generally about decision-making, risk-taking, and public health. Space flight is risky and expensive, though perhaps no more expensive than many other human activities (other branches of science and technology, museums, the National Football League season, or the National Basketball Association season), and no more risky that activities such as skydiving or mountain climbing.

So I don't subscribe to the view that these are unjustified risks or expenses. However, space flight brings many public health issues, and particularly the precautionary principle, into sharp focus. Either the shuttle flies and the crew make it back or they don't. It's digital (a dichotomy). Much of public health is more analog (continuous). We continually make decisions, influenced by political and economic pressures, but it is rare to have disasters as spectacular as the Challenger. Instead, we do better or worse at preventing smoking, air pollution, road accidents, COVID-19, or the health effects of climate change. For example, in the first year of the pandemic, the United States and the United Kingdom had COVID-19 death rates among the highest in the world.[3] This is not seen as such an extreme event as the Challenger, even though a lot more people died. But the underlying principles remain the same. If you cut corners, it catches up with you. It was Ernest Hemingway who, when asked "How did you go bankrupt?" answered "Two ways. Gradually, then suddenly."[4]

The Rogers Report[5] made nine major recommendations, including a redesign of the joints in the solid rockets, changes in the management and regulation of NASA, and the introduction of a new escape mechanism for the astronauts. Other well-known problems were not addressed. In particular, it was already known that there could be damage to the heat-resistant tiles during launch, and this is exactly what happened to the space shuttle Colombia, 17 years later in 2003. NASA engineers three times requested that the suspect area of the left wing be examined by spy satellites, but two requests were rejected and the third was lost in the system. The Colombia broke up on reentry, the second of the four shuttles to be lost.

So what of the future? NASA has new challenges in the return to the moon, a possible human mission to Mars, and also the return of rock and soil samples from Mars. All of these raise issues of the acceptable level of safety—the first two involve the safety of astronauts, whereas the third involves the safety of the planet.[6] All of this can be done at an acceptable level of risk, provided the precautionary principle is followed and available evidence is acted on. But for this to happen, we need much more recognition and discussion of the key pressures and issues involved. How do we communicate uncertainty and risk, and withstand the external pressures from vested interests? How do we act in the presence of uncertainty? What is a reasonable level of risk? The Challenger disaster, and Higginbotham's excellent book, is a great place to start in grappling with these familiar public health issues. AJPH

CORRESPONDENCE

Correspondence should be sent to Professor Neil Pearce, Department of Medical Statistics, London School of Hygiene and Tropical Medicine, Keppel Street, London WC1E 7HT, United Kingdom (e-mail: Neil.pearce@lshtm.ac.uk). Reprints can be ordered at https://www.ajph.org by clicking the "Reprints" link.

PUBLICATION INFORMATION

Full Citation: Pearce N. The Challenger disaster: NASA, public health, and the precautionary principle. *Am J Public Health*. 2025;115(4):448–450.

Acceptance Date: December 23, 2024.

DOI: https://doi.org/10.2105/AJPH.2025.308005

ORCID iD:

Neil Pearce https://orcid.org/0000-0002-9938-7852

CONFLICTS OF INTEREST

The author was a member of a NASA/ESA Committee that produced a report on the safety aspects of the Mars Sample Return.[6]

REFERENCES

1. World Commission on the Ethics of Scientific Knowledge and Technology (COMEST). *The Precautionary Principle.* Paris, France: United Nations Educational, Scientific and Cultural Organization (UNESCO); 2005.
2. Higginbotham A. *Midnight in Chernobyl.* New York, NY: Simon and Schuster; 2019.
3. Vandenbroucke JP, Pearce N. Excess mortality calculations to assess the impact of the COVID-19 pandemic: concepts and methodological issues. *Am J Public Health.* 2024;114(6):593–598. https://doi.org/10.2105/AJPH.2024.307572
4. Hemingway E. *The Sun Also Rises.* New York, NY: Scribners; 1926.
5. *Report to the President: Actions to Implement the Recommendations of the Presidential Commission on the Space Shuttle Challenger Accident.* Washington, DC: National Aeronautics and Space Administration; 1986.
6. Kminek G, Benardini JN, Brenker FE, et al. COSPAR Sample Safety Assessment Framework (SSAF). *Astrobiology.* 2022;22(S1):S186–S216. https://doi.org/10.1089/ast.2022.0017

Benefits of Masks as a School-Based Prevention Intervention Outweigh the Risks

Chloe A. Teasdale, PhD, and Sasha A. Fleary, PhD

ABOUT THE AUTHORS

Chloe A. Teasdale and Sasha A. Fleary are with the City University of New York Graduate School of Public Health and Health Policy, New York, NY.

See also Fielding-Miller et al., p. 519.

In their new study published in this edition of *AJPH*, Fielding-Miller et al. (p. 519) report that mask wearing by children at 10 elementary schools in California was associated with a 10% decrease in severe acute respiratory syndrome coronavirus 2 (SARS-CoV-2) infections as measured in school wastewater. The observational study is one of several demonstrating that masking in schools may be an effective method to reduce COVID-19 transmission.[1–4]

This new study is notable for several reasons. Rather than using self-reported mask use or comparing schools with and without mask mandates (as a proxy for exposure to mask wearing), Fielding-Miller et al. used researcher-observed mask wearing among children at schools, which was correlated with wastewater detection of SARS-CoV-2 five days after observation. The study is unique in selecting schools serving children from historically marginalized communities, which experienced higher burden during the COVID-19 pandemic. It also accounted for important confounders including school size, community COVID-19 infections, and vaccination, and included communities with low (38%) and high (93%) coverage of COVID-19 vaccination.

Another strength of the study was use of wastewater to measure outcomes rather than routinely reported testing data, which were no longer accurate for quantifying disease burden in 2022 because of expanded access to home testing.[5] Wastewater has become essential for ongoing monitoring of COVID-19, as well as other infectious diseases including measles and polio.[6] As shown in this study, wastewater is also a valuable tool for measuring outcomes for impact evaluations of infection mitigation strategies.

While the Fielding-Miller et al. study provides some evidence of the role that masks worn in schools may play in reducing COVID-19 transmission, even with low masking adherence and in settings with varying vaccination coverage, it also has limitations, including that the investigators only examined mask wearing among children and not teachers and other school staff. The study also could not account for mask use outside of schools. Further studies that account for these factors are needed to more fully characterize the impact of masking in schools for COVID-19 prevention.

REFLECTING ON MASK USE

As of November 2024, available data from wastewater monitoring indicate low numbers of COVID-19 infections, as well as lower proportions of hospitalizations and deaths attributed to COVID-19 compared with a year ago.[7] However, concerns remain about the emergence of more transmissible or pathogenic COVID-19 variants, and there are additional threats from other pathogens capable of causing a global pandemic, including the highly lethal influenza virus H5N1, which has already been detected in wastewater in four US states.[8] There is also the increasing worry that in the near future we may see localized outbreaks of vaccine-preventable infections like pertussis and measles as a result of declining vaccination coverage in US children.[9] Unlike with SARS-CoV-2, children are at high risk for serious illness and severe complications from these infections, as well as from influenza, for which vaccination rates have also decreased since 2020. Given these potential threats, the findings in this article, while specific to prevention of COVID-19, provide evidence that masking may be an important mitigation strategy for outbreaks of respiratory infections.

In light of the potential utility of masks as a school-based prevention intervention for future epidemics, we found limited evidence on the impact of masking on development and learning in school-aged children, including long-term studies to understand lasting impact. The available data from a number of studies conducted during the COVID-19 pandemic indicate that masks did not pose a threat to the physical health of children, despite concerns about impaired breathing or other serious health problems.[4] There are, however, mixed findings on possible developmental and cognitive effects of mask use for this age group.

The main areas of research on masking have been focused on potential impairment of social and communicative skills development in children, mainly emotion recognition. A review of the existing evidence suggests that while school-aged children demonstrated lower ability to recognize emotions on masked faces, use of masks did not appear to have had a detrimental effect on learning, language processing, or the ability of children to describe different types of emotions.[10–12] For instance, a US study found that children aged 7 to 12 years were less able to recognize emotions displayed in images of adults with masks compared with those without masks.[10] The same study also found that the effect of masking was most pronounced in children whose families reported more social disruption during the pandemic, suggesting that other factors may explain some of the impairment attributed to masking.

In one of the only randomized controlled trials conducted on mask use in schools, a study from Germany found that among seventh graders randomized to either masks or no masks, there were no differences in cognitive performance between the groups, nor did masks appear to influence attention or executive function.[11] A US study of children aged 4 to 8 years found that while masks did appear to affect emotion recognition, they did not interfere with language processing skills. There are also limited findings with regard to the ability of adults to correctly identify emotions on the faces of children wearing masks, but masks did not impair the ability of adults to conduct assessments, nor did they negatively influence the performance of kindergarteners on oral language measures.[13]

Further studies are needed to understand whether specific groups of children have higher risk of emotion recognition impairment from masks, including those with autism or other neurologic or physical disabilities, as well as to measure any lasting effects and to identify strategies and to improve design characteristics to reduce the risk of any potential negative impact from masking.

MASKS FOR FUTURE EPIDEMICS

Consistent with a public health harm reduction approach, we must consider the best strategies for keeping the public safe during future outbreaks of infectious respiratory infections, whether they are local or global, while also protecting the public's overall well-being and respecting individual rights. Early in the COVID-19 pandemic, there was very little relevant evidence on masking or other interventions, including school closures, to inform guidelines development. We have the opportunity now to use available evidence to reflect and inform more optimal policies for future pandemics.

We feel that there is a strong case to be made for using masks as an effective, albeit imperfect, school-based prevention intervention that aligns with other harm reduction approaches to public health. In light of the available data and weighed against other options that may have more negative consequences—specifically, school closings—masks should be considered an evidence-driven and acceptable intervention. A recent systematic review of studies assessing the effectiveness of school closures on COVID-19 transmission found that while closing schools appears to have prevented infections, it also increased anxiety, depression, and obesity in school-aged children and adolescents.[14] School closures may also have had a negative impact on learning and contributed to widening achievements gaps for some groups of children.[14,15] As highlighted in Fielding-Miller et al., masking in schools may reduce transmission risk from respiratory infections, which could lessen the need for school closures, quarantining, and other mitigation strategies that lead to more profound social disruptions. AJPH

CORRESPONDENCE

Correspondence should be sent to Chloe A. Teasdale, 55 W 125th St, New York, NY 10027 (e-mail: chloe.teasdale@sph.cuny.edu). Reprints can be ordered at https://www.ajph.org by clicking the "Reprints" link.

PUBLICATION INFORMATION

Full Citation: Teasdale CA, Fleary SA. Benefits of masks as a school-based prevention intervention outweigh the risks. *Am J Public Health*. 2025; 115(4):451–453.

Acceptance Date: December 20, 2024.

DOI: https://doi.org/10.2105/AJPH.2024.307999

ORCID iDs:

Chloe A. Teasdale https://orcid.org/0000-0001-9165-8972

Sasha A. Fleary https://orcid.org/0000-0001-9237-2407

CONTRIBUTORS

C. A. Teasdale and S. A. Fleary contributed to reviewing evidence and drafting and reviewing the article.

CONFLICTS OF INTEREST

The authors have no conflicts of interest to declare.

REFERENCES

1. Viera L. Effect of face mask on lowering COVID-19 incidence in school settings: a systematic review. *J Sch Health*. 2024;94(9):878–888. https://doi.org/10.1111/josh.13483
2. DeJonge PM, Pray IW, Gangnon R, McCoy K, Tomasallo C, Meiman J. School district prevention policies and risk of COVID-19 among in-person K-12 educators, Wisconsin, 2021. *Am J Public Health*. 2022;112(12):1791–1799. https://doi.org/10.2105/AJPH.2022.307095
3. Hughes AE, Medford RJ, Perl TM, Basit MA, Kapinos KA. District-level universal masking policies and COVID-19 incidence during the first 8 weeks of school in Texas. *Am J Public Health*. 2022;112(6):871–875. https://doi.org/10.2105/AJPH.2022.306769
4. Greenhalgh T, MacIntyre CR, Baker MG, et al. Masks and respirators for prevention of

respiratory infections: a state of the science review. *Clin Microbiol Rev.* 2024;37(2):e0012423. https://doi.org/10.1128/cmr.00124-23

5. Qasmieh SA, Robertson MM, Teasdale CA, Kulkarni SG, Nash D. Estimating the period prevalence of severe acute respiratory syndrome coronavirus 2 (SARS-CoV-2) infection during the omicron (BA.1) surge in New York City (NYC), 1 January to 16 March 2022. *Clin Infect Dis.* 2023; 76(3):e499–e502. https://doi.org/10.1093/cid/ciac644
6. Keenum I, Lin NJ, Logan-Jackson A, et al. Optimizing wastewater surveillance: the necessity of standardized reporting and proficiency for public health. *Am J Public Health.* 2024;114(9):859–863. https://doi.org/10.2105/AJPH.2024.307760
7. US Centers for Disease Control and Prevention. COVID Data Tracker. Available at: https://covid.cdc.gov/covid-data-tracker/#datatracker-home. Accessed November 26, 2024.
8. Louis S, Mark-Carew M, Biggerstaff M, et al. Wastewater surveillance for influenza A virus and H5 subtype concurrent with the highly pathogenic avian influenza A(H5N1) virus outbreak in cattle and poultry and associated human cases—United States, May 12–July 13, 2024. *MMWR Morb Mortal Wkly Rep.* 2024;73(37):804–809. https://doi.org/10.15585/mmwr.mm7337a1
9. Seither R. Coverage with selected vaccines and exemption from school vaccine requirements among children in kindergarten—United States, 2022–23 school year. *MMWR Morb Mortal Wkly Rep.* 2023;72(45):1217–1224. https://doi.org/10.15585/mmwr.mm7245a2
10. Chester M, Plate RC, Powell T, Rodriguez Y, Wagner NJ, Waller R. The COVID-19 pandemic, mask-wearing, and emotion recognition during late-childhood. *Soc Dev.* 2022;32(1):315–328. https://doi.org/10.1111/sode.12631
11. Schlegtendal A, Eitner L, Falkenstein M, et al. To mask or not to mask—evaluation of cognitive performance in children wearing face masks during school lessons (MasKids). *Children (Basel).* 2022;9(1):95. https://doi.org/10.3390/children9010095
12. Bourke L, Lingwood J, Gallagher-Mitchell T, López-Pérez B. The effect of face mask wearing on language processing and emotion recognition in young children. *J Exp Child Psychol.* 2023; 226:105580. https://doi.org/10.1016/j.jecp.2022.105580
13. Surrain S, Mesa MP, Assel MA, Zucker TA. Does assessor masking affect kindergartners' performance on oral language measures? A COVID-19 era experiment with children from diverse home language backgrounds. *Lang Speech Hear Serv Sch.* 2023;54(4):1323–1332. https://doi.org/10.1044/2023_LSHSS-22-00197
14. Hume S, Brown SR, Mahtani KR. School closures during COVID-19: an overview of systematic reviews. *BMJ Evid Based Med.* 2023;28(3):164–174. https://doi.org/10.1136/bmjebm-2022-112085
15. Gee KA, Asmundson V, Vang T. Educational impacts of the COVID-19 pandemic in the United States: inequities by race, ethnicity, and socioeconomic status. *Curr Opin Psychol.* 2023;52:101643. https://doi.org/10.1016/j.copsyc.2023.101643

Using Surveillance Data to Estimate Infectious Disease Burden: Opportunities and Challenges

Harry Hochheiser, PhD, and Praveen Kumar, PhD

ABOUT THE AUTHORS

Harry Hochheiser is with the Department of Biomedical Informatics, School of Medicine, University of Pittsburgh, Pittsburgh, PA. Praveen Kumar is with the Department of Health Policy and Management, School of Public Health, University of Pittsburgh, Pittsburgh, PA.

See also Couture et al., p. 546

AJPH April 2025, Vol. 115, No. 4

Public health responses to infectious disease outbreaks rely on accurate counts of parameters that are often unavailable or even impossible to measure directly. Numbers of cases, timing of epidemic peaks, incubation times, transmissibility, vaccine efficacy, and numerous other parameters can be expensive (or impossible) to measure reliably. In developing infectious disease models capable of providing estimates of these quantities, modelers are often faced with recursive instances of the initial problem, as they review existing data to identify gaps and determine which needed quantities might be estimated and how. These estimations often require painstaking review of data from disparate sources and the eventual harmonization of those data. Given the expense of these efforts and the importance of their outputs, it is imperative that the public health community learns from this work, improves available data, and increases the reproducibility of modeling efforts.

ESTIMATING INFLUENZA HOSPITALIZATION BURDEN

These challenges are illustrated in the work of Couture et al. (p. 546) on the estimations of influenza hospitalization burden during 2022 to 2023 in the United States. Noting both the lack of robust state-level data on hospitalization owing to influenza and the limits that case ascertainment difficulties place on the accuracy of counts that are collected, Couture et al. adapted a modeling approach previously used for similar work on COVID-19.[1]

To generate influenza estimates, they started with the best available data: FluSurv-Net (the Influenza Hospitalization Surveillance Network of the Centers for Disease Control and Prevention [CDC]) counts of hospitalizations in 13 states, adjusted for underreporting. They then used nine federal data sources together with data from more than 20 states to estimate covariates, including rates of positive influenza tests, percentages of deaths attributed to influenza, influenza vaccination rates, percentages of outpatient visits for influenza-like illness, and percentages of influenza patients among intensive care unit patients, along with demographic variables including racial/ethnic representation, rural–urban distributions, social vulnerabilities, and measurements of behavior risks. Couture et al. used these data to generate a Bayesian hierarchical model expressing state-level hospitalizations in terms of unobserved "true" hospitalization rates, which were in turn determined by covariates.[1] The resulting models stratified estimated hospitalization counts by age group, month, and state. Comparison of adjusted estimates for FluSurv-NET states to model outputs demonstrates the accuracy of the proposed approach.

APPLICATIONS AND LIMITATIONS OF THE MODEL

The contributions of this effort include both the immediate practical hospitalization estimates and numerous potential applications of the generalized approach. Beyond obvious extensions to case or death counts, one might imagine finer-grained examination of hospitalizations of different severities, possibly including those requiring intensive care unit admission or ventilator usage. Given appropriate data, these strategies might be adapted to other outbreaks or extended to address challenges with different data availability profiles.

Couture et al. provide a useful discussion of the potential pitfalls of using information from multiple, diverse sources to fill gaps in available data. Acknowledged limitations include the limited coverage of FluSurv-NET, the related difficulty of extrapolating to states not participating in FluSurv-NET, and gaps in data used to generate key covariates. Given known variations in influenza burden between states, these concerns could have a substantial impact on resulting estimates. Although broader participation in FluSurv-NET might reduce or eliminate this problem, expansion of surveillance efforts seems an unlikely prospect, thus ensuring the relevance of estimation efforts.

INNOVATIVE MODELING APPROACHES

Fortunately, the flexibility of the framework used by Couture et al. suggests approaches that might address these limitations and open new possibilities, As the authors acknowledge, their approach might be readily adapted to reflect new signals that may become available in the future, such as wastewater data surveillance, which might be seen as an attractive and inexpensive alternative to broad-based surveillance.[2] Electronic health record data on virology tests and admitting diagnoses have previously been used to inform hospitalization burden.[3] More fine-grained insights on differing impacts across racial/ethnic groups might be achieved through integration of available data on influenza vaccination rates.[4] Although any of these data sources might be added to the Bayesian hierarchical model, they all raise caveats of their own. For example, data on wastewater or vaccination rates might be hard to incorporate, particularly if those data came from a subset of states.

The approach used by Couture et al. is just one example of the recent explosion of innovation in infectious disease modeling research motivated largely (although not exclusively) by the COVID-19 pandemic. Recent efforts have explored the use of time series neural networks,[5] novel sampling techniques designed to reduce bias,[6] and Bayesian approaches for estimating latent variables.[7,8] These and numerous related advances present the potential of improved models capable of providing public health practitioners with more precise information about future outbreaks.

ENCOURAGING OPEN SCIENCE PRACTICES

To fully realize the utility of these and similar infectious disease modeling efforts, epidemiologists responsible for initial data collection and dissemination and modelers who use those data must work together to adopt modern data science techniques. On the data side, this means working toward compliance with the Findable, Accessible, Interoperable, and Reusable (FAIR) data vision of data sharing.[9] FAIR strategies include the use of unique and persistent identifiers, rich and accessible metadata based on shared vocabularies and representations, clear descriptions of licenses and usage description, and detailed provenance describing the derivation of data sets. For modelers, these approaches would provide increased confidence that any of the multiple data sources used by Couture et al. to derive covariates would be readily available for future reanalyses.

Improved data practices are only one side of the story. Modelers should work to adopt open science practices, which have made huge impacts in bioinformatics, physics, and many other fields. Proposed reporting checklists aimed at supporting increased reproducibility of infectious disease modeling efforts specify extensive information, including the types of data used, how those data were processed, evaluation methods, the source code used to build the model, and other relevant details.[10,11] The modeling community might also adopt the expectation that modeling code be shared as open-source code built on open platforms and available on public code-sharing platforms as prerequisites for publication.

TOWARD GREATER TRANSPARENCY AND COLLABORATION

Increased data and code sharing for infectious disease modeling is complicated by organizational and privacy concerns. Many data sets cannot be shared easily, because of data use requirements or restrictive or ambiguous licenses that may not allow redistribution in altered forms. Similarly, code sharing may be limited by organizations that have not fully adopted open science principles. Recent federal initiatives, such as the CDC's move toward increased data sharing[12] and the National Institutes of Health's data-sharing policies, provide some encouragement for increased openness. In the meantime, imperfect transparency in published work can have immediate effects. For efforts such as the estimates of influenza hospitalization burden by Couture et al., this might mean sharing the code used to harmonize data sources and derive covariate matrices, even if the underlying data could not be shared.

BUILDING A SHARING AND ADAPTABILITY CULTURE

The effective use of modeling to inform responses to infectious disease outbreaks is likely to continue to require learning to quickly adapt existing methods to new conditions in the face of incomplete data. Couture et al. have developed a model that might be adapted to rise to this challenge. Establishing a culture of data and code sharing is an important step to help modelers learn from this and similarly instructive examples. AJPH

CORRESPONDENCE

Correspondence should be sent to Harry Hochheiser, PhD, 5607 Baum Blvd, Pittsburgh, PA 15206 (e-mail: harryh@pitt.edu). Reprints can be ordered at https://www.ajph.org by clicking the "Reprints" link.

PUBLICATION INFORMATION

Full Citation: Hochheiser H, Kumar P. Using surveillance data to estimate infectious disease burden: opportunities and challenges. *Am J Public Health*. 2025;115(4):454–456.

Acceptance Date: January 6, 2024.

DOI: https://doi.org/10.2105/AJPH.2025.308023

ORCID iDs:

Harry Hochheiser https://orcid.org/0000-0001-8793-9982

Praveen Kumar https://orcid.org/0000-0003-4948-968X

CONTRIBUTORS

Both authors conceptualized, drafted, and revised the editorial.

ACKNOWLEDGMENTS

H. Hochheiser and P. Kumar are supported by the National Institutes of Health (NIH; grant R24GM153920).

Note. The content of this editorial is solely the responsibility of the authors and does not necessarily represent the official views of the NIH.

CONFLICTS OF INTEREST

The authors report no potential or actual conflicts of interest from funding- or affiliation-related activities pertinent to this editorial.

REFERENCES

1. Couture A, Iuliano AD, Chang HH, et al. Estimating COVID-19 hospitalizations in the United States with surveillance data using a Bayesian hierarchical model: modeling study. *JMIR Public Health Surveill*. 2022;8(6):e34296. https://doi.org/10.2196/34296
2. Diamond MB, Keshaviah A, Bento AI, et al. Wastewater surveillance of pathogens can inform public health responses. *Nat Med*. 2022;28(10):1992–1995. https://doi.org/10.1038/s41591-022-01940-x
3. Zimmerman RK, Balasubramani GK, D'Agostino HEA, et al. Population-based hospitalization burden estimates for respiratory viruses, 2015–2019. *Influenza Other Respir Viruses*. 2022;16(6):1133–1140. https://doi.org/10.1111/irv.13040
4. Centers for Disease Control and Prevention. Flu vaccination coverage, United States, 2023–24 influenza season. September 20, 2024. Available at: https://www.cdc.gov/fluvaxview/coverage-by-season/2023-2024.html. Accessed December 3, 2024.
5. Aiken EL, Nguyen AT, Viboud C, Santillana M. Toward the use of neural networks for influenza prediction at multiple spatial resolutions. *Sci Adv*. 2021;7(25):eabb1237. https://doi.org/10.1126/sciadv.abb1237
6. Howa AC, Zhu Y, Wyatt D, et al. Estimating the burden of influenza hospitalizations across multiple seasons using capture–recapture. *J Infect Dis*. 2024;229(6):1823–1829. https://doi.org/10.1093/infdis/jiad417
7. Aravamuthan S, Mandujano Reyes JF, Dopfer D. Real-time estimation and forecasting of COVID-19 cases and hospitalizations in Wisconsin HERC regions for public health decision making processes. *Int J Infect Dis*. 2022;116:S28–S29. https://doi.org/10.1016/j.ijid.2021.12.068
8. Chitwood MH, Russi M, Gunasekera K, et al. Reconstructing the course of the COVID-19 epidemic over 2020 for US states and counties: results of a Bayesian evidence synthesis model. *PLoS Comput Biol*. 2022;18(8):e1010465. https://doi.org/10.1371/journal.pcbi.1010465
9. Wilkinson MD, Dumontier M, Aalbersberg IJ, et al. The FAIR guiding principles for scientific data management and stewardship. *Sci Data*. 2016;3:160018. https://doi.org/10.1038/sdata.2016.18
10. Pollett S, Johansson MA, Reich NG, et al. Recommended reporting items for epidemic forecasting and prediction research: the EPIFORGE 2020 guidelines. *PLoS Med*. 2021;18(10):e1003793. https://doi.org/10.1371/journal.pmed.1003793
11. Pokutnaya D, Childers B, Arcury-Quandt AE, Hochheiser H, Van Panhuis WG. An implementation framework to improve the transparency and reproducibility of computational models of infectious diseases. *PLoS Comput Biol*. 2023;19(3):e1010856. https://doi.org/10.1371/journal.pcbi.1010856
12. Wiltz JL, Lee B, Kaufmann R, Carney TJ, Davis K, Briss PA. Modernizing CDC's practices and culture for better data sharing, impact, and transparency. *Prev Chronic Dis*. 2024;21:E18. https://doi.org/10.5888/pcd21.230200

The Evolving Overdose Crisis: United States Needs Robust Policy Change to Address the Fourth Wave

Shoshana V. Aronowitz, PhD, MSN, MSHP, and Megan K. Reed, PhD, MPH

ABOUT THE AUTHORS

Shoshana V. Aronowitz is with the Department of Family and Community Health, University of Pennsylvania School of Nursing, Philadelphia, PA. Megan K. Reed is with the Department of Emergency Medicine and the Center for Connected Care at Sidney Kimmel Medical College, and the College of Population Health, Thomas Jefferson University, Philadelphia.

See also Diekhans et al., p. 555.

After a year-over-year increase since 2018, the United States saw a small dip in overdose deaths in 2023. Despite this slight reduction in fatal overdoses, driven primarily by fewer deaths caused by opioids, deaths from stimulants like amphetamines and cocaine increased, and some communities across the country suffered significantly more overdoses than in 2022.[1] Specifically, fatal overdose rates among non-Hispanic Black, Native Hawaiian, and other Pacific Islander populations rose dramatically during this time period.[1] In addition, newer substances like nitazenes, xylazine, and novel fentanyl analogs are rapidly entering the drug supply across the country, with each region of the United States experiencing these changes differently.[2,3]

Rather than view the small overall reduction in overdoses as a sign that the crisis is abating, many experts believe we have entered the fourth "wave" of the 21st century overdose crisis.[4] This wave is marked by polysubstance use—specifically, the use of both fentanyl and stimulants. In this issue, Diekhans et al. (p. 555) describe a study that analyzed drug residue and paraphernalia found at the scenes of fentanyl-involved fatal overdoses in San Francisco, California, in 2022. Their findings add to a growing body of evidence supporting an evolving drug supply, an increase in stimulant-involved fatal overdoses, and a shift among some people who use drugs toward different modes of use beyond injection.

THE CHANGING DRUG SUPPLY

The US drug supply is heterogeneous. Previous research highlights how fentanyl and xylazine first emerged on the East Coast before making their way west.[2,5] For example, we conduct research in Philadelphia, Pennsylvania, a city where new trends in the drug supply often emerge. The city's opioid supply shifted almost completely from heroin to fentanyl by 2015. Newer substances in the local supply include medetomidine—similar to but more potent than xylazine—and the sedative etomidate, and 99% of the street opioid supply contained xylazine in the first half of 2023.[6,7] By contrast, Diekhans et al. found xylazine in only 10% of their study's included cases in San Francisco and a stimulant supply of methamphetamine and cocaine. In their study, methamphetamine was typically found alone, whereas cocaine was detected more frequently alongside fentanyl.

These trends and differences have important implications for public health responses. The United States has not systematically invested in scaled-up drug checking, obscuring the data needed to implement public health interventions. These data are critical on two fronts: to aggregate results to better understand a comprehensive picture of the composition of a locality's drug supply and to provide real-time data to people who use drugs about the drugs they are buying and using so they can make more informed decisions about their use.

In addition to supporting the assertion that the overdose crisis is now in its fourth wave, the findings from Diekhans et al. also underscore how our policy responses to the constantly evolving crisis are often a step behind. Information about the drug supply notwithstanding, drug use patterns are driven at least in part by the unregulated supply of drugs even when some information about the supply is known. The authors note that more than half of overdose decedents in their included cases test positive for at least one stimulant in addition to fentanyl. This is a noteworthy hallmark of the fourth wave of the overdose crisis and mirrors trends of polysubstance use and overdoses seen across the country.[1]

AJPH April 2025, Vol. 115, No. 4

Likewise, some preliminary data from our research in Philadelphia indicate that more people are using stimulants to counter the sedating impacts of xylazine. Increased stimulant use is especially pronounced among unhoused people who use drugs, a population more structurally vulnerable to both violence while sedated and fatal overdoses. Polysubstance use of stimulants and opioids requires a different treatment approach than that for solely opioids.[4] For example, there is no gold-standard medication treatment of stimulant-use disorders as there is for opioid use disorder. Research about effective treatment of polysubstance use lags that of opioids alone, and current regulations inhibit the accessibility of an evidence-based behavioral treatment of stimulant use disorder.[4] As long as the drug supply continues to be unregulated, drug-related morbidity and mortality will remain elevated, and their patterns will shift ahead of our ability to have robust public health and treatment responses.

SHIFTS IN ROUTES OF ADMINISTRATION

Finally, this study adds to the body of evidence reporting a shift toward smoking and snorting among many people who use drugs, which may offer some (although in many cases not sufficient) protection from overdose and skin and soft tissue infections.[8,9] People who choose smoking or snorting instead of injecting report making the change in an attempt to mitigate risks in the face of an increasingly unpredictable drug supply and, in some cases, because the drug supply has already led to wounds and scarring that have made injection more difficult.[8]

Given this shift, it is imperative that harm reduction programs are able to offer appropriate supplies, and providing alternatives to injection—like pipes and other smoking and snorting equipment—may increase participant engagement with the litany of services these programs provide, including overdose prevention resources such as naloxone distribution.[10] Unfortunately, safer smoking supplies are notoriously difficult for many programs to obtain given a ban on using federal funds to cover distribution,[11] and harm reduction programs have faced increasing scrutiny and pushback despite strong evidence that they provide a litany of vital services including overdose reversal, wound care, and opioid use disorder treatment.[12] While the findings of this study and many others highlight the need for expanded harm reduction services, these programs and other evidence-based substance use disorder interventions are increasingly under attack.[12]

As highlighted recently by this journal, the impacts of the overdose crisis are far reaching; more than 1.4 million US children have lost a family member.[13] Despite headlines celebrating a small dip in fatal overdoses, the yearly death toll remains shockingly and unacceptably high. Until we take pragmatic action, which should include all evidence-based approaches including overdose prevention sites, expanding available medications for opioid use disorder, investing in effective treatments for stimulant and polysubstance use disorders, and exploring options for a safer supply of substances, we will not be able to make substantial progress in stemming the overdose crisis and improving the health outcomes of people who use drugs. AJPH

CORRESPONDENCE

Correspondence should be sent to Shoshana V. Aronowitz, 418 Curie Blvd, Philadelphia, PA 19104 (e-mail: visho@nursing.upenn.edu). Reprints can be ordered at https://www.ajph.org by clicking the "Reprints" link.

PUBLICATION INFORMATION

Full Citation: Aronowitz SV, Reed MK. The evolving overdose crisis: United States needs robust policy change to address the fourth wave. *Am J Public Health*. 2025;115(4):457–459.

Acceptance Date: January 23, 2025.

DOI: https://doi.org/10.2105/AJPH.2025.308041

ORCID iDs:

Shoshana V. Aronowitz https://orcid.org/0000-0003-2169-9562

Megan K. Reed https://orcid.org/0000-0002-4367-7076

CONTRIBUTORS

Both authors contributed equally to this editorial.

ACKNOWLEDGMENTS

S.V. Aronowitz's efforts were supported by National Institute on Drug Abuse of the National Institutes of Health under award K23DA057528. M.K. Reed's efforts were supported by National Institute on Drug Abuse of the National Institutes of Health under awards R21DA058582 and R21DA056790.

Note. This sponsor had no role in the writing of the viewpoint nor in the decision to submit it for publication.

CONFLICTS OF INTEREST

The authors report no conflicts of interest.

REFERENCES

1. Garnett M, Minino A. *Drug Overdose Deaths in the United State, 2003–2023*. National Center for Health Statistics. 2024. Available at: https://www.cdc.gov/nchs/products/databriefs/db522.htm. Accessed January 4, 2025.
2. Shover CL, Falasinnu TO, Dwyer CL, et al. Steep increases in fentanyl-related mortality west of the Mississippi River: recent evidence from county and state surveillance. *Drug Alcohol Depend*. 2020;216:108314. https://doi.org/10.1016/j.drugalcdep.2020.108314
3. Armenian P, Vo K, Barr-Walker J, Lynch K. Fentanyl, fentanyl analogs and novel synthetic opioids: a comprehensive review. *Neuropharmacology*. 2018;134(ptA):121–132. https://doi.org/10.1016/j.neuropharm.2017.10.016
4. Rawson RA, Erath TG, Clark HW. The fourth wave of the overdose crisis: examining the prominent role of psychomotor stimulants with and without fentanyl. *Prev Med*. 2023;176:107625. https://doi.org/10.1016/j.ypmed.2023.107625
5. Cano M, Daniulaityte R, Marsiglia F. Xylazine in overdose deaths and forensic drug reports in US states, 2019–2022. *JAMA Netw Open*. 2024;7(1):

e2350630. https://doi.org/10.1001/jamanetworkopen.2023.50630

6. Philadelphia Department of Public Health, Division of Substance Use Prevention and Harm Reduction. Etomidate detected in Philadelphia's drug supply and involved in overdose deaths. 2024. Available at: https://hip.phila.gov/document/4686/PDPH-HAN-429U-Etomidate-08.12.2024-1.pdf. Accessed August 19, 2024.
7. The Center for Forensic Science Research and Education. Drug Checking Report: Quarter 1 and Quarter 2 2023, Philadelphia. 2023. Available at: https://www.cfsre.org/images/content/reports/drug_checking/2023_Q1_and_Q2_Drug_Checking_Quarterly_Report_CFSRE_NPS_Discovery.pdf. Accessed January 4, 2025.
8. Kral AH, Lambdin BH, Browne EN, et al. Transition from injecting opioids to smoking fentanyl in San Francisco, California. *Drug Alcohol Depend.* 2021;227:109003. https://doi.org/10.1016/j.drugalcdep.2021.109003
9. Tanz LJ, Gladden R, Dinwiddie A, et al. Routes of drug use among drug overdose deaths—United States, 2020–2022. *MMWR Morb Mortal Wkly Rep.* 2024;73(6):124–130. https://doi.org/10.15585/mmwr.mm7306a2
10. Chung EO, Patel SV, Wenger LD, et al. Distributing safer smoking pipes increases engagement with harm reduction services in the United States: findings from the National Survey of Syringe Services Programs. Posted online January 1, 2024: medRxiv 2024.06.28.24309683. https://doi.org/10.1101/2024.06.28.24309683
11. Dunham K, Shihipar A, Marshall BDL. Shifting to smoking: adapting policy to changing patterns of substance use. *Health Affairs Forefront.* June 25, 2024. https://doi.org/10.1377/forefront.20240621.217485
12. Aronowitz SV, Reed MK. Regressive policing, a return to the War on Drugs, and the need for qualitative and ethnographic policy evaluations. *Int J Drug Policy.* 2024;133:104565. https://doi.org/10.1016/j.drugpo.2024.104565
13. Verdery AM, Ryan-Claytor C, Smith-Greenaway E, Sarkar N, Livings M. More than 1.4 million US children have lost a family member to drug overdose. *Am J Public Health.* 2024;114(12):1394–1397. https://doi.org/10.2105/AJPH.2024.307847

Considering the Complexity of Professional Identity for Public Health Nurse Workforce Enumeration

Shawn M. Kneipp, PhD, RN, ANP, PHNA-BC

ABOUT THE AUTHOR

Shawn M. Kneipp is the Sarah Frances Russell Distinguished Term Professor in the School of Nursing and adjunct associate professor in the Gillings School of Global Public Health at The University of North Carolina at Chapel Hill. She is past chair of the American Public Health Association's Public Health Nursing Section, and currently serves as a member of the Editorial Board for the American Journal of Public Health.

See also Bekemeier et al., p. 536.

AJPH April 2025, Vol. 115, No. 4

Enumerating the public health workforce has been an ongoing project in the United States since the early 1900s.[1] At the most basic level, to achieve national health goals, obtaining an accurate account of the public health workforce is required; yet, accuracy has been a formidable aspect of enumeration efforts.[2–4] In this issue, Bekemeier et al. (p. 536) add to these efforts in an attempt to more precisely determine the scope of the public health nurse (PHN) governmental workforce in the United States.

ESTIMATES OF THE WORKFORCE BY DIFFERENT METHODS

Extending beyond employment setting or organization type to determine the PHN workforce, the authors also applied nurses' self-reported specialty area to identify PHNs among the registered nurse (RN) workforce across three traditionally governmental public health settings: public health agencies, correctional facilities, and schools. With this approach, two group estimates were generated: a broad governmental PHN group that includes a wider range of specialty areas comprising 3.7% of all RNs, and a restricted governmental group based on specialty areas most aligned with public health, comprising a mere 1.8% of all RNs. Their findings are consistent with other recent enumerations showing declines in the PHN workforce,[5] including a 36% drop in PHNs over the decade immediately preceding COVID-19[6]—a trend that both put the American people in harm's way of the pandemic and hamstrung improving population health during conventional times.

NURSE IDENTITY AS A POTENTIAL SOURCE FOR LACK OF CLARITY

Their findings also highlight the need for more attention to how nurses view their professional identities, and to strengthen the conceptual ground and measurement of public health functions in future enumeration studies. Based on data from Table 1 (p. 539), among the broad governmental PHN group, 53% of nurses in a school health setting, 46% in a correctional health setting, and 13% in a public health setting self-identified as belonging to an "unspecified" rather than "public health" or "community health" specialty area. The authors explain this finding through state-specific responses from Alaska, given that its PHN workforce more readily aligns with the objectives of Public Health 3.0.[7] They speculate that the high proportion of nurses identifying with the "unspecified" specialty option may be because PHNs in Alaska see themselves in a generalist role given their breadth of practice roles in that state, and extend this as a possible explanation for why respondents across their sample similarly selected this option.

How PHNs perceive themselves, and the processes that inform how they identify their specialty area of practice within public health contexts, however, is far more complex. From their qualitative inquiry into how PHNs produce, understand, and maintain their professional identity, Drevdahl and Canales[8] describe this complexity within the overarching themes of narrative self-identity, mandated identity, and identity as struggle. In their trajectory of developing a narrative self-identity as a professional nurse, PHNs in the sample used by Bekemeier et al. trained as RNs first. Through higher educational systems and ongoing public expectations of what nurses in the United States do, the training of RNs has been, and largely remains, steeped in an ideology that defines a nurse's role as providing clinical care to individuals, rather than populations. Even in cases where someone with an advanced public health education later becomes an RN, that individual's primary identity formation as a nurse precedes integrating any practice specialty as a nurse—such as that required to competently assume all aspects of the PHN scope of practice.[9]

Despite accounting for the largest proportion of the public health workforce, not all PHNs pursue jobs that are population focused with intentionality; several may inadvertently accept positions within governmental or other public health systems based on other appealing characteristics of the position (such as weekday and regular business hours). Particularly for nurses in the latter scenario, explicit communication that the position requires a population health practice perspective is necessary to bring this aspect of one's responsibilities to the fore, although such communication is unlikely to occur as nurses seek new jobs. In a study of 161 PHN position descriptions in local health departments, for example, Polivka and Chaudry[10] found that 78% included task-oriented statements that were disconnected from role expectations that reflect PHN professional competencies or that were described within the context of fulfilling one or more public health essential services. Coupled with supervisor expectations that a PHN's scope of practice is confined to carrying out solely "clinical" care tasks to individuals seeking direct health care services, this messaging reflects the mandated identity described by Drevdahl and Canales[8] that nurses in PHN roles feel required to assume.

For nurses in the PHN workforce who are aware of these externally imposed ideological limitations placed on their ability to function at the population level of practice they desire, professional identity as struggle[8] emerges as a theme in their day-to-day work, and contributes to burnout and nurse attrition from the public health workforce. Many other nurses working in PHN roles, however, cling to what is often their primary socialization in nursing—an identity that must be grounded in providing individual clinical care—while rejecting (at worst) or marginalizing (at best) the population-level focus that defines the PHN specialty. Thus, the high number of PHNs within each of the three public health settings in the authors' study who see themselves belonging to an "unspecified" specialty, rather than one defined by "public health" or "community health," may be rooted in identity struggles that go beyond seeing themselves as nurse generalists within the PHN practice space.

MORE PRECISE DATA NEEDED FOR FUTURE RESEARCH

Finally, Bekemeier et al. note that using "specialty area" as a proxy for the multifaceted and nuanced roles, functions, and job tasks carried out by PHNs was a limitation imposed by the National Council of State Boards of Nursing data—one of few data sources available to conduct this type of research.[4] Adding this proxy variable to the analysis did advance enumeration estimates beyond those defined solely by practice setting; however, as national initiatives prompt health care organizations outside the governmental public health sphere to expand services that include some aspects of population health, workforce enumeration will become even more difficult. In 2022, my colleagues and I articulated the discrepancies between professional definitions of and guidelines for PHN practice, and how both the nursing and public health disciplines approach enumerating the PHN workforce in national surveys.[4] We also recommended specific paths forward for being able to account for PHN roles, functions, and tasks in enumeration efforts to guide future research in this area.[4] In their discussion, Bekemeier et al. acknowledge the need for advancing research in this area, noting "more precise data are clearly needed to understand the specific functions and activities of the PHN workforce" (p. 543). Although parsimony is an important consideration for measurement development and constructing workforce surveys, we are at a juncture where accuracy may matter more. Without a PHN workforce with an identity firmly grounded in the population health–level functions, or the ability to quantify how much of a PHN's practice is operating at the individual or population level, much of our public health planning efforts in the service of protecting the public's health may indeed be in vain. AJPH

CORRESPONDENCE

Correspondence should be sent to Shawn M. Kneipp, PhD, RN, ANP, PHNA-BC, Sarah Frances Russell Distinguished Term Professor, The University of North Carolina at Chapel Hill School of Nursing, Carrington Hall CB #7460, Office #5012, Chapel Hill, NC 27599-7460 (e-mail: skneipp@email.unc.edu). Reprints can be ordered at https://www.ajph.org by clicking the "Reprints" link.

PUBLICATION INFORMATION

Full Citation: Kneipp SM. Considering the complexity of professional identity for public health nurse workforce enumeration. *Am J Public Health*. 2025;115(4):460–462.

Acceptance Date: January 15, 2025.

DOI: https://doi.org/10.2105/AJPH.2025.308033

ORCID iD:

Shawn M. Kneipp https://orcid.org/0000-0002-8907-0587

ACKNOWLEDGMENTS

I thank the many public health nursing scholars and researchers whose work elicited or informed this editorial.

CONFLICTS OF INTEREST

There are no potential or actual conflicts of interest from funding or affiliation-related activities.

REFERENCES

1. Merrill J, Btoush R, Gupta M, Gebbie K. A history of public health workforce enumeration. *J Public Health Manag Pract.* 2003;9(6):459–470. https://doi.org/10.1097/00124784-200311000-00005
2. Sumaya CV. Enumeration and composition of the public health workforce: challenges and strategies. *Am J Public Health.* 2012;102(3):469–474. https://doi.org/10.2105/AJPH.2011.300388
3. Froeb K, Weinberg S, Adam A, Cope E. A research agenda for an evolving public health system: directions for the field of public health services and systems research. January 24, 2024. Available at: https://academyhealth.org/publications/2024-01/report-identifies-directions-field-public-health-services-and-systems-research. Accessed December 28, 2024.
4. Kneipp SM, Edmonds JK, Cooper J, Campbell LA, Little SH, Mix AK. Enumeration of public health nurses in the United States: limits of current standards. *Am J Public Health.* 2022;112(S3):S292–S297. https://doi.org/10.2105/AJPH.2022.306782
5. Pittman P, Park J. Rebuilding community-based and public health nursing in the wake of COVID-19. *Online J Issues Nurs.* 2021;26(2). https://doi.org/10.3912/OJIN.Vol26No02Man07
6. National Association of County & City Health Officials. NACCHO's 2019 profile study: changes in local health department workforce and finance capacity since 2008. May 2020. Available at: https://www.naccho.org/uploads/downloadable-resources/2019-Profile-Workforce-and-Finance-Capacity.pdf. Accessed December 28, 2024.
7. DeSalvo KB, Wang YC, Harris A, Auerbach J, Koo D, O'Carroll P. Public Health 3.0: a call to action for public health to meet the challenges of the 21st century. *Prev Chronic Dis.* 2017;14:E78. https://doi.org/10.5888/pcd14.170017
8. Drevdahl DJ, Canales MK. Being a real nurse: a secondary qualitative analysis of how public health nurses rework their work identities. *Nurs Inq.* 2020;27(4):e12360. https://doi.org/10.1111/nin.12360
9. *Public Health Nursing: Scope and Standards of Practice.* 3rd ed. Silver Spring, MD: American Nurses Association; 2022.
10. Polivka BJ, Chaudry RV. Public health nursing position descriptions congruence with ANA standards, public health essential services, and quad council domains. *Public Health Nurs.* 2015;32(5):532–542. https://doi.org/10.1111/phn.12148

Can "Food Is Medicine" Interventions Be Positioned to Combat the Historical Effects of Racism in Black Communities Deprived of Food Resources?

Chelsea R. Singleton, PhD, MPH

ABOUT THE AUTHOR

The author is with the Celia Scott Weatherhead School of Public Health & Tropical Medicine, Tulane University, New Orleans, LA.

See also Nicholson-Robinson et al., p. 528.

In the United States, Black Americans continue to disproportionately carry the burden of poor nutritional outcomes (e.g., food insecurity, obesity, type 2 diabetes) and be more likely to live in a community deprived of health-supporting food resources (e.g., supermarkets, grocery stores).[1,2] Several studies have linked these nutritional inequities to current and historical manifestations of structural racism.[2] Structural racism, which refers to racist systems, policies, structures, and social norms, is widely accepted as a root cause of racialized health inequities in the United States.[3]

These racialized inequities are particularly pronounced in the Deep South, where states such as Mississippi, Alabama, Louisiana, Georgia, and South Carolina have obesity prevalence rates that exceed 43% for Black-identifying adults.[4] Health interventions have not moved the needle toward addressing the nutritional and health concerns of Black Americans, despite the field's steadfast emphasis on cultural tailoring and community-based health programming.[5]

In this issue of *AJPH*, Nicholson-Robinson et al. (p. 528) provide readers a necessary lesson on the importance of centering the lived experiences of a target population when designing and implementing health interventions. In their work, which highlights the voices of Black people living in three food-deprived rural counties of the Mississippi Delta, they argue that Food Is Medicine (FIM) interventions, in particular, should be fashioned in a manner that accounts for the historical trauma caused by structural racism and racial violence. Such interventions would thus be better positioned to foster community acceptability, equitable implementation, and long-term sustainability.

The FIM movement has gained much traction in recent years.[6,7] In 2024, the US Department of Health and Human Services published its FIM landscape summary, which underscored growing interest in FIM as a solution to the nation's most pressing nutritional challenges.[7] FIM, as a concept, recognizes that providing people with stable access to affordable nutritious foods is vital to chronic disease prevention and treatment.[6] Collaboration between local entities invested in community health (e.g., public health offices, health care systems, community organizations) is necessary to build capacity, organize resources, and effectively implement FIM interventions.

A recent narrative review conducted by Houghtaling et al. identified several barriers to FIM intervention implementation, particularly in health care settings.[7] The authors recognized that an FIM intervention may be harmful to members of the target population if the organization leading the charge has a history of racist practices, policies, and priorities.[7] The recommendation checklist they provided to those working in health care settings recognized the need for organizations to face and address their racist past. But what about the community's past? Many health care organizations serve communities that have endured generations of structural racism and racial violence, leaving these areas deprived of food resources. Nicholson-Robinson et al. emphasize the importance of addressing the economic, environmental, and, most important, psychosocial effects of racism to promote racial equity in FIM programming.

In this editorial, I briefly summarize key points made by Nicholson-Robinson et al., which were informed by an impactful qualitative study they conducted in the Mississippi Delta region. In addition, I offer my thoughts on what else is needed to position FIM

AJPH April 2025, Vol. 115, No. 4

interventions as a strategy to combat the historical effects of racism in food-deprived Black communities.

ACKNOWLEDGING THE PAST

Nicholson-Robinson and colleagues' work stresses the importance of acknowledging how the historical effects of racism can challenge FIM intervention design, implementation, and evaluation. First, they describe how structural racism and racial violence can negatively influence all components of the local food system (i.e., production, processing, distribution, procurement).[8] FIM interventions, particularly those that supply the target population with health-supporting food resources (e.g., nutrition incentives, produce prescriptions), often rely on partnerships with local growers.

Unfortunately, many Black communities in the United States have stories that are similar to those of the rural counties of the Mississippi Delta. Black people have faced disenfranchisement, often at the hands of government agencies, which has hindered their ability to own farmland and obtain relevant resources such as loans, grants, and subsidies.[9] As a result, there continues to be a dearth of Black growers across the United States. If FIM interventions are to address racial inequities, they must support Black people's endeavors to become vocal and active contributors to their community's food system.

Second, Nicholson-Robinson et al. describe how historical mistrust of new health programs often stems from Black communities being overtaxed by ambitious research teams that lack the intention to provide sustainable solutions and resources. In addition to medical maltreatment, low-income and racially marginalized populations have endured the negative effects of helicopter research and health equity tourism, which can undermine efforts to create health programs that center racial equity.[10,11] FIM interventions must be developed by individuals and organizations that are invested in the community's social, political, and economic well-being and intend to offer viable solutions for food resource deprivation.

Lastly, Nicholson-Robinson et al. reiterate the importance of building community–academic partnerships that elevate and advance the target population's beliefs and preferences pertaining to food. This requires doing the formative work of connecting like-minded local change makers and studying the target population's lived experiences, beliefs, and preferences through innovative qualitative methodologies.[5] Researchers, practitioners, and, most important, funding agencies should prioritize this formative work when seeking to support FIM interventions in low-resourced Black communities. This will ensure that FIM interventions are being conducted through strong community–academic partnerships comprising individuals and groups that lack paternalistic views on the community's beliefs and preferences.

CHARTING A NEW COURSE

Nicholson-Robinson et al. provide readers with six recommendations to effectively implement FIM interventions in communities historically affected by racism. I believe that all individuals and organizations working in the FIM space should study these recommendations and allow them to chart a new course in FIM intervention design, implementation, and evaluation moving forward.

Other recommendations to consider pertain to the training of future generations of health leaders and the research priorities of funding agencies. The fields of nutrition and public health must push to create antiracist curricula and training, especially in programs that train students to develop health interventions. In recent years, several frameworks and tools for teaching students about racism have been introduced to the scientific literature, demonstrating the growing demand for these resources among educators.[12,13] By strengthening the training of nutrition and public health students, we will empower future generations of leaders to work alongside low-resourced Black communities to develop FIM interventions.

According to Nicholson-Robinson et al., funding agencies seeking to support FIM interventions must be prepared to financially invest in local agriculture and food resources. I strongly agree with this sentiment and implore funding agencies to also rethink their research and evaluation expectations for grantees. Many of the traditional sources of funding for health programming stress the need to document changes in health behaviors and health outcomes at the individual level (e.g., dietary intake, weight). If FIM interventions are to be positioned to combat historical trauma caused by racism, funding agencies must allow researchers to prioritize the measurement and evaluation of upstream factors that represent social and commercial determinants of health, for example perceived access to healthy food, the financial stability of local food businesses, and chronic disinvestment.[14] This is essential to ensuring that FIM interventions being introduced to historically low-resourced Black communities are working to address the underlying determinants of racial inequities in nutrition and health.

In summary, as FIM programming continues to expand in the United States, the need for effective FIM interventions that serve low-resourced Black communities will grow. To ensure that these interventions are feasible, acceptable, and sustainable, they must be designed and implemented in a manner that combats the historical effects of racism. AJPH

CORRESPONDENCE

Correspondence should be sent to Chelsea R. Singleton, PhD, MPH, Department of Social, Behavioral, and Population Sciences, Celia Scott Weatherhead School of Public Health & Tropical Medicine, Tulane University, 1440 Canal St, Suite 2200-20, New Orleans, LA 70112 (e-mail: csingle1@tulane.edu). Reprints can be ordered at https://www.ajph.org by clicking the "Reprints" link.

PUBLICATION INFORMATION

Full Citation: Singleton CR. Can "Food Is Medicine" interventions be positioned to combat the historical effects of racism in Black communities deprived of food resources? *Am J Public Health*. 2025;115(4):463–465.

Acceptance Date: January 23, 2025.

DOI: https://doi.org/10.2105/AJPH.2025.308042

ORCID iD:

Chelsea R. Singleton https://orcid.org/0000-0002-4494-157X

ACKNOWLEDGMENTS

I acknowledge Vanessa Nicholson-Robinson and her colleagues for writing a compelling article about the current and historical effects of racism on food and nutrition in Mississippi. Their work should be read by all experts and entities seeking to develop nutrition interventions that target Black communities.

CONFLICTS OF INTEREST

The author reports no conflicts of interest.

REFERENCES

1. Bell CN, Thorpe RJ, Bowie JV, LaVeist TA. Race disparities in cardiovascular disease risk factors within socioeconomic status strata. *Ann Epidemiol*. 2018;28(3):147–152. https://doi.org/10.1016/j.annepidem.2017.12.007
2. Singleton CR, Wright LA, McDonald M, et al. Structural racism and geographic access to food retailers in the United States: a scoping review. *Health Place*. 2023;83:103089. https://doi.org/10.1016/j.healthplace.2023.103089
3. Bailey ZD, Feldman JM, Bassett MT. How structural racism works - racist policies as a root cause of U.S. racial health inequities. *N Engl J Med*. 2021;384(8):768–773. https://doi.org/10.1056/NEJMms2025396
4. Centers for Disease Control and Prevention. Adult obesity prevalence. Available at: https://www.cdc.gov/obesity/data-and-statistics/adult-obesity-prevalence-maps.html. Accessed January 13, 2025.
5. Greene M, Houghtaling B, Sadeghzadeh C, et al. African Americans' perceptions of nutrition interventions: a scoping review. *Nutr Res Rev*. 2023;36(2):320–339. https://doi.org/10.1017/S0954422422000099
6. US Department of Health and Human Services. Food Is Medicine: landscape summary. Available at: https://odphp.health.gov/foodismedicine/understanding-food-medicine/exploring-food-medicine-landscape. Accessed January 7, 2025.
7. Houghtaling B, Short E, Byker Shanks C, et al. Implementation of Food Is Medicine programs in healthcare settings: a narrative review. *J Gen Intern Med*. 2024;39(14):2797–2805. https://doi.org/10.1007/s11606-024-08768-w
8. Freedman DA, Clark JK, Lounsbury DW, et al. Food system dynamics structuring nutrition equity in racialized urban neighborhoods. *Am J Clin Nutr*. 2022;115(4):1027–1038. https://doi.org/10.1093/ajcn/nqab380
9. Tshabalala P. A brief history of discrimination against black farmers including by the USDA. Available at: https://blog.ucsusa.org/precious-tshabalala/a-brief-history-of-discrimination-against-black-farmers-including-by-the-usda. Accessed January 15, 2024.
10. Lett E, Adekunle D, McMurray P, et al. Health equity tourism: ravaging the justice landscape. *J Med Syst*. 2022;46(3):17. https://doi.org/10.1007/s10916-022-01803-5
11. Lambert WM, Camacho-Rivera M, Boutin-Foster C, Salifu M, Riley WJ. Ending "domestic helicopter research." *Cell*. 2024;187(8):1823–1827. https://doi.org/10.1016/j.cell.2024.02.027
12. Metzl JM, Petty J, Olowajoba OV. Using a structural competency framework to teach structural racism in pre-health education. *Soc Sci Med*. 2018;199:189–201. https://doi.org/10.1016/j.socscimed.2017.06.029
13. Santoro CM, Farmer M, Lobato G, James M, Herring SJ. Antiracism training for nutrition professionals in the Special Supplemental Nutrition Program for Women, Infants, and Children (WIC): a promising strategy to improve attitudes, awareness, and actions. *J Racial Ethn Health Disparities*. 2022;10(6):2882–2889. https://doi.org/10.1007/s40615-022-01465-6
14. Freudenberg N. Integrating social, political and commercial determinants of health frameworks to advance public health in the twenty-first century. Available at: https://journals.sagepub.com/doi/10.1177/00207314221125151?url_ver=Z39.88-2003&rfr_id=ori:rid:crossref.org&rfr_dat=cr_pub%20%200pubmed. Accessed January 15, 2024.

How US Grassroots Organizations Confront the Global Anti-LGBTQ+ Crisis and Support LGBTQ+ Asylum Seekers

Chioma Nnaji, MPH, MEd, Al Green, BS, and Nathalie J. Weeks, LMSW, MBA

ABOUT THE AUTHORS

Chioma Nnaji is with the Multicultural AIDS Coalition, Boston, MA. Al Green is with the LGBT Asylum Task Force, Worcester, MA. Nathalie J. Weeks is with the African Services Committee, New York, NY.

AJPH April 2025, Vol. 115, No. 4

A rise in anti-LGBTQ+ (lesbian, gay, bisexual, transgender, queer, and additional sexual and gender expansive individuals) legislation in African and Caribbean countries has compelled many LGBTQ+ individuals to seek refuge in the United States. There is limited data on the exact number. However, from 2012 to 2017, an estimated 4000 out of 30 900 LGBTQ+ asylum applicants cited persecution due to their sexual orientation or gender identity.[1] For Black LGBTQ+ asylum seekers, the journey is particularly challenging. They must navigate a complex US immigration system while dealing with dual layers of discrimination—racial inequities and anti-LGBTQ+ stigma.[2,3] This compounded marginalization not only heightens the trauma of their migration but also creates significant barriers to resettlement, restricting access to employment, housing, and social support within both broader society and their own ethnic communities.[4,5]

Grassroots community-based organizations—many founded by immigrants—are essential for Black LGBTQ+ asylum seekers to find stability. Despite limited resources, they provide crucial services like housing, legal aid, health information, and mental health support. These organizations are often the only trusted source, offering both immediate relief and a sense of community, safety, and belonging.

Two individuals working at the frontlines of this crisis were interviewed. Al Green (A. G.) is the ministry director of the LGBT Asylum Task Force. In 2008, L. C., a young gay man from Jamaica seeking asylum, was referred to Hadwen Park Congregational Church for spiritual and housing support. This led him and the church's pastor to cofound the LGBT Asylum Task Force. Since its inception, the Task Force has supported over 400 LGBTQ+ asylum seekers from more than 30 countries. Nathalie J. Weeks, LMSW, MBA (N. W.) is a mental health counselor and coordinator of behavioral health services at African Services Committee, an organization founded 43 years ago by an Ethiopian refugee. It was initially created to support newly arrived immigrants needing basic support services. Soon after being established, it expanded to address HIV/AIDS among African and Caribbean immigrants.

TRUST SYSTEMS AND INDIVIDUAL FEARS

For many Black LGBTQ+ asylum seekers, the process of migration is deeply traumatic because of rejection and violence. This trauma often breaks their trust in both family and society, leading to ongoing psychological distress and fear of exposure. We asked A. G. and N. W., "What migration stories have your clients shared with you?"

A. G.: I've spoken with a woman who endured corrective gang rape. She was told by her family—her parents and brothers—that if she didn't go through with it, she wouldn't be cured of being queer or a lesbian. The belief was that having sex with a man would somehow make her straight. I've also seen people sell everything they own—their farms, cattle, and all their possessions—just to afford a ticket to come to the United States. Some people, for better or worse, form partnerships with older White men in the United States who pay their fare, but then expect sexual favors in return once they arrive. This happens quite frequently. Some have shared stories of traveling through South America, moving through Central America, crossing the Rio Grande, and witnessing people being exploited and drowning beside them. Many have nearly drowned themselves. Once in the United States, they've been treated like cattle—shipped around and used as political pawns, before eventually finding safety and reaching us.

N. W.: One of the things I've seen is the constant pressure on these individuals—cultural, religious, and legal. From an early age, they face mocking, beatings, and betrayal from their families, teachers, and communities. Their natural systems of trust are destroyed or nonexistent. There is constant fear of being found out, guilt, and anger. Many have endured horrific practices like being thrown out on the streets naked to be beaten by the community or being forced into marriage to produce grandchildren. On top of that, they face the ultimate consequences: arrest, rape, beatings, or, ultimately, even murder.

LIFETIME TRAUMA

Seeking asylum creates compounding layers of trauma, from persecution in one's home country to systemic barriers in the United States that hinder access to stability and safety. To better understand these challenges, we asked A. G. and N. W. to describe the barriers Black LGBTQ+ immigrants seeking asylum face.

A. G.: Once they arrive in the United States, there's often a lack of understanding about the asylum process. While the US government has a website detailing the process, it's still hard to navigate, even for someone like me who has been doing this work for a long time. For asylum seekers without this experience, it's incredibly challenging to know what documentation they need to provide or what they need to prove. On top of that, finding a lawyer to help them decipher everything and prepare their case is difficult, as legal support is in very short supply.

N. W.: I've been calling what people experienced as ongoing PTSD [post-traumatic stress disorder]. Because PTSD can refer to those earliest childhood experiences of betrayal, to that time when in fact you were attacked by a mob of five men, because you were kissing or walking on the street with another person of the same sex. . . . And having to flee, and then having the nightmare experience of coming up to the US border through South and Central American . . . to being detained by the US Border Patrol, you have no idea how long you're going to be detained. Then, you get out and are sent to New York City. Then, what have you got? A New York City shelter where you are harassed, threatened, robbed. Then you learn about the stringent rules here. You can't work. You've got to find a lawyer. There are no lawyers . . . how much trauma can you manage in your lifetime?

WORSENING CONDITIONS

Although anti-LGBTQ+ persecution has long forced individuals to flee, recent legislative crackdowns have exacerbated the crisis, increasing the number of asylum seekers while straining the resources of organizations that support them. We asked A. G. and N. W., "How has the global rise in anti-LGBTQ+ legislation impacted your organization?" and "How are your clients coping with resettling in the United States?"

Effect of Anti-LGBTQ+ Legislation

A. G.: Recently we've seen an uptick in asylum seekers reaching out to us because conditions in their home countries have worsened. I mean, they've always been bad, but they're getting worse. Just look at the recent laws enacted in Uganda and the shifting situations in places like Swaziland, Nigeria, and Kenya. We've had a significant increase in people contacting us—about 50% more this year alone. And it's not just online inquiries; people are showing up at our doorstep with nowhere else to go. There are so few alternative resources to redirect people to. No other organization is equipped to handle this, and even if there were, they're not suitable conditions for LGBTQ+ asylum seekers. This has put an enormous strain on our already limited resources.

N. W.: I'd say it's impacted us positively because we've been able to welcome LGBTQ persons who otherwise wouldn't have a place in the city. While there are some pockets of support elsewhere, what we offer here is the real deal. We've developed a strong queer presence in the agency, and keep in mind, the vast majority of the staff are from the countries that wanted to kill these people. So what kind of impact do you think we are having over time? The number of queer staff who've been hired gets higher all the time. This visibility has normalized being queer within the agency.

Dealing With A New Environment

A. G.: Clients cope in a number of ways. Most take advantage of the opportunities presented to them, such as activities the Task Force offers—whether it be trips, social gatherings, or other events. There are some who attend all of these, while others stay isolated and locked up in their rooms as their way of coping. Some turn to substances, and we try our best to help them through that. Unfortunately, there are also those who engage in sex acts as a way to feel some sort of connection or belonging with another human being.

COMMUNITY SUPPORT

The presence of community plays a critical role in shaping the resettlement experiences of Black LGBTQ+ asylum seekers. Social support networks not only provide immediate resources but also foster a sense of belonging. We asked A. G. and N. W. to discuss how their organizations provide refuge and access to services, and what they view as markers of success in their work.

Providing Refuge and Access to Services

A. G.: We provide housing and resources for LGBTQ+ asylum seekers during the up to two years that it takes after arriving in the United States before an asylum seeker is able to have their papers processed and get their work permit. . . . As of this month, we're able to guarantee asylum seekers in our housing a free lawyer. We also get them signed up for health insurance, open a bank account, and connect them with educational opportunities and career mentorship.

N. W.: We provide a safe, trusted space. . . . Every Tuesday evening, we offer food, social gatherings, and professionally facilitated support group meetings. We take members on community outings to places like the Botanical Gardens, the aquarium, museums, and parks to show them the city and give them a sense of belonging.

Impact on Organizations

A. G.: With the Task Force, 100% of our folks have gone on to receive asylum. And that just speaks even more to the fact that having a community behind you, having access to resources, can significantly increase or influence your outcomes.

N. W.: Members of LGBTQ+ communities who have escaped their countries come to African Services not necessarily knowing that they will be welcomed or served here. But once they're here, they are welcomed. And because now we're known throughout the city by a significant number of organizations, people are referred here specifically for the LGBTQ program.

CONCLUSION

In conclusion, the interviews highlight the profound challenges African and Caribbean LGBTQ+ asylum seekers face, from the trauma of fleeing persecution to navigating a complex and often discriminatory asylum process. Yet, they also showcase the resilience of these individuals and the vital role that community-driven efforts play in providing not only immediate relief, but also long-term support. As the global anti-LGBTQ+ crisis worsens, the work of organizations like the LGBT Asylum Task Force and African Services Committee becomes even more crucial. We must continue to support and amplify the efforts of grassroots organizations while advocating for the dismantling of current immigration policies that disproportionately harm Black LGBTQ+ immigrants and exacerbate their vulnerability to systemic inequities. AJPH

CORRESPONDENCE

Correspondence should be sent to Chioma Nnaji, 7 Palmer St, Roxbury, MA 02119 (e-mail: chioma.nnaji@gmail.com). Reprints can be ordered at https://www.ajph.org by clicking the "Reprints" link.

PUBLICATION INFORMATION

Full Citation: Nnaji C, Green A, Weeks NJ. How US grassroots organizations confront the global anti-LGBTQ+ crisis and support LGBTQ+ asylum seekers. *Am J Public Health*. 2025;115(4):466–468.

Acceptance Date: November 17, 2024.

DOI: https://doi.org/10.2105/AJPH.2024.307949

ORCID iD:

Chioma Nnaji https://orcid.org/0000-0001-8512-7913

CONTRIBUTORS

C. Nnaji conceptualized the editorial, conducted the interviews, and led the writing, including revisions. A. Green and N. J. Weeks contributed to reviewing and editing.

CONFLICTS OF INTEREST

The authors have no conflicts of interest to declare.

REFERENCES

1. Conron KJ, Luhur W. *Asylum Applications to the US by LGBT People*. Los Angeles, CA: The Williams Institute, UCLA; 2021.
2. Center for American Progress. Black LGBTQ individuals experience heightened levels of discrimination. Center for American Progress. July 13, 2021. Available at: https://www.americanprogress.org/article/black-lgbtq-individuals-experience-heightened-levels-discrimination. Accessed October 17, 2024.
3. Lasowski P, Moscicki O, Liu CZ, Katzenstein C, Singer EK, Baranowski KA. Persecution and migration experiences of lesbian, gay, bisexual, transgender, queer/questioning, and other sexual and gender minority asylum seekers. *J Trauma Stress*. 2023;36(3):605–616. https://doi.org/10.1002/jts.22932
4. Weiss D. Persecuted and marginalized: black LGBTQ migrants face unique challenges. ABA Journal. October 2, 2023. Available at: https://www.abajournal.com/web/article/persecuted-and-marginalized-Black-LGBTQ-migrants-face-unique-challenges. Accessed October 17, 2024.
5. PBS. Oluchi Omeoga and the Black LGBTQIA+ Migrant Project. Chasing the Dream. October 2023. Available at: https://www.pbs.org/wnet/chasing-the-dream/2023/10/oluchi-omeoga-black-lgbtqia-migrant-project. Accessed October 17, 2024.

Better Together: Implementation of a Public Health Learning Community During the COVID-19 Pandemic

Kristen M. Brown, PhD, MS, Brigette Courtot, MPH, Zara Porter, BA, and Sofia Hinojosa, BA

The Centers for Disease Control and Prevention's Partnering for Vaccine Equity program was developed during the COVID-19 public health emergency to fund more than 500 community-based organizations working to improve vaccine equity. Organizations were supported by a virtual learning community where members received tailored learning content, peer-to-peer learning opportunities, and resources that facilitated deployment of vaccine-related programming during a dynamic pandemic. Process evaluation metrics indicate successful implementation of the learning community. The virtual learning community model can be duplicated to address other public health issues. (*Am J Public Health*. 2025;115(4):469–472. https://doi.org/10.2105/AJPH.2024.307965)

AJPH April 2025, Vol. 115, No. 4

When COVID-19 vaccinations became available in the United States under emergency use authorization, an estimated 343 845 people had already died from COVID-19 in the country.[1] Longstanding racial, ethnic, and socioeconomic inequities; differential access to a trustworthy health care system; and unequal exposure to the virus for essential workers who are disproportionally people of color raised concerns about the equitable distribution of vaccines, even before they were available.[2,3]

INTERVENTION AND IMPLEMENTATION

In summer 2020, the Centers for Disease Control and Prevention (CDC) convened a diverse group of leaders to discuss strategies for ensuring that vaccines reached racial and ethnic minoritized populations. Based on this session, the Partnering for Vaccine Equity (P4VE) program was established to equip community-based organizations with knowledge and resources that could be dispersed locally.[4] These organizations used P4VE funding to plan and host community outreach events and vaccine clinics, train trusted messengers, develop educational materials and communication campaigns, and evaluate and disseminate best practices. They were supported by a learning community infrastructure that had three main objectives: (1) connect members to subject matter experts for tailored learning content, (2) provide forums for members to share knowledge with each other, and (3) build a set of resources to support longer-term vaccine equity efforts.

The P4VE learning community was supported by a team of Urban Institute researchers that served as its group learning manager. All organizations with P4VE funding were considered members. Four primary components facilitated collective learning opportunities (Table 1). The group learning manager hosted virtual learning events in various formats including webinars (45-minute presentations by subject matter experts with a question-and-answer segment), capacity-building workshops (90-minute sessions for learning a technical skill), coworking sessions (two-hour sessions to work virtually on a common task, with subject matter experts available for individual assistance), and "ask the expert" office hours (sessions with 10-minute time slots for one-on-one technical assistance). Webinars covered topics such as vaccine science and understanding vaccine hesitancy, and workshops focused on topics such as optimizing social media and motivational interviewing.

The second component, Communities of Practice (COP) groups, gave members a forum for peer-to-peer information sharing. Learning community members determined the three COP groups that were formed, based on the common priority populations they served: (1) African American/African

TABLE 1— Objectives of the Partnering for Vaccine Equity Learning Community and Corresponding Program Activities

	Events: Virtual Group Learning Events Hosted in Various Formats (e.g., Webinars, Workshops, Coworking Sessions, Office Hours)	Web Site: Online Platform That Included Searchable Member Directory, Discussion Board, Events Calendar, Resource Library	Communities of Practice: Forum for Peer-to-Peer Information Sharing With Other Organizations Who Served the Same Priority Population	Promising Practices: Subgrants Provided to 18 Organizations to Implement Tailored Strategies to Advance Vaccine Equity and Uptake
Objective 1: Connect members to subject matter experts for tailored learning content.	√			√
Objective 2: Provide forums for members to share knowledge and expertise with each other.	√	√	√	√
Objective 3: Build a set of resources to support longer-term vaccine equity efforts.	√			√

Diaspora, (2) Hispanic/Latinx, and (3) Asian American, Native Hawaiian, Pacific Islander, American Indian, and Alaska Native.

The third component of the P4VE learning community was the members-only Community Connector Web site. It included a searchable peer directory, group discussion board, events calendar, and a library of materials from past events and resources such as toolkits and fact sheets. The final component was the Promising Practices initiative under which Urban Institute provided $25,000 subgrants to 18 P4VE-funded organizations to develop, implement, and evaluate the effectiveness of a promising practice in one of three areas: (1) media-based outreach, (2) community-based outreach, and (3) vaccine events and partnerships.[5]

PLACE, TIME, AND PERSONS

The CDC contracted with the Urban Institute to manage the P4VE Learning Community from April 2021 through April 2024. The virtual P4VE learning community supported information sharing among more than 500 community-based organizations throughout the United States who received P4VE funding from the CDC, and participation was voluntary. The societal reliance on technology, especially virtual meetings, that increased during the pandemic supported application of an online learning community structure that was available to people in various geographies, minimized training costs, and permitted inclusion of members with diverse perspectives and resource-limited organizations.

PURPOSE

Vaccines were a critical component of the COVID-19 pandemic response, and distribution needed to occur quickly and equitably to combat the raging, highly infectious virus. Previous literature demonstrates the effectiveness of community-based organizations in implementing public health programming in local areas of influence.[6,7] These organizations understand local culture including assets and obstacles (e.g., transportation, work environments, health care facilities) for accessing health-promoting resources (e.g., testing, vaccinations). Therefore, they are well-positioned to design and implement culturally and linguistically appropriate programming that can play a critical role in affecting health behaviors (e.g., vaccine uptake) of the community members they serve.

Numerous initiatives focus on increasing vaccination among racially and ethnically minoritized populations, but programmatic efforts often miss opportunities to build in collaboration that facilitates efficient use of resources. The P4VE Learning Community fostered an information-sharing network for organizations focused on vaccine equity to enhance their collective societal impact, and this coordination supported a time-sensitive response to the COVID-19 pandemic.

EVALUATION AND ADVERSE EFFECTS

More than 500 organizations, representing 52 US states and territories, were part of the P4VE partner network. This included 404 nonprofits (nonmedical associations), 64 federally qualified health centers (FQHCs), 34 health departments, 16 community health centers (non-FQHCs), 16 universities, 11 nonprofit medical associations, six social media partners, and two city governments.[4]

The Urban Institute conducted a process evaluation of learning community activities as part of quarterly and annual reporting to the CDC; performance indicators were based on self-reported data from the group learning team and P4VE-funded organizations. These indicators demonstrated that the learning community was a valuable component of the P4VE program and helped its members conduct program activities. The learning community team hosted a total of 149 learning events, and, for each reporting period, on average at least 95% of event attendees agreed or strongly agreed that they learned something during the event that enhanced their P4VE program work.

The COP groups served as a space for learning community members to build relationships for peer-to-peer information sharing. According to COP facilitators, members engaged in timely discussions such as cultural influence on the perception of vaccines, messaging for new variants, and managing changing funding allotments. In total, 129 people joined the African American/African Diaspora group, 100 people joined Hispanic/Latinx group, and 50 people joined the Asian American, Native Hawaiian, Pacific Islander, American Indian, Alaska Native group. The Community Connector Web site was used for communication and asynchronous learning. There were 1014 logins, 1969 resources downloaded, and 1985 total discussion posts. The Promising Practices initiative provided an opportunity for organizations to test an initiative that addressed vaccine equity within a cohort structure and with group-learning team support on implementation and evaluation. All 18 organizations completed the six-month performance period and submitted data evaluating their efforts as well as final reports. The success of this component of the learning community has been previously described.[5]

In total, between the program's launch and April 2024, P4VE funded organizations and their partners trained 410 000 trusted messengers to conduct community outreach, engaged more than 4 million people at promotional events, reached 572 000 clinicians, launched 674 educational campaigns in 45 languages, and administered 2.4 million COVID-19 and influenza vaccines.[8]

SUSTAINABILITY

The COVID-19 pandemic created the opportunity to establish a network of organizations to make a tangible public health impact, and several factors make P4VE sustainable. The organizations that comprised the learning community are committed to the people their work serves. In fact, most organizations were engaging in health-promoting activities before joining the P4VE learning community and were selected for funding because they were already well-connected to the communities the initiative prioritized. Feedback survey results indicate learning community participation helped members connect and learn from other organizations with similar missions and priority populations, making their programming more efficient. Secondly, the group learning team developed a large repository that includes hundreds of resources such as recorded webinars, fact sheets, and social media materials that can be used to guide future programmatic efforts. They also developed protocols (e.g., online event planning, implementing a subgrant program) to guide learning community operations that can be used as a foundation for ongoing and new programs. Finally, COP members made relationships with other organizations that can be sustained.

PUBLIC HEALTH SIGNIFICANCE

Community-based organizations that possess knowledge of the local culture and have community trust are well-positioned to address public health issues. A network that facilitates strategy sharing can enhance productivity and impact. While the P4VE learning community was implemented during the COVID-19 public health emergency, the network can be employed to address longstanding health inequities. For example, the National Institutes of Health's Community Engagement Alliance program (NIH-CEAL), which had similar goals to P4VE at its inception, is leveraging the partnerships built during the COVID-19 pandemic to understand long COVID and other chronic diseases as well as the social, structural, and environmental factors that lead to health inequities.[9] Like NIH-CEAL, the P4VE Learning Community provides evidence of (1) the power of community-level efforts to have a positive impact on the health of residents when properly resourced and (2) the strength of operating in a network of organizations with aligned goals.

In addition to vaccinations, there are well-documented inequities in social determinants such as food access, transportation, education quality, job opportunities, and myriad health outcomes including cancer, diabetes, and cardiovascular disease that organizations of varying sizes can work within a network to efficiently address. The relationships and strategies established by P4VE learning community members to promote the rapid uptake of the COVID-19 vaccine can be sustained and expanded to address a wider range of vaccinations, long COVID, and other diseases that have persistent inequities. AJPH

ABOUT THE AUTHORS

Kristen M. Brown, Brigette Courtot, Zara Porter, and Sofia Hinojosa are with the Health Policy Center, Urban Institute, Washington, DC.

CORRESPONDENCE

Correspondence should be sent to Kristen M. Brown, PhD, MS, 500 L'Enfant Plaza SW, Washington, DC 20024 (e-mail: krbrown@urban.org). Reprints can be ordered at https://www.ajph.org by clicking the "Reprints" link.

PUBLICATION INFORMATION

Full Citation: Brown KM, Courtot B, Porter Z, Hinojosa S. Better together: implementation of a public health learning community during the COVID-19 pandemic. *Am J Public Health*. 2025;115(4):469–472.

Acceptance Date: November 26, 2024.

DOI: https://doi.org/10.2105/AJPH.2024.307965

ORCID iDs:

Kristen M. Brown https://orcid.org/0000-0002-9955-0568

Brigette Courtot https://orcid.org/0000-0001-9374-6781

Zara Porter https://orcid.org/0009-0002-5779-0050

CONTRIBUTORS

K. M. Brown and B. Courtot conceptualized the article. All authors contributed to implementation and writing.

ACKNOWLEDGMENTS

The Partnering for Vaccine Equity learning community was funded by the Centers for Disease Control and Prevention (CDC) within the US Department of Health and Human Services (HHS).

The authors acknowledge thoughtful review by Lisa Dubay, PhD.

Note. The findings and conclusions reported here are those of the authors and do not necessarily represent the official views of, nor an endorsement, by CDC, HHS, or the US government.

CONFLICTS OF INTEREST

The authors report no conflicts of interest.

HUMAN PARTICIPANT PROTECTION

This work was exempted from institutional review because it did not involve human participant research.

REFERENCES

1. Centers for Disease Control and Prevention. COVID Data Tracker: Trends by geographic area. Available at: https://covid.cdc.gov/covid-data-tracker/#trends_weeklydeaths_select_00. Accessed September 4, 2023.
2. Gayle HD, Childress JF. Race, racism, and structural injustice: equitable allocation and distribution of vaccines for the COVID-19. *Am J Bioeth*. 2021;21(3):4–7. https://doi.org/10.1080/15265161.2021.1877011
3. Webb Hooper M, Nápoles AM, Pérez-Stable EJ. No populations left behind: vaccine hesitancy and equitable diffusion of effective COVID-19 vaccines. *J Gen Intern Med*. 2021;36(7):2130–2133. https://doi.org/10.1007/s11606-021-06698-5
4. Centers for Disease Control and Prevention. Partnering for vaccine equity. Available at: https://www.cdc.gov/vaccines/health-equity/index.html. Accessed August 28, 2023.
5. Hill I, Porter Z, Mayer J, Verdeflor A, Brown K, Lawrence D. Building the evidence base for advancing vaccine equity. Findings from the P4VE Promising Practices Project. Urban Institute. September 19, 2023. Available at: https://www.urban.org/research/publication/building-evidence-base-advancing-vaccine-equity. Accessed January 27, 2025.
6. Administration for Strategic Preparedness and Response. Promising practices for reaching at-risk individuals for COVID-19 vaccination and information. Available at: https://aspr.hhs.gov/at-risk/Pages/engaging_CBO.aspx. Accessed May 6, 2024.
7. Korin MR, Araya F, Idris MY, Brown H, Claudio L. Community-based organizations as effective partners in the battle against misinformation. *Front Public Health*. 2022;10:853736. https://doi.org/10.3389/fpubh.2022.853736
8. Centers for Disease Control and Prevention. Partnering for Vaccine Equity (P4VE) Program. Available at: https://www.cdc.gov/vaccine-equity/php/about/index.html. Accessed January 7, 2025.
9. Mensah GA, Johnson LE. Community Engagement Alliance (CEAL): leveraging the power of communities during public health emergencies. *Am J Public Health*. 2024;114(S1):S18–S21. https://doi.org/10.2105/AJPH.2023.307507

Outreach to Adolescents in Crisis on Social Media, YouthLine's Safe Social Spaces, 2019 to 2024

Craig Leets, MA, Angela Nielsen, MS, MA, Meghan Buchanan, BA, Ayah Zirikly, PhD, Mark Dredze, PhD, Leslie Miller, MD, Holly C. Wilcox, PhD, and Carlos Gallo, PhD

YouthLine developed Safe Social Spaces (SSS), a program that trains young adult crisis specialists to identify and assist youths expressing suicidal thoughts and behaviors on social media platforms. Crisis specialists contacted 3868 youths in crisis from across the United States through social media private messaging from 2019 to 2024. Fifty-six percent of youths responded to outreach by SSS. SSS is a scalable program, created to meet youths where they are—on social media and online. (*Am J Public Health*. 2025;115(4):473–476. https://doi.org/10.2105/AJPH.2024.307970)

AJPH April 2025, Vol. 115, No. 4

Most crisis centers do not provide outreach and intervention to adolescents on social media.[1] The crisis response system typically waits for individuals to reach out for help. Unfortunately, most people who die by suicide never seek out and receive mental health services.[2]

INTERVENTION AND IMPLEMENTATION

YouthLine's Safe Social Spaces (SSS) crisis specialists identify and intervene with adolescents in crisis on social media. When youths post about distress, self-harm, or suicidal thoughts, the SSS team provides support, de-escalation, and resource referrals by private message. SSS is an innovative outreach program, meeting youths where they are, on social media apps.[3,4] Herein we highlight a crisis center–academic research partnership established to scale SSS to serve more youths by introducing computational implementation science approaches.

PLACE, TIME, AND PERSONS

SSS was developed in 2017 by the YouthLine program at Lines for Life in Portland, Oregon. The Oregon Health Authority's Youth Suicide Intervention and Prevention Plan in 2016[5] sought recommendations for online interventions for youth suicidal and self-injurious behaviors, given the prevalence of technology in adolescents' lives. YouthLine, in collaboration with partners Youth ERA and Reachout.com, drafted a plan for online crisis intervention that resulted in funding for SSS in 2018. YouthLine's program director, seeing the need to proactively reach youths on social media who were posting about their suicidal thoughts and behaviors, created SSS. Although youths may be engaging in help-seeking by posting about their mental health crises, social media apps do not have the policies, procedures, or staff to provide personalized support from a crisis specialist. Consequently, SSS began in 2019 with seed money from the Oregon Health Authority to YouthLine to provide support to youths in crisis by proactively identifying young people on social media apps who need support.

From January 2019 to May 2024, SSS directly messaged 3868 youths across the United States. A total of 527 (14%) of the youths declined conversation (Table 1); 2167 (56%) responded to messages from crisis responders; 1640 (42%) directly engaged in online conversation with SSS, 328 of whom successfully engaged in de-escalation strategies intended to prevent suicide and self-injuries. A total of 3810 youths (99%) received personalized resources; 58 (1%) did not receive resources, because (1) SSS staff was blocked before resources could be sent or (2) the conversation occurred when outcomes were not tracked. A total of 1010 youths (26%) responded within an SSS staff shift of four or five hours, during which time most conversations start and end.

TABLE 1— Responses of Youths Contacted by Safe Social Spaces (SSS) Outreach: United States, January 2019–May 2024

Youth Did the Following	No. (%)
Responded to SSS	2167 (56)
And engaged immediately	1010 (26)
And engaged at a later date	630 (16)
And declined SSS outreach	527 (14)
Did not respond to SSS	1701 (44)
And resources were provided	1643 (43)
And resources were not provided	58 (1)
Total	3868 (100)

PURPOSE

Suicide is the second leading cause of death for people aged 10 to 14 years and 25 to 34 years.[6] Although effective interventions for suicidal thoughts and behaviors exist, most individuals who die by suicide do so before making contact with a mental health professional.[7] Because youths are increasingly engaged in online social media platforms, this medium offers a unique opportunity to engage youths experiencing a mental health crisis who may not otherwise reach out for professional help.

The Biden–Harris administration made an investment of nearly $1 billion to support the 988 Suicide and Crisis Lifeline and infrastructure to build up crisis center capacity. Despite this investment, research shows that some people contemplating suicide will not call 988 through lack of awareness of these services, stigma, or other reasons.[8] SSS fills a gap in existing crisis intervention approaches by proactively outreaching to youths in crisis through social media. SSS specialists are trained in de-escalation techniques, Youth Mental Health First Aid, and safeTALK and are supervised by highly experienced crisis response staff. These specialists monitor posts on TalkLife, Discord, Vent, Tumblr, Amino, and Wisdo. These social media apps are mental health oriented and have direct messaging features. These elements, not present on all platforms, are essential to provide proactive and confidential crisis support. Once specialists identify youth posts discussing suicide, self-harm, and related emotions, such as hopelessness and despair, they send direct messages to those youths. The personalized support can include de-escalation techniques, safety planning, and resource referral. If staff determine that emergency services are needed, a rescue call is initiated in cooperation with the youth. If the location is known, SSS staff engage with the local emergency services and report the post to the social media app.

EVALUATION AND ADVERSE EFFECTS

SSS developed a rubric to assess risk and safety. The risk score is based on acuity of thoughts, plans, access to lethal means, and suicide intent expressed in the initial post content and the conversation. The safety score measures the specificity of the safety plan and the receptivity to resources delivered by SSS staff. Following the conversation, staff use a scoring matrix to determine whether suicide or self-injury was possibly averted as a result of the interaction. This de-escalation score is generated by comparing the difference between the risk score and the safety score. Suicide or self-injury was de-escalated and possibly prevented when the youth agreed to stay safe and reach out for help if future support was needed. Demographic characteristics were collected when volunteered by the youth (62% of the time) and were not a requirement to receive services. The mean age was 19.4 years (SD = 2.8 years). Gender ranged from cisgender man (9%), cisgender woman (18%), nonbinary (4%), transgender man (3%), transgender woman (1%), and unknown (61%). Here are two examples of phrases that triggered SSS intervention: "I have nobody in my life" and "I'm so pointless that nobody talks to me, if I disappeared nobody is noticing." Although it is possible for youths to use hyperbole,[9] SSS treats every distressing post as genuine. Previous research has found that there is no added risk but actual benefit in asking individuals whether they feel suicidal.[10] SSS staff could not always distinguish whether posts were hyperbolic or genuine, so more research is needed on this issue.

Evaluation has focused on refining crisis intervention approaches and assessing the most effective and efficient ways to intervene online with youths in crisis. SSS staff have been online on various days and times throughout the week to determine when they receive the highest rate of response from youths. Future research is necessary to evaluate the effectiveness of SSS on mental health service utilization and the prevention of recurrence of suicidal thoughts and behaviors. In our previous work with the evaluation of Crisis Text Line,[11] we found that the majority of help-seekers benefited from immediate de-escalation. We are seeking funding for a hybrid implementation trial that will test the effectiveness of SSS while measuring implementation outcomes (e.g., reach and fidelity) and assessing the best strategies for scaling the program to help more youths in crisis.

SSS staff have explored multiple social media apps, resulting in a program presence on apps with more posts about self-injury and suicide and with greater response rates from youths contacted. Also, SSS staff share successful engagement approaches with each other in an effort to identify which strategies are most impactful. Importantly, SSS is currently addressing an unmet need in adolescent mental health services and helping to address Internet safety standards.

One possible adverse effect of SSS is the potential for vicarious trauma and adverse effects on the specialists' mental well-being; as such, staff only work 20 hours per week and are required to work in an office setting where they can get immediate support from a supervisor to help co-support a youth in crisis or to support their own wellness. SSS staff have encountered some youths who were disappointed with the short-term nature of the intervention. SSS is a crisis service that has the ability to reach out to many youths and provide immediate support. However, it is beyond the scope of the service to provide ongoing follow-up contact and mental health support. Some youths express the desire to become friends with the crisis specialists. The specialists are required to set boundaries and clarify expectations with the youths.

SCALABILITY

SSS continues to partner with additional social media platforms and refine protocols and best practices for this innovative intervention approach. The SSS team has partnered with public health and computer science researchers to develop social informatics methods for identifying youths at risk to expand capacity.[12] Additionally, staff are currently adapting computational tools to assess fidelity to the program protocol in an automated fashion.[13] This will increase the sustainability and scalability of SSS while ensuring fidelity during scaling out.

PUBLIC HEALTH IMPLICATIONS

Although SSS is not currently part of the Protecting Kids on Social Media Act, public health policy that incentivizes and promotes such partnerships with social media platforms and mental health crisis services has the potential to save lives. The SSS team envisions a future where major apps, like TikTok, Instagram, and Discord, incorporate proactive mental health safety measures involving outreach by a human and the provision of personalized resources, as well as national legislation creating a safer Internet culture for youths. The SSS team also encouraged apps to increase transparency in their safety practices and adopt policies that keep youths safe. SSS staff have reached out to establish formal partnerships with these apps to better support youths in crisis. AJPH

ABOUT THE AUTHORS

Craig Leets, Angela Nielsen, and Meghan Buchanan are with YouthLine, Lines for Life, Portland, OR. Ayah Zirikly is with the Malone Center for Engineering in Healthcare and the Center for Language and Speech Processing, Whiting School of Engineering, Johns Hopkins University, Baltimore, MD. Mark Dredze is with the Malone Center for Engineering in Healthcare and the Department of Computer Science, Johns Hopkins University, Baltimore. Leslie Miller is with the Department of Psychiatry and Behavioral Sciences, Johns Hopkins University School of Medicine, Baltimore. Holly C. Wilcox is with the Department of Psychiatry and Behavioral Sciences, Johns Hopkins University School of Medicine, and the Department of Mental Health, Johns Hopkins Bloomberg School of Public Health, Baltimore. Carlos Gallo is with the Department of Psychiatry and Behavioral Sciences, Northwestern University, Chicago, IL.

CORRESPONDENCE

Correspondence should be sent to Carlos Gallo, Research Faculty, Northwestern University, 750 North Lake Shore, Drive Floor 10th, Psych and Behavioral Dept, Chicago, IL 60611 (e-mail: carlos.gallo@northwestern.edu). Reprints can be ordered at https://www.ajph.org by clicking the "Reprints" link.

PUBLICATION INFORMATION

Full Citation: Leets C, Nielsen A, Buchanan M, et al. Outreach to adolescents in crisis on social media, YouthLine's Safe Social Spaces, 2019 to 2024. *Am J Public Health*. 2025;115(4):473–476.

Acceptance Date: December 3, 2024.

DOI: https://doi.org/10.2105/AJPH.2024.307970

ORCID iDs:

Ayah Zirikly https://orcid.org/0000-0002-8441-1741

Holly C. Wilcox https://orcid.org/0000-0003-2624-0654

Carlos Gallo https://orcid.org/0000-0003-3270-8786

CONTRIBUTORS

All authors conceptualized and designed the study, analyzed and interpreted data, drafted or revised the manuscript, and approved the final version.

ACKNOWLEDGMENTS

We acknowledge funding from the National Institute of Mental Health, which supported this research in part (5R01MH117598).

CONFLICTS OF INTEREST

The authors report no conflicts of interest.

HUMAN PARTICIPANT PROTECTION

This study is not human participant research and was exempt from institutional review board review.

REFERENCES

1. Mann JJ, Michel CA, Auerbach RP. Improving suicide prevention through evidence-based strategies: a systematic review. *Focus Am Psychiatr Publ*. 2023;21(2):182–196. https://doi.org/10.1176/appi.focus.23021004
2. Tang S, Reily NM, Arena AF, et al. People who die by suicide without receiving mental health services: a systematic review. *Front Public Health*.

2022;9:736948. https://doi.org/10.3389/fpubh.2021.736948

3. Anderson M, Jiang J. Teens' social media habits and experiences. Pew Research Center. 2018. Available at: https://www.pewresearch.org/internet/wp-content/uploads/sites/9/2018/11/PI_2018.11.28_teens-social-media_FINAL4.pdf. Accessed July 1, 2024.
4. Vogels EA, Gelles-Watnick R, Massarat N. Teens, social media and technology 2022. Available at: https://www.pewresearch.org/internet/2022/08/10/teens-social-media-and-technology-2022. Accessed July 1, 2024.
5. Oregon Health Authority. Youth suicide intervention and prevention plan annual report. 2017. Available at: https://sharedsystems.dhsoha.state.or.us/DHSForms/Served/le8874c.pdf. Accessed January 31, 2024.
6. National Vital Statistics System. Mortality 2018–2022 on CDC WONDER Online Database, released in 2024. Data are from the Multiple Cause of Death Files, 2018–2022, as compiled from data provided by the 57 vital statistics jurisdictions through the Vital Statistics Cooperative Program. Available at: http://wonder.cdc.gov/mcd-icd10-expanded.html. Accessed April 23, 2024.
7. National Research Council (US) and Institute of Medicine (US) Committee on the Prevention of Mental Disorders and Substance Abuse Among Children, Youth, and Young Adults: Research Advances and Promising Interventions. *Preventing Mental, Emotional, and Behavioral Disorders Among Young People: Progress and Possibilities.* M. E. O'Connell, T. Boat, K. E. Warner, eds. Washington, DC: National Academies Press; 2009.
8. Roth KB, Szlyk HS. Hotline use in the United States: results from the Collaborative Psychiatric Epidemiology Surveys. *Adm Policy Ment Health.* 2021;48(3):564–578. https://doi.org/10.1007/s10488-020-01089-0
9. Ali N, Qadir S, Alsoubai A, De Choudhury M, Razi A, Wisniewski P. "I'm gonna KMS": from imminent risk to youth joking about suicide and self-harm via social media. In: *CHI '24: Proceedings of the CHI Conference on Human Factors in Computing Systems.* New York, NY: Association for Computing Machinery; 2024:Article 999, 1–18. https://doi.org/10.1145/3613904.3642489
10. Gould MS, Marrocco FA, Kleinman M, et al. Evaluating iatrogenic risk of youth suicide screening programs: a randomized controlled trial. *JAMA.* 2005;293(13):1635–1643. https://doi.org/10.1001/jama.293.13.1635
11. Gould MS, Pisani A, Gallo C, et al. Crisis text-line interventions: evaluation of texters' perceptions of effectiveness. *Suicide Life Threat Behav.* 2022;52(3):583–595. https://doi.org/10.1111/sltb.12873
12. Gallo C, Berkel C, Mauricio A, et al. Implementation methodology from a social systems informatics and engineering perspective applied to a parenting training program. *Fam Syst Health.* 2021;39(1):7–18. https://doi.org/10.1037/fsh0000590
13. Gallo C, Pantin H, Villamar J, et al. Blending qualitative and computational linguistics methods for fidelity assessment: experience with the Familias Unidas preventive intervention. *Adm Policy Ment Health.* 2015;42(5):574–585. https://doi.org/10.1007/s10488-014-0538-4

A Novel Reentry Hotline Led by Community Health Workers to Address the Health Needs of People Returning From Incarceration: Transitions Clinic Network, California, June 2020–June 2023

Bethany Divakaran, DNP, MPH, Anna Steiner, MSW, MPH, Sidney Lin, BA, Sharon Fennix, CADC, and Shira Shavit, MD

Community members returning from incarceration experience serious health disparities, which intensified during the COVID-19 pandemic. In response, community health workers with lived experience of incarceration in the Transitions Clinic Network established a California reentry health care hotline to support time-sensitive linkages to postrelease medical care. From June 2020 to June 2023, the hotline supported 1276 people transitioning from incarceration. Lessons from this peer-led public health intervention are relevant for states utilizing Medicaid waivers to improve health equity for justice-involved populations. (*Am J Public Health*. 2025;115(4):477–480. https://doi.org/10.2105/AJPH.2024.307969)

AJPH April 2025, Vol. 115, No. 4

Community reentry following incarceration is perilous—people face worsened health, high rates of acute care utilization, and risk of death after release.[1] In California, hundreds of thousands of people are released from prisons and jails annually.[2]

INTERVENTION AND IMPLEMENTATION

Transitions Clinic Network (TCN) is a community-based nonprofit organization addressing the health and social needs of people returning from incarceration. TCN improves community health systems nationally by embedding community health workers (CHWs) with lived experience of incarceration onto teams in primary care clinics. The evidence-based TCN model improves engagement in primary care and reduces emergency department and preventable hospital visits for returning community members.[3–5] Since 2006, TCN has been building a robust network of community clinics that implemented the TCN model in California, spanning 21 health systems across 14 counties.

With the COVID-19 pandemic emerging, TCN's formerly incarcerated CHWs watched with concern as the virus exploded in overcrowded prisons and jails. Communication with incarcerated peers became difficult as institutions halted programming and visitation.[6] At the urging of health professionals and advocates, releases were expedited to depopulate prisons, but people came home to communities with health and social services severely disrupted by the pandemic, exacerbating the challenges returning community members face with securing basic needs. TCN CHWs acted to support people inside and coming home during this public health crisis by developing a reentry health care hotline in California. This hotline was staffed by TCN CHWs with lived experience of incarceration and leveraged TCN's existing network of community clinics to support linkages to medical care.

The CHWs received calls through a third-party phone system, with TCN assuming the cost of calls from carceral institutions. Hotline CHWs documented caller attributes and needs in an online hotline log. TCN disseminated flyers advertising the hotline to jails, prisons, probation and parole officers, and community-based partners.

PLACE, TIME, AND PERSONS

The reentry health care hotline is a statewide intervention in California. The hotline went live in June 2020 amid the emerging pandemic, which had a disproportionate impact on incarcerated populations.[6] A team of 10 CHWs who worked for TCN-affiliated clinics staffed the hotline on weekday shifts with support from TCN's organizational staff.

PURPOSE

TCN's hotline was created to reach people preparing for and recently released from incarceration to support medical care linkages and reentry resources. Because community and carceral systems are disjointed, it is difficult for health professionals in the community to reach people while incarcerated for prerelease care coordination. Returning community members experience barriers accessing health insurance coverage, primary and specialty care in the community, timely refills of medications, and their medical records.[7] In California, systems and resources vary by county, requiring local expertise to navigate fragmented community services. CHWs working in primary care systems used their lived experience of reentry and rich knowledge of community resources to provide real-time peer support on the hotline.

Hotline CHWs assisted callers with navigating county-based Medicaid enrollment; identifying local community clinics (including TCN-affiliated clinics) that provide primary care, mental health, and substance use treatment services (including medications for opioid use disorder); and locating resources to address social determinants of health. By utilizing an already existing network of TCN-affiliated clinics, hotline CHWs could connect callers directly with other supportive TCN CHWs in their local communities to help navigate these complex systems.

The hotline was a vital resource in a chaotic time, a line of communication to people behind prison walls and a safety net to those who needed guidance navigating release. Given the unique and complex needs of the reentry population, CHWs with lived experience are best suited to serve their peers with competency and empathy.[4,8] Many callers reached out in crisis, having recently been reintroduced into society, and the real-time peer support offered by hotline CHWs was a source of connection and hope.

Furthermore, TCN identified systems-level challenges by hearing from callers across the state. For instance, hotline CHWs heard reports from people released into COVID-19 isolation hotels that they were lacking regular meals. TCN advocated for these clients to the entity overseeing the isolation housing to successfully address the problem.

EVALUATION AND ADVERSE EFFECTS

From June 2020 through June 2023, hotline CHWs logged 1333 hotline interactions from 1275 unique callers. Of these unique callers, 93% were calling for themselves, and 7% were calling on behalf of others (e.g., family). Hotline CHWs tracked caller incarceration status and type: 30% were currently incarcerated, while 69% were recently released to the community (1% unknown); 93% were incarcerated by the state prison system, 4% by local jail systems, and 3% unknown. Of those calling after release, 36% called within one week of release, and 76% called within one month (Figure A, available as a supplement to the online version of this article at https://ajph.org).

Hotline CHWs supported callers with many needs, primarily with finding a clinic in the community, navigating Medicaid enrollment, accessing medications for opioid use disorder and other medications, and addressing social determinants of health (e.g., housing, transportation, food; Table 1). Hotline CHWs supported callers with resources for 46 of 58 California counties.

There were no known adverse effects to this intervention. One possible unintended impact is callers having negative experiences with resources offered on the hotline—it is difficult to ensure the cultural competencies or daily capacity of every resource, especially in under-resourced regions. One surprising outcome was that most callers utilized the hotline in the community after release, despite the original intent to reach people inside prisons and jails.

SUSTAINABILITY

As the pandemic stabilized, hotline CHWs resumed in-person clinic responsibilities, leading to hotline staffing challenges. Sustainable staffing has been achieved through providing stipends to hotline CHWs who volunteer beyond their clinic responsibilities. In addition, TCN staffs a full-time CHW hotline coordinator.

Sustainable funding is the greatest challenge. The hotline was started with

TABLE 1— Health Care Needs of Hotline Callers Transitioning From Incarceration: Transitions Clinic Network, California, June 2020–June 2023

Need Identified	Callers, No. (%)
Health clinic	967 (75.8)
Medicaid navigation	345 (27.1)
Social determinants	337 (26.4)
Medications for opioid use disorder (MOUD)[a]	177 (13.9)
Medication refills (not MOUD)	111 (8.7)
Letters to support parole	67 (5.3)

Note. The sample size was n = 1275.
[a]MOUD was added to the hotline log in June 2021, so this count is limited.

COVID-19 relief funds and sustained through grants but lacks a consistent funding stream. Current Medicaid payment models, even for CHW services, do not support such population-level interventions.

One policy positively impacting TCN's hotline was legislation making phone calls from state prisons free, which was implemented by the state prison system in January 2023.[9]

PUBLIC HEALTH SIGNIFICANCE

There are thousands of public health hotlines, and the pandemic generated more telephonic resources for health education and navigation.[10] CHWs played critical roles in serving vulnerable populations during the COVID-19 pandemic.[11] Nonetheless, there are scarce examples of hotlines staffed by CHWs[12] or targeting incarcerated or reentry populations.[13] There are no published examples known to these authors of hotlines staffed by formerly incarcerated CHWs supporting reentry health care.

Beyond the pandemic, TCN's novel peer-support hotline remains relevant for service delivery to this high-risk population. Our data indicate that returning community members will utilize a reentry health hotline, most often within a month after release when needs are most urgent. Furthermore, the intervention fills a systems-level gap for monitoring statewide reentry challenges, allowing TCN to report community concerns back to carceral partners. This hotline is now a staple resource included in discharge packets for all people leaving California prisons.

Novel interventions for the reentry population are significant for states undergoing Medicaid reform through Section 1115 waivers. California's model waiver, called California Advancing and Innovating Medicaid, will serve the "justice-involved" population with prerelease care coordination and enhanced community services.[14] Even with more proactive and collaborative release planning, safety-net supports are still needed for when clients need the most support following release. Many returning community members experience homelessness or transience making them even harder to reach and engage in care.[15] A statewide hotline is a critical resource clients can use on their own behalf no matter where they land in the community. Medicaid reforms that target this population should create mechanisms to pay for population-level interventions. Investments are needed to build strong community health and social services infrastructures, as hotline navigation services are only as effective as the strength of the resources available with which to connect people in need.

Furthermore, services provided for the reentry population must be tailored to their unique needs, and investments in reentry services should prioritize programs and interventions led by people with lived experience of incarceration. Because people impacted by incarceration often have negative health care experiences that impede engagement in care, community-driven and culturally appropriate public health strategies like this hotline are critical for reaching people who need services and for garnering trust. States utilizing Section 1115 waivers to improve health equity for justice-involved populations have a prime opportunity to improve patient engagement in community health care resources both before and after release, promote collaboration between carceral and community entities, and prioritize the experience and expertise of people with lived experience to show us what works. More broadly, investments in and supports for a strong CHW workforce are needed to meet the most vital needs of the most vulnerable populations. AJPH

ABOUT THE AUTHORS

Bethany Divakaran, Anna Steiner, Sharon Fennix, and Shira Shavit are with the Transitions Clinic Network (TCN), a project of the San Francisco Public Health Foundation. Shira Shavit is also with the University of California San Francisco Department of Family and Community Medicine. Sidney Lin is with the University of California San Diego School of Medicine.

CORRESPONDENCE

Correspondence should be sent to Bethany Divakaran, 1855 Folsom St, San Francisco, CA 94103 (e-mail: tcninfo@ucsf.edu). Reprints can be ordered at https://www.ajph.org by clicking the "Reprints" link.

PUBLICATION INFORMATION

Full Citation: Divakaran B, Steiner A, Lin S, Fennix S, Shavit S. A novel reentry hotline led by community health workers to address the health needs of people returning from incarceration: Transitions Clinic Network, California, June 2020–June 2023. *Am J Public Health*. 2025;115(4):477–480.

Acceptance Date: December 3, 2024.

DOI: https://doi.org/10.2105/AJPH.2024.307969

ORCID iD:
Bethany Divakaran https://orcid.org/0009-0009-7906-9302

CONTRIBUTORS

All authors contributed to the conceptualization or implementation of the hotline and to the writing of this article.

ACKNOWLEDGMENTS

Thank you to our past and present funders for collaborating with TCN, including the Governor's Returning Home Well Initiative, the Molina Cares Foundation, the California Health Care Foundation, and the Board of State and Community Corrections.

We acknowledge the ongoing collaboration with our TCN clinic partners in the community, especially the innovative community health workers who have gone above and beyond to establish and staff this hotline. We acknowledge current and former TCN staff who were instrumental in the creation of the hotline. Most importantly, we acknowledge all those who have been impacted by mass incarceration who offer their experiences and expertise.

CONFLICTS OF INTEREST

The authors have no conflicts of interest to disclose.

HUMAN PARTICIPANT PROTECTION

This study underwent expedited review by the institutional review board (IRB) at the University of California San Francisco and was approved. The IRB approved a waiver of informed consent.

REFERENCES

1. Binswanger IA, Stern M, Deyo R, et al. Release from prison—a high risk of death for former inmates. *N Engl J Med*. 2007;356(2):157–165. https://doi.org/10.1056/NEJMsa064115
2. Sawyer W. Since you asked: how many people are released from each state's prisons and jails every year? Prison Policy Initiative. August 25, 2022. Available at: https://www.prisonpolicy.org/blog/2022/08/25/releasesbystate. Accessed March 13, 2024.
3. Wang EA, Wang Y, Krumholz HM. A high risk of hospitalization following release from correctional facilities in Medicare beneficiaries: a retrospective matched cohort study, 2002 to 2010. *JAMA Intern Med*. 2013;173(17):1621–1628. https://doi.org/10.1001/jamainternmed.2013.9008
4. Wang EA, Hong C, Shavit S, Sanders R, Kessell E, Kushel M. Engaging individuals recently released from prison into primary care: a randomized trial. *Am J Public Health*. 2012;102(9):e22–e29. https://doi.org/10.2105/AJPH.2012.300894
5. Wang EA, Lin W, Aminawung J, et al. Propensity-matched study of enhanced primary care on contact with the criminal justice system among individuals recently released from prison to New Haven. *BMJ Open*. 2019;9(5):e028097. https://doi.org/10.1136/bmjopen-2018-028097
6. Kwan A, Sears D, Bertozzi SM, Williams B, eds. *California State Prisons During the COVID-19: A Report by the CalPROTECT Project*. 2022. Available at: https://amend.us/wp-content/uploads/2022/05/2022-0501-CalPROTECT-Report.pdf. Accessed December 18, 2023.
7. California Department of Corrections and Rehabilitation. CDCR launches free audio calls. December 30, 2022. Available at: https://www.cdcr.ca.gov/news/2022/12/30/cdcr-launching-free-audio-calls-for-incarcerated-population. Accessed February 8, 2024.
8. Tan R. In an era of quarantine, crisis hotlines face growing—and urgent—demand. *Washington Post*. March 23, 2020. Available at: https://www.washingtonpost.com/local/crisis-hotline-quarantine-coronavirus-mental-health/2020/03/23/632e2d7c-6abe-11ea-9923-57073adce27c_story.html. Accessed December 5, 2023.
9. Peretz PJ, Islam N, Matiz L. Community health workers and the Covid-19 pandemic—addressing social determinants of health in times of crisis and beyond. *N Engl J Med*. 2020;383(19):e108. https://doi.org/10.1056/NEJMp2022641
10. Wewers ME, Shoben A, Conroy S, et al. Effectiveness of two community health worker models of tobacco dependence treatment among community residents of Ohio Appalachia. *Nicotine Tob Res*. 2017;19(12):1499–1507.
11. Komaromy M, Tomanovich M, Taylor J, et al. Adaptation of a system of treatment for substance use disorders during the COVID-19 pandemic. *J Addict Med*. 2021;15(6):448–451. https://doi.org/10.1097/ADM.0000000000000791
12. Puglisi L, Kroboth L, Shavit S. Public health behind bars; In: Greifinger RB. *Public Health Behind Bars*, Ed. 1. New York, NY: Springer Nature; 2021:429–443:
13. Patel K, Boutwell A, Brockmann BW, Rich JD. Integrating correctional and community health care for formerly incarcerated people who are eligible for Medicaid. *Health Aff (Millwood)*. 2014;33(3):468–473. https://doi.org/10.1377/hlthaff.2013.1164
14. California Department of Health Care Services. CalAIM Justice-Involved Initiative. 2024. Available at: https://www.dhcs.ca.gov/CalAIM/Justice-Involved-Initiative/Pages/home.aspx. Accessed November 30, 2023.
15. Couloute L. Nowhere to go: homelessness among formerly incarcerated people. Prison Policy Initiative. August 2018. Available at: https://www.prisonpolicy.org/reports/housing.html. Accessed January 14, 2024.

Building Common Ground for Public Health: Perspectives and Practice Experiences

William J. Kassler, MD, MPH, Howard Rodenberg, MD, MPH, and Steven C. Fiala, MPH

ABOUT THE AUTHORS

William J. Kassler was formerly the state health officer and medical director, New Hampshire Department of Health and Human Services, Concord, NH. Howard Rodenberg was formerly the state health officer, Kansas Department of Health and Environment, Topeka, KS. Steven C. Fiala is the AJPH deputy editor for open access supplements, and is with the Oregon Public Health Division, Portland, OR.

See also Common Ground, pp. 484–518.

Common ground is found when people or groups at odds with each other unite to find areas of agreement. Building common ground has always been challenging in public health policy, but the need to do so is especially critical today given the acute political and ideological divides in the United States. The inaugural special section On Building Common Ground, the brainchild of former state health officers serving both Democratic and Republican administrations, appeared in the October 2023 issue of *AJPH*.[1] This ongoing effort builds on earlier work by presenting perspectives and practice experiences that inform the consensus-building process required to protect the health and safety of all people in the United States.

EROSION OF TRUST IN PUBLIC HEALTH

As we write this preface, tectonic shifts in public health policy are under way—part of a larger global trend of populism on the right and left, driven by large groups of people who no longer feel government is working for them. This populism is characterized by skepticism toward the elite, mistrust of expertise, and lost confidence in governmental institutions.[2] We see the effects of this in our communities, including troubling rollbacks of progress on water fluoridation and childhood vaccination.[3,4] This erosion of trust—which traditional, science-based public health practice has become caught up in—has resulted in partisan political polarization and created fertile ground for alternative narratives to arise that reject science-based practices.[5] Narratives that are amplified on social media are often the product of misinformation campaigns by foreign adversaries with the intent to destabilize democracies.[6] This places an increased burden on public health practitioners to reach out to those who disagree with us to build bridges so we might effectively engage with those who fear or mistrust us and seek common ground in support of the public's health.

As we explore this topic in the special section, it might be worthwhile to take a step back to consider how we came to this state of affairs. In public health there is inherent tension between individual liberty and economic freedom and community-level population-based interventions. These simmering tensions often boil over into conflict when the police powers of public health are exercised. This is certainly not unique to the recent pushback on COVID-19 mandates and lockdowns. Similar conflicts arose in the early HIV epidemic, with ill-fated attempts to close bathhouses in New York City and San Francisco, California.[7] Going back to the 1918 pandemic, there was considerable large-scale opposition and outright resistance to disease control measures.[8]

Unfortunately, the public health field appears to have forgotten those earlier experiences. We were caught off guard in our COVID-19 response and struggled to communicate scientific uncertainty while simultaneously enforcing widely dislocating and unpopular social-distancing measures. The pandemic collided with the budding populist movement and created a perfect storm in which an already polarized society readily fused their ideological beliefs and political affiliation to opposing narratives of public health. To date, there has not been a post–COVID-19 rapprochement.

BRIDGING DIVIDES VIA DIALOGUE AND ENGAGEMENT

Indeed, recent events indicate that the lines have hardened. So how do we go forward? We feel that today's challenge is to look critically at our profession to see how we might regain trust and influence. Revamping the way we tell the story of public health and how we interact outside our institutions is critical. Public health agencies and professionals should be looking for evidence-based interventions and best practices to build bridges and create consensus on key aspects of health. Tone and content matter, and an adversarial approach to advocacy seems only to entrench opposition on both sides of the political spectrum.

As we seek to counter alternative narratives, it is fitting to look to communication science and lead this special section with the work of Chou et al., "Public Health Communication Approaches for Building Common Ground" (p. 511). Their article explains how communication strategies can use existing common ground by appealing to shared values and identities and can cultivate further links through trust-focused work. Crucially, the authors identify and warn about communications that drive wedges between groups and have done distinct harm to our efforts. We are happy to feature this important work as a foundational piece for those that follow.

Further articles in this special section discuss different techniques for building bridges. Guided dialogue focused on decreasing political polarization as a means to advance public health infrastructure is key to several practice-based articles. The Civity Project (Strand and Kopell, p. 506) uses shared storytelling to increase social trust and decrease social distance in communities, building connections through the exchange of lived experiences. Outside analysis found that the Civity Project was highly ranked among efforts aimed at reducing animosity across the political spectrum.

The Milbank Foundation works to depolarize conflict through their Emerging Leaders Program at the city, county, and state levels and the Milbank Fellows Program for senior leaders in state executive agencies and legislative chairs. Participants noted that they bettered their knowledge of the importance of partnerships; of how a focus on diversity, equity, and inclusion improved communications through awareness of adverse language and assumptions; and of how policy goals are advanced through coalition building and systemic problem-solving.

Bosché et al. (p. 500) describe the process of democratic deliberation. Involving community members in exercises such as citizen panels, citizen juries, consensus conferences, and scenario workshops, democratic deliberation strives to further consensus building, knowledge exchange, and participation of underrepresented populations in the public sphere.

Where ground may be reclaimed in the public sphere, it may be best accomplished by taking small bites of the apple. Projects with uniform appeal may represent those first steps. The Move with the Mayor effort described by Waugh et al. (p. 495) uses the noncontroversial goal of increasing physical activity in the community to build coalitions of support for future health policies and programs.

Outreach to new communities is crucial as well. Former surgeon general Jerome Adams mentors new professionals, who describe the positive impact that outreach and dialogue with youths can have on public health policy. In reaching out to new communities, we must heed the warning of Chou et al. that effective communication is not just a set of processes and procedures: it requires empathy and a deeper understanding of the ties that bind us through shared values. It is with this in mind that we conclude the special section with the thoughts of Gunderson et al. (article forthcoming in the May issue) on the vital connection between religion and public health.

These articles are a representative sample of the state of the art in building common ground. But we have yet to see the public health community truly come to grips with the role of populist movements on both the left and the right and with the roles of outside actors and deliberate misinformation. We suspect that this is because these topics necessarily involve reflection on our own ignorance and errors, which is a difficult proposition in the best of times. However, we believe that if we are to respond to this challenge, the literature must reflect an awareness and analysis of these seismic events.

MEASURING SUCCESS IN BUILDING COMMON GROUND

Finally, the unspoken caveat to many of the interventions described in this section is that it is difficult to quantify results. Although process objectives—things you can measure following a dialogue, meeting, or project—may be positive, the proof of the pudding comes when concrete outcomes are shaped and influenced by these efforts. In an accompanying editorial to the 2023 special section, the editors hoped "future articles (and, perhaps, future special sections) will tell the stories of successful and unsuccessful attempts to build common ground, highlighting best practices and using rigorous evaluation methodology."[1(p1094)]

This year, we are gratified to see further development in the field as reflected in these excellent articles, but we observe that the field is still in relative infancy with the ongoing need for methodologically rigorous evaluation of efficacy, sustainability, scalability, and impact. There is admittedly a certain degree of naivety in believing that somehow we can all just get along, but one needs to start somewhere. We hope this collection of work serves as a lighthouse to guide us forward. It has been our privilege to support these authors and perhaps help add a candle or two to the beacon atop the tower. AJPH

CORRESPONDENCE

Correspondence should be sent to Steven C. Fiala, 800 NE Oregon St, Portland, OR 97232 (e-mail: steve.fiala@gmail.com). Reprints can be ordered at https://www.ajph.org by clicking the "Reprints" link.

PUBLICATION INFORMATION

Full Citation: Kassler WJ, Rodenberg H, Fiala SC. Building common ground for public health: perspectives and practice experiences. *Am J Public Health*. 2025;115(4):481–483.

Acceptance Date: January 27, 2025.

DOI: https://doi.org/10.2105/AJPH.2025.308044

ORCID iD:
Steven C. Fiala https://orcid.org/0000-0001-8881-5762

CONTRIBUTORS

W. J. Kassler and H. Rodenberg drafted the editorial. S. C. Fiala critically reviewed and edited the editorial.

ACKNOWLEDGMENTS

We acknowledge our Association of State and Territorial Health Officials alumni colleagues, particularly those who helped draft the call for articles, and the *AJPH* editorial staff.

CONFLICTS OF INTEREST

The authors have no conflicts of interest to declare.

REFERENCES

1. Fine M, Kassler WJ, LeBlanc TT. On building common ground: an *AJPH* special section. *Am J Public Health*. 2023;113(10):1093–1095. https://doi.org/10.2105/AJPH.2023.307399
2. Saad L. Historically low faith in US institutions continues. *Gallup*. July 6, 2023. Available at: https://news.gallup.com/poll/508169/historically-low-faith-institutions-continues.aspx. Accessed January 29, 2025.
3. Florida Department of Health. State surgeon general Dr. Joseph A. Ladapo issues community water fluoridation guidance. November 22, 2024. Available at: https://www.floridahealth.gov/newsroom/2024/11/20241122-fluoridation-guidance.pr.html. Accessed January 29, 2025.
4. Centers for Disease Control and Prevention. Coverage with selected vaccines and exemption rates among children in kindergarten—United States, 2023–24 school year. *MMWR Morb Mortal Wkly Rep*. 2024;73(41):925–932. https://doi.org/10.15585/mmwr.mm7341a3
5. US Government Accountability Office. Foreign disinformation: defining and detecting threats. September 26, 2024. Available at: https://www.gao.gov/assets/gao-24-107600.pdf. Accessed January 29, 2025.
6. Harvard T.H. Chan School of Public Health; Robert Wood Johnson Foundation. The public's perspective on the United States public health system. May 2021. Available at: https://hsph.harvard.edu/wp-content/uploads/2024/10/RWJF-Harvard-Report_FINAL-051321.pdf. Accessed January 29, 2025.
7. Disman C. The San Francisco bathhouse battles of 1984: civil liberties, AIDS risk, and shifts in health policy. *J Homosex*. 2003;44(3–4):71–129. https://doi.org/10.1300/J082v44n03_05
8. Navarro JA, Markel H. Politics, pushback, and pandemics: challenges to public health orders in the 1918 influenza pandemic. *Am J Public Health*. 2021;111(3):416–422. https://doi.org/10.2105/AJPH.2020.305958

Depolarization Through Public-Sector Leadership Development: Emerging Leaders and Fellows Programs, United States, 2015–2024

Morgan F. McDonald, MD

See also Common Ground, pp. 481–518.

Directing depolarization efforts toward those with authority over public health funding and population health policies has great potential to improve health outcomes. Two nonpartisan legislative and executive branch state leadership programs demonstrated personal growth and mutual respect among participants necessary for depolarization that was evidenced by cross-state and cross-party policy implementation. Intentional cohort selection of politically and demographically diverse participants, ground rules based on fundamental values, and curriculum emphasizing collective problem-solving built trust and curiosity despite differing viewpoints. (*Am J Public Health*. 2025;115(4):484–488. https://doi.org/10.2105/AJPH.2025.308004)

AJPH April 2025, Vol. 115, No. 4

This article describes two distinct year-long leadership programs for executive and legislative branch state and large city and county health policymakers.

INTERVENTION AND IMPLEMENTATION

The Emerging Leaders Program (ELP) hosts early and midcareer executive branch professionals and state legislators with up to five years in office. The Fellows program hosts senior state executives and legislative committee chairs. Key elements of the programs include recruitment strategy, trust and relationship building through guided listening and mutual interest in complex population health problems, and a curriculum built on adaptive leadership that requires participants to practice shifting their own values to find solutions on new ground when common ground does not exist.[1]

Recruitment occurs primarily via nomination for Fellows and application for ELP, prioritizing growth mindset and commitment to improving the health of communities they serve. Alumni recommendation, directed outreach, and emphasis on demographic representation in recruitment materials results in annual cohorts that are intentionally diverse in race and ethnicity, gender identity and sexual orientation, physical abilities, government sector, political affiliation, and geography.

The core competencies of the programs are rooted in the Public Sector Leadership Framework[2] designed by a collaborative of entities working with Medicaid and public health officials. Those competencies are housed in the overarching pedagogy of adaptive leadership, which distinguishes technical problems that can be solved with the right resources and skills from adaptive problems that are complex and require learning, collaboration, and creativity as well as shifts in values and mindsets. The ability to build trust and shift one's own set of values to enable new solutions is at the core of adaptive leadership and also depolarization.

Programming consists of three in-person two-day meetings with agendas that balance skills building, policy briefings, and experience sharing. This is supplemented with monthly interactive virtual sessions and regular communications. Content delivery was best received via conversational interviews with invited experts rather than formal presentations. Small group discussion following those interviews allows deeper exploration and relationship development. ELP participants found participant-directed mentor matching, exploration of their own leadership styles with standardized tools and tactical skill building on negotiation, strategic communications, and team management to be most useful for personal growth and as a starting point for more difficult conversations. Fellows were often previously exposed to those skills and found policy discussions and sharing high-stakes political and administrative or budgetary decision-making of most value in their curriculum. A curricular path of person–role–system begins with sharing personal drivers of public service, then trading successes and mutual frustrations, then sharing policies on bipartisan priorities like mental health.

Cohort facilitation mirrors reciprocal group reflection as described by Baron et al.: "Depolarization [in group reflection] is especially effective when it includes both informational and emotional components, such that [citizens] who are moved to empathize with outgroup members become more likely to internalize new information about them."[3(p1)] Dialogue and relationship building emphasize common values at the outset to create emotional linkage. Once participants build relational trust, they are asked to bring their own complex problems to discuss as adaptive challenges with the assistance of their colleagues across the political spectrum.

By virtue of its long-standing commitments to evidence-based policymaking and bipartisanism and its honest and transparent experience confronting how its own actions have perpetuated injustice,[4] Milbank Memorial Fund has been a trusted and credible convener for this work. The use of such a facilitator willing to take a first step in vulnerability models the ground rules and self-reflection needed for personal growth.

PLACE, TIME, AND PERSONS

As of summer 2024, there were more than 200 graduates of the two leadership programs. ELP was implemented in 2015 and has graduated seven cohorts. The Fellows program began in 2021 and has graduated three cohorts. Forty-five percent of participants from the last five years identify as people of color. Fifteen percent of recent participants self-identify as lesbian, gay, bisexual, transgender, queer/questioning, intersex, or asexual (LGBTQIA). Participants are evenly representative of geography, legislative or executive branch, and party affiliation across 49 states and the District of Columbia.

PURPOSE

The need for public-sector leaders committed to and skilled in population health continues to grow, as evidenced by the poor performance[5] of the US health care system on virtually every measure of population health and health equity and the widening gap in the performance among individual states. The rapid turnover in state houses and among executive branch leaders has made relationship building difficult, leading more state officials to sequester in political and administrative silos. Meanwhile, the political polarization of the US public is widening.[6] As polarization increased, the ability of government to pass and implement legislation slowed.[7] Just as concerning, polarization has been correlated with negative physical[8] and mental health[9] impacts on individuals.

Approaches to depolarization have been proposed and studied. These include multiple vote electoral systems,[10] consensus-based democratic governance,[11] and even artificial intelligence–generated media interventions.[12] The leadership program approach is consistent with recommendations from Alberti et al. to "intentionally connect local, state, and national action and create professional development opportunities that span the three."[13(p3)]

EVALUATION AND ADVERSE EFFECTS

Seventy-seven percent of alumni are still working in state service. Of those still in state service, 30% have been promoted since their participation in the program. Evaluation elements in both programs include meeting feedback forms, midprogram interviews, and pre- and postprogram surveys administered to participants. The Colorado Health Institute conducted a formal qualitative analysis of participant data in 2023 and 2024. Participants were asked to reflect on the impact of the program on their leadership, knowledge, and creation of meaningful connections. The thematic analysis revealed several key themes reflective of depolarization:

- Intentional connection and collaboration with leaders across the country and across the aisle provided opportunities to learn new strategies and equipped participants to examine issues from various points of view.
- Focus on diversity, equity, and inclusion improved communication with colleagues and the public by encouraging awareness of Fellows' language and their assumptions of others.
- Fellows are better equipped to effect change at the state and local level as a result of the knowledge gained on consensus building, adaptive leadership techniques, and cross-system collaboration strategies.

In the words of one participant, "the presentations about diversity, equity,

TABLE 1— Likert Scale Responses to Postprogram Survey Items Related to Emerging Leaders Program (ELP) Participant Outcomes Among Cohort 7 (2023–2024) Participants: United States

Survey Item	No.	Mean ±SD
ELP equipped me with skills for depolarization that assist with effective policy implementation.	13	1.92 ±0.64
ELP increased my capacity to advance population health.	13	1.54 ±0.66
ELP improved my leadership skills.	13	1.46 ±0.66
ELP increased my capacity to work with others who have different values, motivations, and lived experience/political perspectives than my own.	13	1.46 ±0.52
ELP helped me utilize evidence to advance population health decision-making.	13	1.85 ±0.69
ELP helped me utilize a network of colleagues from across the country to advance my work.	13	1.23 ±0.44

Note. Postprogram survey respondents rated their agreement with each survey item on a scale from 1 (strongly agree) to 5 (strongly disagree). The sample size was n = 27.

and inclusion issues created a fundamental shift in thinking for me and helped me better understand the resistance some colleagues and community members have. That will help me rethink language, assumptions, and discussions to hopefully help break the barriers."

Postprogram survey results from the 2023–2024 Fellows and ELP cohorts indicate that both leadership programs equip participants with skills for depolarization. Postprogram surveys asked participants to rate their agreement with the following statement using a scale of 1 (strong agreement) to 5 (strong disagreement): ELP or Fellows equipped me with skills for depolarization that assist with effective policy implementation. On average, ELP participants (Tables 1 and 2; mean = 1.92; SD = 0.64) and Fellows (Tables 2 and 3; mean = 1.23; SD = 0.44) who completed the postprogram survey strongly agreed or agreed with the statement. Participants also reported policies they implemented across states and across political parties. These included behavioral health school-based interventions, suicide and firearm injury prevention, regulatory changes to manage health care costs, and Medicaid investments. One state legislative committee chair said of another from the opposing party, "I really never thought I'd be so happy to work with him again!"

TABLE 2— Likert Scale Responses to Postprogram Survey Depolarization Item Among Cohort 3 (2023–2024) Fellows Program (FP) and Cohort 7 (2023–2024) Emerging Leaders Program (ELP) Participants: United States

Please Rate Your Agreement With the Following Statement: FP or ELP Equipped Me With Skills for Depolarization That Assist With Effective Policy Implementation	No.	Mean ±SD
Leadership program		
ELP and FP	26	1.58 ±0.64
FP only	13	1.23 ±0.44
ELP only	13	1.92 ±0.64

Note. Postprogram survey respondents rated their agreement with each survey item on a scale from 1 (strongly agree) to 5 (strongly disagree). The sample size was n = 51.

Not all feedback was positive. One applicant left the program for political reasons. Virtual session participation across programs waned over time. This was improved somewhat by virtual small-group breakout sessions, including social conversation, having peers discuss their work, and using virtual engagement tools. In early cohorts, group projects were found to be a time-consuming "add on" and not as useful as peer coaching for their current priority initiatives, and so curricula adjusted to only include the latter.

SUSTAINABILITY

The described cohort building and adaptive leadership emphasis in cross-branch, cross-party, and cross-state leadership development could be scaled as a strategy for depolarization and bipartisanship in the public sector. Both programs are sustained by independent funding from an endowed operating fund. This transparent funding strategy enabled the programs to maintain a nonpartisan approach that has helped recruit legislators and executive branch officials from both political parties. Demand for the programs has been demonstrated with nearly three times the number of applications as

TABLE 3— Likert Scale Responses to Postprogram Survey Items Related to Fellows Program (FP) Participant Outcomes Among Cohort 3 (2023–2024) Fellows: United States

Survey Item	No.	Mean ±SD
FP equipped me with skills for depolarization that assist with effective policy implementation.	13	1.23 ±0.44
FP increased my knowledge on population health issues.	13	1.54 ±0.66
FP increased my knowledge on interdisciplinary health and human services systems.	13	1.38 ±0.65
FP increased my knowledge on evidence-based approaches to improve population health.	13	1.69 ±0.63
FP increased my capacity to articulate and drive forward a public health vision and agenda.	13	1.31 ±0.48
FP increased my access to resources and relationships that support taking action in my state or tribe.	13	1.31 ±0.48

Note. Postprogram survey respondents rated their agreement with each survey item on a scale from 1 (strongly agree) to 5 (strongly disagree). The sample size was n = 24.

capacity over the last two years. Additional funding from private or public sources could scale the program to several times its current size, and successful elements of the programs are applicable to other leadership programs desiring depolarization as an outcome.

PUBLIC HEALTH SIGNIFICANCE

Given deepening political divides in the United States, the resulting antagonism toward public health, and the negative impact on health outcomes resulting from both trends, it is increasingly important to implement strategies directed at depolarization. Likewise, directing those efforts to individuals with authority over public health funding and population health policies has great potential to improve those health outcomes.[14] Initial evaluation of these cross-branch and cross-party executive leadership programs is promising and indicates a potentially scalable model to increase investment in public health and evidence-based health policy with a health equity lens. *AJPH*

ABOUT THE AUTHOR

Morgan McDonald is the National Director for Population Health and Health Equity Leadership at the Milbank Memorial Fund, New York, NY.

CORRESPONDENCE

Correspondence should be sent to Morgan McDonald, Milbank Memorial Fund, 645 Madison Ave, 15th Floor, New York, NY 10022 (e-mail: mmcdonald@milbank.org). Reprints can be ordered at https://www.ajph.org by clicking the "Reprints" link.

PUBLICATION INFORMATION

Full Citation: McDonald MF. Depolarization through public-sector leadership development: emerging leaders and fellows programs, United States, 2015–2024. *Am J Public Health*. 2025;115(4):484–488.

Acceptance Date: January 2, 2025.

DOI: https://doi.org/10.2105/AJPH.2025.308004

ORCID iD:

Morgan F. McDonald https://orcid.org/0009-0002-1516-4385

ACKNOWLEDGMENTS

This publication represents the work of M. McDonald and the Milbank Memorial Fund, which is the sole and independent funder of the described programs.

M. McDonald would like to acknowledge the contributions of program officers Erica Brown, Trina Gonzalez, Michelle Alletto, and Kate McEvoy as well as our consultants in the construction and evaluation of the programs. They are Rich Callahan of TAP International, Gretchen Hammer of Public Leadership Group, Kenneth W. Kizer, and Karam Ahmad and Alyssa Sloan of the Colorado Health Institute.

CONFLICTS OF INTEREST

The author reports no conflicts of interest.

HUMAN PARTICIPANT PROTECTION

Educational evaluation data was gathered using de-identified surveys, interviews, and public comment and was analyzed in aggregate.

REFERENCES

1. Nelson T, Squires V. Addressing complex challenges through adaptive leadership: a promising approach to collaborative problem solving. *J Leadersh Educ.* 2017;16(4):111–123. https://doi.org/10.12806/V16/I4/T2
2. National Association of Medicaid Directors. Public Sector Leadership Framework. September 15, 2020. Available at: https://medicaiddirectors.org/resource/public-sector-leadership-framework. Accessed June 14, 2024.
3. Baron H, Blair R, Choi DD, et al. Couples therapy for a divided America: assessing the effects of reciprocal group reflection on partisan polarization. Brown University. May 8, 2021. Available at: https://osf.io/preprints/osf/3x7z8_v1. Accessed June 14, 2024.
4. Milbank Memorial Fund. 2025 Racial Equity Statement of Purpose. January 9, 2025. Available at: https://www.milbank.org/about/racial-equity-statement-of-purpose. Accessed January 9, 2025.
5. Radley D, Shah A, Collins S, Powe N, Zephyrin L. Advancing racial equity in US health care: The Commonwealth Fund 2024 State Health Disparities Report. Commonwealth Fund. April 18, 2024. Available at: https://www.commonwealthfund.org/publications/fund-reports/2024/apr/advancing-racial-equity-us-health-care. Accessed June 14, 2024.
6. Oberlander J. Polarization, partisanship, and health in the United States. *J Health Polit Policy Law.* 2024;49(3):329–350. https://doi.org/10.1215/03616878-11075609
7. LoCascio J, Siegel B, Pereira I. 118th Congress on track to become one of the least productive in US history. ABC News. January 10, 2024. Available at: https://abcnews.go.com/Politics/118th-congress-track-become-productive-us-history/story?id=106254012. Accessed June 14, 2024.
8. Fraser T, Aldrich D, Panagopoulos C, Hummel D, Kim D. The harmful effects of partisan polarization on health. *PNAS Nexus.* 2022;1(1):pgac011. https://doi.org/10.1093/pnasnexus/pgac011
9. Nayak SS, Fraser T, Panagopoulos C, Aldrich D, Kim D. Is divisive politics making Americans sick? Associations of perceived partisan polarization with physical and mental health outcomes among adults in the United States. *Soc Sci Med.* 2021;284:113976. https://doi.org/10.1016/j.socscimed.2021.113976

10. Crosson J, Tsebelis G. Multiple vote electoral systems: a remedy for political polarization. *J Eur Public Policy.* 2021;29(6):932–952. https://doi.org/10.1080/13501763.2021.1901962

11. Bernaerts K, Blanckaert B, Caluwaerts D. Institutional design and polarization: do consensus democracies fare better in fighting polarization than majoritarian democracies? *Democratization.* 2022;30(2):153–172. https://doi.org/10.1080/13510347.2022.2117300

12. Liu R, Wang L, Jia C, Vosoughi S. Political depolarization of news articles using attribute-aware word embeddings. *Proceedings of the International AAAI Conference on Web and Social Media.* 2021;15:385–396. https://doi.org/10.1609/icwsm.v15i1.18069

13. Alberti PM, Orgera K, Alvarado CS. Generation Z challenges partisan divides for health equity. *Am J Public Health.* 2023;113(10):1114–1115. https://doi.org/10.2105/AJPH.2023.307391

14. McDonald M, Sparer L, Brown L. Top 10 ways to build bipartisan support for public health infrastructure. Milbank Memorial Fund. October 10, 2023. Available at: https://www.milbank.org/2023/10/top-10-ways-to-build-bipartisan-support-for-public-health-infrastructure. Accessed June 14, 2024.

Depolarizing Health Policy Through Intergenerational Conversations

Bhav Jain, John C. Lin, and Jerome M. Adams, MD, MPH

ABOUT THE AUTHORS

Bhav Jain is with the Stanford University School of Medicine, Stanford, CA. John C. Lin is with the Perelman School of Medicine, University of Pennsylvania, Philadelphia. Jerome M. Adams is with the Center for Community Health Enhancement and Learning, Purdue University, West Lafayette, IN.

See also Common Ground, pp. 481–518.

Over the past two decades, health care has increasingly dominated national politics. More than 70% of US adults believe that the modern American health care system is failing to meet their needs.[1] Whereas most Americans consistently share concerns about certain issues such as the high costs of health care and prescription drugs, others—including the COVID-19 response, access to gender-affirming and reproductive care, and gun violence—remain highly controversial. As current medical students and the former nation's doctor, we advocate for leveraging intergenerational dialogue to address these contentious issues and depolarize health care discussions as the nation exits a critical election cycle.

EMPOWERING YOUTH: BUILDING BRIDGES ACROSS GENERATIONS

First, health care leaders and policymakers should more actively engage the younger generation, which is often directly affected by public health crises and less attached to political interests. Youths have novel approaches to understanding issues and advocating for solutions as well as unique abilities to drive movements forward. Indeed, young people have played pivotal roles across most social movements in modern history,[2] ranging from the civil rights movement of the mid–20th century and its student leaders such as Diane Nash to the modern-day climate movement led by teenage activists such as Greta Thunberg.

Moreover, youths generally exhibit a higher level of consensus than their older peers that health care reform is needed on polarizing issues such as gun violence and health insurance coverage.[3] This is not necessarily surprising, as gun violence became the leading cause of death among children and adolescents in the United States in 2020 and young adults continue to have the lowest rate of health insurance coverage of any age group.[4,5] Given these lived experiences, young people can approach legislators and drive bipartisan change.

For instance, one of the authors (J. C. L.) is a young Asian American who personally survived a hate crime during the early months of the COVID-19 pandemic. When he later served as a legislative staffer in the Texas House of Representatives, he was intimately familiar with rising violence against Asian American children and elderly adults that was causing serious hospitalizations at a time when hospitals were already at capacity. For months, no Texas legislators wrote legislation to address this high-stakes issue. Inspired by his experiences and his community's struggles, Lin proposed and worked with Representative Hubert Vo to draft House Resolution 538, which condemned these hate crimes and directed law enforcement to actively address them.

Despite initial doubt among even advocates that passing this resolution was possible, Lin worked with community organizations, researchers, and both Republican and Democratic representatives from all ages and backgrounds. Their coalition was ultimately able to help secure bipartisan, unanimous support for the legislation—a rarity in such a polarized era. This success was possible only because of the coalition's intergenerational and intercommunity partnerships that showed why this issue was so important for public health and safety.

In addition, health care leaders can collaborate with youths to build grassroots movements that engage multiple generations in solving shared challenges. During the onset of the COVID-19 pandemic, another author (B. J.) launched The Connected Foundation, a national nonprofit that sought to address the social isolation faced by youths and older adults alike by building virtual intergenerational connections. By offering patient advocacy, educational engagement, and mentorship programming with the support of physicians across more than 20 states, the foundation provided an opportunity for high school-age and college-age students to engage with older adults to share their stories and form lifelong bonds. Similarly, in late 2023, current US Surgeon General Vivek Murthy launched his "We Are Made to Connect" national tour to connect with college students and address the loneliness, social isolation, and mental health epidemics disproportionately affecting young Americans. His efforts underscore the potential for addressing health care challenges by focusing on improving the collective well-being and societal resilience of youths through intergenerational engagement.

Young people can also collaborate with the more than 70 Gen Z legislators across state and federal governments to ensure that their voices are heard on health care issues affecting the nation. Similar to the youth advisory boards established by organizations such as the United Nations and World Health Organization, the American Medical Association, (which benefits from robust contributions from student, resident, and young physician sections) and the National Academy of Medicine can establish forums to facilitate this process. Those involved in such forums can learn from similar efforts already established at the local and state levels as well, including the Collective of Youth Leaders at Children's Hospital Los Angeles and the Governor's Youth Advisory Council in Massachusetts. Although these next steps will require concerted efforts on the part of both youth and established leaders, they may prove fruitful in achieving an unprecedented level of health reform.

A CULTURE OF SCIENCE AND EVIDENCE-BASED DECISION MAKING

Second, current leaders have an opportunity to collaborate with youths to set a precedent for evidence-based decision making, shaping a culture that future generations can follow. At the core of depolarizing health care is a steadfast commitment to leveraging scientific inquiry and evidence-based practices. When another of the authors, former US Surgeon General Jerome M. Adams, served as Indiana state health commissioner, there was an outbreak of HIV and viral hepatitis resulting from opioid and injection drug use. The outbreak, which occurred in early 2015, had disproportionate impacts among young people 16 to 24 years of age.[6] Despite initial community resistance to a syringe exchange program, Adams's outreach to and empowerment of affected young people in Scott County led to the state authorizing these emergency programs, effectively controlling the outbreak. Within one year, nearly 90% of people who inject drugs used the program, and rates of infection returned to near baseline.[7]

Subsequently, Indiana passed legislation extending these temporary authorizations, and what started as a moral quandary eventually garnered bipartisan support. Since then, organizations such as CEASe of Scott County and the EMPOWER Youth Coalition have been regularly hosting events with students in the community to work toward the elimination of substance abuse. This example demonstrates the importance of health care professionals engaging with youths and setting politics aside during public health crises to provide objective recommendations that save lives. To be sure, health care issues are inherently political, and addressing them requires adopting an intergenerational approach to engaging with communities and political representatives.

BUILDING BRIDGES ACROSS POLITICAL DIVIDES

Finally, efforts to address ongoing crises in health care can be communicated with language that resonates with more Americans, independent of political affiliation. Given their less partisan perspectives, youths are particularly well positioned to lead these bipartisan communication efforts. For example, although climate change remains controversial among older generations, an international study from 2021 showed that nearly 62% of youths and young adults experience climate anxiety.[8] As such, youth leaders can reframe the crisis in terms of job creation and economic development. After federal and state subsidies have been taken into account, renewable energy sources such as wind and solar not only outcompete fossil fuels in cost but also promise to generate millions of new jobs, offering a tangible path toward economic revitalization in the decades ahead.[9,10]

In addition, the debate surrounding Medicaid expansion presents a ripe opportunity for reframing challenges in bipartisan terms. Expansion is still pending in 10 states, despite sound evidence that it improves health outcomes and socioeconomic status among low-income families and unemployed workers, reduces uncompensated care for hospitals, and is a proven economic stimulus for states.[11] Given these cost savings for individuals and governments, expanding insurance coverage can be reframed by emphasizing shared values of fiscal conservatism, as demonstrated by supermajority Republican–led Indiana's decision in 2015 to expand coverage. Indiana's recent monumental increase in public health funding by 1500%, coupled with Governor Eric Holcomb's emphasis on benefits for businesses and the workforce, further underscores the viability of this approach.[12]

Furthermore, during the COVID-19 pandemic, discourse surrounding masking, vaccination, and testing guidance could have been enhanced by placing greater emphasis on their potential effects on the economy and workforce[13] rather than purely focusing on individual behaviors and moral considerations. In a polarized political landscape, the imperative to bridge divides and prioritize the collective well-being of all Americans has never been more urgent.

CONCLUSION

Although health care issues continue to be highly politicized in the United States, there are opportunities to depolarize these challenges and achieve tangible reform in creative ways. By engaging youths in shaping policy, fostering evidence-based decision making, and reframing crises through bipartisan lenses, we can build a more unified and effective health care system. As the next generation continues to engage in social movements and navigate politically loaded issues, it will become increasingly necessary to build a culture wherein all Americans can have open debates and civil discussions grounded in science and individual values. AJPH

CORRESPONDENCE

Correspondence should be sent to Jerome M. Adams, MD, MPH, Purdue University, 610 Purdue Mall, West Lafayette, IN 47907 (e-mail: adams616@purdue.edu). Reprints can be ordered at https://www.ajph.org by clicking the "Reprints" link.

PUBLICATION INFORMATION

Full Citation: Jain B, Lin JC, Adams JM. Depolarizing health policy through intergenerational conversations. *Am J Public Health*. 2025;115(4):489–491.

Acceptance Date: December 5, 2024.

DOI: https://doi.org/10.2105/AJPH.2024.307971

ORCID iDs:

Bhav Jain https://orcid.org/0000-0003-2648-4894

John C. Lin https://orcid.org/0000-0002-1976-0574

Jerome M. Adams https://orcid.org/0009-0001-3231-937X

CONTRIBUTORS

All of the authors drafted and revised the article.

CONFLICTS OF INTEREST

The authors declare no conflicts of interest.

REFERENCES

1. Ducharme J. Most Americans say the health care system fails them. Available at: https://time.com/6279937/us-health-care-system-attitudes. Accessed August 12, 2024.
2. Costanza-Chock S. Youth and social movements: key lessons for allies. Available at: https://cyber.harvard.edu/sites/cyber.harvard.edu/files/KBWYouthandSocialMovements2012_0.pdf. Accessed August 12, 2024.
3. Alberti PM, Orgera K, Alvarado CS. Generation Z challenges partisan divides for health equity. *Am J Public Health*. 2023;113(10):1114–1115. https://doi.org/10.2105/AJPH.2023.307391
4. Goldstick JE, Cunningham RM, Carter PM. Current causes of death in children and adolescents in the United States. *N Engl J Med*. 2022;386(20):1955–1956. https://doi.org/10.1056/NEJMc2201761
5. Conway D. Health insurance coverage among young adults aged 19 to 34: 2018 and 2019. Available at: https://www.census.gov/library/publications/2020/acs/acsbr20-02.html. Accessed August 12, 2024.
6. The Health Foundation of Greater Indianapolis. Community Health Improvement Initiative. Available at: https://www.in.gov/health/hiv-std-viral-hepatitis/files/CHII-Adolescents-Executive-Summary-Final.pdf. Accessed August 12, 2024.
7. Dasgupta S, Broz D, Tanner M, et al. Changes in reported injection behaviors following the public health response to an HIV outbreak among people who inject drugs: Indiana, 2016. *AIDS Behav*. 2019;23(12):3257–3266. https://doi.org/10.1007/s10461-019-02600-x
8. Hickman C, Marks E, Pihkala P, et al. Climate anxiety in children and young people and their beliefs about government responses to climate change: a global survey. *Lancet Planet Health*. 2021;5(12):e863–e873. https://doi.org/10.1016/S2542-5196(21)00278-3
9. Lazard. Levelized cost of energy+. Available at: https://www.lazard.com/media/xemfey0k/lazards-lcoeplus-june-2024-_vf.pdf. Accessed November 24, 2024.
10. International Renewable Energy Agency. Renewable energy and jobs: annual review 2024. Available at: https://www.irena.org/-/media/Files/IRENA/Agency/Publication/2024/Oct/IRENA_Renewable_energy_and_jobs_2024.pdf. Accessed November 24, 2024.
11. Buchmueller TC, Cliff BQ, Levy H. The benefits of Medicaid expansion. *JAMA Health Forum*. 2020;1(7):e200879. https://doi.org/10.1001/jamahealthforum.2020.0879
12. Messerly M. A red state boosted public health funding by 1,500 percent. This is how they did it. Available at: https://www.politico.com/news/2023/07/13/red-state-public-health-funding-indiana-00105982. Accessed April 2, 2024.
13. Bollyky TJ, Castro E, Aravkin AY, et al. Assessing COVID-19 pandemic policies and behaviours and their economic and educational trade-offs across US states from Jan 1, 2020, to July 31, 2022: an observational analysis. *Lancet*. 2023;401(10385):1341–1360. https://doi.org/10.1016/S0140-6736(23)00461-0

Toward Common Ground: Rethinking Both Public Health and Religion, Together

Gary Gunderson, DMin, MDiv, James R. Cochrane, PhD, MDiv, and Teresa Cutts, PhD

ABOUT THE AUTHORS

Gary Gunderson is with the School of Divinity, Wake Forest University, Winston-Salem, NC. James R. Cochrane is professor emeritus of the School of Public Health, University of Cape Town, Cape Town, South Africa. Teresa Cutts is with the Public Health Sciences Division, School of Medicine, Wake Forest University, Winston-Salem, NC.

See also Common Ground, pp. 481–518.

AJPH April 2025, Vol. 115, No. 4

In his foreword to the *Handbook on Religion and Health: Pathways for a Turbulent Future*, former dean of Emory University Rollins School of Public Health Jim Curran writes:

> Approaching religion and public health simultaneously is not without risk. We are all advised to avoid discussion of religion (and politics) in public. But to ignore the relationship between religion and health places society at even greater peril and misses so many opportunities for better lives. The mission of public health is closely aligned to the nearly universal social mission of most religions—We are in this together.[1]

THE COMPLEX RELIGION–PUBLIC HEALTH RELATIONSHIP

Jeff Levin writes in the *Annals of Epidemiology* that public health and faith have a long and well-documented relationship that is understood with increasing nuance by researchers, if not all medical or public health providers, much less the lay public.[2] *AJPH* has reported on this long relationship for at least a century, as noted in an extensive special edition in March 2019, particularly in the comments from the editor.[3] It is not a simple relationship. The necessary nuance about how religion functions at personal, social, and public scales to protect against disease and encourage health is easily lost when the political moment is served by teasing science and religion into opposing camps. Although epidemiologists would generally agree that religion correlates positively with good health over a lifespan,[2] political scientists would note that religion is easily weaponized to undermine public health support and practice. The most basic responsibility of partners in such times is to come to the aid of each other when under attack.

THE FAITH–SCIENCE POLITICAL DIVIDE

A recent example occurred during the height of the COVID-19 pandemic when religious arguments were brought before the US Supreme Court to undermine basic public health legal practices. The Supreme Court chose not to pay attention to the scientific arguments, deciding instead to protect religious privilege.[4,5] Religious leaders of sufficient depth and standing, although themselves doing much to promote public health efforts (e.g., the National Council of Churches encouraged good practice[6]), did not in this case come to the defense of their social justice partners. This left a gap easily exploited by those wishing to split religion from science, not only in court but also in the larger domain of public discourse. Both science and faith were left weaker in their role of protecting the well-being of the most vulnerable amid the pandemic.

STRENGTHENING FAITH–PUBLIC HEALTH PARTNERSHIPS

Why was or is this support not forthcoming? Collaborative partnerships between faith groups and public health or health care bodies have, after all, been significant over the past decade or more.[7–9] Although no longer facing an active pandemic, our public square, including the weaponization of religious faith to attack science, remains contentious. One factor is a loss of trust in public institutions in the battle over how private and public goods are distributed (or not)—including the benefits of 21st-century public health. It is always wise to follow the money, as science, like religion, is easily bent to serve whoever pays for it. Equally, just as science tends to reinforce the power dynamics of those wealthy enough to pay for its research, so are preachers and prophets all too often paid, with uncanny predictability, to call the worst deviations from justice as blessed by divine law. In the

American South, tobacco companies commonly gave their employees free cigarettes to ensure they were among those addicted. And rural churches often had an acre of tobacco and thus ensured their own addiction to a leading cause of death—the body by cancer, the spirit by complicity.

In short, interests and ideology easily combine. The times demand deeper and more multifaceted alignment, not just collaborations on this or that project. Any entity that wants more than its share of wealth, education, voice, social standing, political power, or privileges gains from inequality and will oppose social justice as the path toward health for all. This is political practice that is willing to use any argument—including religious ones—that serves it, even if the peer-reviewed literature argues the opposite. Tenacious and well resourced, with obvious reasons to undermine the findings of science and the ethics shared by many global faiths,[10] this is a particular challenge today.

LOCAL SUCCESSES AND PATHS FORWARD

There is another way to look at it, a more positive one. Public health and faith are best seen on one's own local ground, where seemingly simple collaborations grow into policy-relevant models that cross boundaries while respecting distinctive roles. Frequently, these sustained collaborations are initiated in a moment of crisis but then sustained through a web of relationships that spread to adjacent opportunities (e.g., starting with vaccination and progressing to social supports). An example of such an enabler of webs from the former tobacco town of Winston-Salem, North Carolina, is Love Out Loud (https://www.loveoutloudws.com), which has become a crucial partner with public health. Its ministry grew out of a conservative evangelical church to become part of the wider civic muscle connecting nearly every sinew and brain cell in the local body politic—exactly what turned out to be needed for COVID-19. In the early days of the pandemic, a local physician, William Satterwhite, saw the possibility of working with the public health community, businesses, and hospitals to "mask the city." Love Out Loud brought great imagination and on-the-ground practicality as civic, not just faith, muscle. Its links, connections, and credibility helped public health scientists and engineers get a third of a million masks into every nook and cranny of local business, church, and civic life.

This success caught the attention of the National Academies of Sciences.[11] Today, Love Out Loud works with the same creative tenacity to support equitable public education to work with another local network, Action4Equity, on a host of antiracist initiatives and, more recently, to adapt the framework of Vital Conditions[12] to an array of health-promoting initiatives. This intentional meshing of religious networks and public health practices is an example of what is possible—and is no doubt happening in many similar places. This should not be a surprise, and it is what we should look for. In the most challenging neighborhoods in the more than 3000 counties of the United States, you will find public health and religion at work. Both earn their way in civic life by their relevance to the most predictable events in personal, social, and political life: birth, death, disease, dependence, and interdependence. At this granular level, it would be more difficult to weaponize faith against public health, for both are morally oriented toward the health and well-being of all. This is the most fundamental basis of common ground.

Among top public health advocates in the United States, there has also been a keen interest in another direction. About a dozen years ago Gene Matthews, Centers for Disease Control and Prevention general counsel for 26 years under numerous administrations, began speaking in public about public health. The Network for Public Health Law would seem the unlikely agent of conciliation, but no collection of public health specialists understands more about how law, policy, and practice are human constructs suspended in a web woven of citizens' language.[13] The Network found itself drawn from the initial work of crafting better, more effective public messages to the uncomfortable task of becoming better messengers.[14] The traditions of Islam and others call this "the work of becoming human in a way that heals the whole." A contemporary example of this principle in action was seen when Ray Baxter, an eminent public health leader and National Academies fellow, was asked during the COVID-19 pandemic by his own Episcopal diocese to guide his church members through the complexities of science. Because he was fluent in both worlds, he could model, not just prescribe, the process of moving with partial knowledge guided by science while being respectful of all faiths.

Because both religion and health are so integral to the sociopolitical fabric, they are easy targets when the fabric frays, the pandemic runs amok, or the people forget how to talk in public about the things that matter most, such as now. We clearly need to "be in this together," as Jim Curran says, but in radically new ways.[1] The *Handbook on Religion and Health*, to which he refers, attempts just this, with more than

30 respected authors writing about the dynamics and fundamental shifts in language and logic we require from both religion and public health, from the local ground to a planetary scale. By now we have assembled a mature enough science—biological, epidemiological, etiological (including religious, social, and environmental determinants)—to see the possibilities that could be released from the ancient actualities of gross, unequal suffering and to recognize that the task of achieving health for all and of the whole is not in fact entirely determined but has everything to do with the choices we make. These include political choices, which, in turn, require responsive, transparent, and deeply accountable governmental systems as integral to the health of the public as is the connectional system that holds muscles to a skeleton. AJPH

CORRESPONDENCE

Correspondence should be sent to Gary Gunderson, DMin, MDiv, Wake Forest University School of Divinity, 502 Tanners Park Ct, Winston-Salem, NC 27101 (e-mail: gary.gunderson@gmail.com). Reprints can be ordered at https://www.ajph.org by clicking the "Reprints" link.

PUBLICATION INFORMATION

Full Citation: Gunderson G, Cochrane JR, Cutts T. Toward common ground: rethinking both public health and religion, together. *Am J Public Health*. 2025;115(4):492–494.

Acceptance Date: January 25, 2025.

DOI: https://doi.org/10.2105/AJPH.2025.308047

ORCID iDs:

Gary Gunderson https://orcid.org/0000-0002-9778-3923

James R. Cochrane https://orcid.org/0000-0001-5995-7227

Teresa Cutts https://orcid.org/0000-0002-5743-3005

CONTRIBUTORS

The authors contributed equally to this editorial.

ACKNOWLEDGMENTS

We appreciate the rich dialogue among Hold.Health and university colleagues leading to this editorial.

CONFLICTS OF INTEREST

The authors have no conflicts of interest to declare.

REFERENCES

1. Curran J. Foreword. In: Cochrane JR, Gunderson GR, Cutts T, eds. *Handbook on Religion and Health: Pathways for a Turbulent Future.* Cheltenham, UK: Edward Elgar Press; 2024:xv–xvii.
2. Levin J. Toward a translational epidemiology of religion: challenges and applications. *Ann Epidemiol*. 2022;75:25–31. https://doi.org/10.1016/j.annepidem.2022.08.053
3. Morabia A. Faith-based organizations and public health: another facet of the public health dialogue. *Am J Public Health*. 2019;109(3):341. https://doi.org/10.2105/AJPH.2018.304935
4. Gostin LO, Parmet WE, Rosenbaum S. The US Supreme Court's rulings on large business and health care worker vaccine mandates: ramifications for the COVID-19 response and the future of federal public health protection. *JAMA*. 2022;327(8):713–714. https://doi.org/10.1001/jama.2022.0852
5. Levin J, Idler EL, VanderWeele TJ. Faith-based organizations and SARS-CoV-2 vaccination: challenges and recommendations. *Public Health Rep*. 2022;137(1):11–16. https://doi.org/10.1177/00333549211054079
6. National Council of the Churches of Christ in the USA. Resources on COVID-19 for churches. December 2021. Available at: https://nationalcouncilofchurches.us/resources-on-covid-19-for-churches. Accessed October 31, 2024.
7. Idler EL, ed. *Religion as a Social Determinant of Public Health.* New York, NY: Oxford University Press; 2014. https://doi.org/10.1093/acprof:oso/9780199362202.001.0001
8. Oman D, ed. *Why Religion and Spirituality Matter for Public Health: Evidence, Implications, and Resources.* Cham, Switzerland: Springer; 2018. https://doi.org/10.1007/978-3-319-73966-3
9. Idler E, Levin J, VanderWeele TJ, Khan A. Partnerships between public health agencies and faith communities. *Am J Public Health*. 2019;109(3):346–347. https://doi.org/10.2105/AJPH.2018.304941
10. Parliament of the World's Religions. Global ethic. Available at: https://parliamentofreligions.org/globalethic. Accessed October 31, 2024.
11. National Academies of Sciences, Engineering, and Medicine. Collaborative webinar: a conversation about employer Covid19 issues and emerging opportunities. Available at: https://www.nationalacademies.org/event/05-22-2020/collaborative-webinar-a-conversation-about-employer-covid19-issues-and-emerging-opportunities. Accessed January 29, 2025.
12. Milstein B, Roulier M, Kelleher C, Hartig E, Wegley S, eds. Thriving together: a springboard for equitable recovery and resilience in communities across America. CDC Foundation and Well Being Trust. July 2020. Available at: https://www.ihi.org/resources/publications/thriving-together-springboard-equitable-recovery-and-resilience-communities. Accessed January 29, 2025.
13. Burris S, Berman ML, Penn M, Ramanthan Holiday T. *The New Public Health Law: A Transdisciplinary Approach to Practice and Advocacy.* New York: Oxford University Press; 2018. https://doi.org/10.1093/oso/9780190681050.001.0001
14. Network for Public Health Law. Becoming better messengers. 2025. Available at: https://www.networkforphl.org/resources/topics/trainings/becoming-better-messengers. Accessed October 31, 2024.

Mobilizing Mayors Across the Political Spectrum to Promote Population Health: The Move With the Mayor Initiative

Emma Waugh, MPH, Jen Childress, MS, MCHES, Michelle Snyder, MPH, Christina Muryn, and John Clymer

ABOUT THE AUTHORS

Emma Waugh, Jen Childress, Michelle Snyder, and John Clymer are with the National Forum for Heart Disease and Stroke Prevention, Washington, DC. Christina Muryn is the mayor of Findlay, OH.

See also Common Ground, pp. 481–518.

Increasing partisanship in the United States was evident even before the COVID-19 pandemic disrupted public life in 2020.[1] As state and national politicians moved toward partisan extremes, Americans struggled to find common ground on basic issues.[2] Agreement on facts and trust of science has declined, partly as a result of increasing amounts of misinformation and disinformation described by the World Health Organization secretary general as an "infodemic."[3–5]

The COVID-19 pandemic exacerbated these trends, making health a partisan issue and eroding confidence in public health.[6] By October 2021, partisanship was the single strongest predictor of COVID-19 vaccination status, surpassing age, geography, education, insurance, and race.[7] This division prolonged the pandemic and led to real health consequences.[8] Other health issues are now being challenged. Legislation has been introduced or passed in 15 states to weaken public health authority, hindering its ability to carry out its basic functions.[9] According to surveys of local health departments conducted in late 2020 and early 2021, 57% of respondents reported at least one type of harassment of their local health officials.[10] It is imperative to find ways to bring people together and reclaim public health as a nonpartisan value.

In stark contrast to these partisan trends, the Move with the Mayor® (MWTM) initiative shows that local elected officials can depoliticize population health, build consensus, and unite stakeholders from the public, private, and civic sectors to advance shared public health goals.

INITIATION OF MOVE WITH THE MAYOR

The National Forum for Heart Disease and Stroke Prevention (hereafter National Forum) launched the MWTM initiative in 2014 with a walking event in Indianapolis, Indiana, led by then-mayor Greg Ballard and first lady Winnie Ballard. They engaged local employers, the city's largest university, multiple local government departments, the city's NFL and NBA teams, and the media to promote the following message: improving health starts with a single step.

After this successful pilot, the National Forum, a nonprofit cofounded by the Centers for Disease Control and Prevention, the American Heart Association, and the Association of State and Territorial Health Officials, expanded MWTM into a national initiative. Over 10 years, 205 mayors from 39 states have participated in MWTM, including 71 Democrats, 27 Republicans, 10 independents, 48 nonpartisan mayors, and 49 mayors with undisclosed parties (it is common in some states for mayors not to disclose their political affiliations). Participating mayors represent diverse communities across all regions of the country, from small, rural farming communities to medium and large suburbs and large cities.

EVOLUTION OF MOVE WITH THE MAYOR

Since beginning as a platform promoting physical activity, MWTM has steadily evolved in scope. In 2024, the initiative empowered mayors to implement evidence-based programs, policies, and infrastructure changes addressing multiple social determinants of health associated with heart disease and stroke risk. Key components of MWTM are described subsequently.

The National Forum provides mayors with messaging resources such as social media posts, graphics, public service announcement scripts, press releases, and proclamations. These resources are e-mailed regularly to mayors and their staff. Social media materials are based on health communication best practices and are reviewed by health scientists and trusted partners at national public health organizations. Messages draw on research and field testing conducted by the Ad Council, Luntz International, the DeBeaumont Foundation, and other organizations.

Mayors are encouraged to complete self-assessment tools developed by the National Forum. These tools help cities identify their strengths and opportunities to equitably improve population health. The National Forum provides evidence-based policy, program, and infrastructure change recommendations to mayors who complete the self-assessment through tailored reports, policy menus, and one-on-one meetings. The National Forum holds virtual briefings to highlight evidence-based policy and program recommendations and assigns mayors dedicated community engagement coordinators who serve as their points of contact throughout their involvement. The coordinators provide resources and develop rapport with mayors and their staff. The National Forum hosts regular webinars for mayors providing opportunities for them to learn from subject matter experts and one another. Mayors who are in geographic proximity have hosted joint events and encouraged neighboring mayors to participate.

These program components are part of MWTM campaigns and challenges that address a variety of risk factors for heart disease and stroke, including vaccination, which has been seen as politically divisive. The National Forum determines MWTM campaign topics on the basis of mayoral input, population health priorities, and timeliness (e.g., flu season).

The MWTM Flu Vaccination Campaign has been ongoing since 2021. Overall, 43 mayors have participated: 18 Democrats, nine Republicans, five independents, two nonpartisans, and nine with unknown affiliations. The MWTM Adult Vaccination Campaign ran from 2021 to 2023 with the goal of encouraging COVID-19 and routine vaccinations (e.g., flu, shingles, pneumonia, and tetanus); 88 mayors participated (44 Democrats, nine Republicans, six independents, 18 nonpartisans, and 11 with unknown affiliations). Nearly half (40) of the participating mayors came from states that voted for the Republican presidential nominee in the 2020 election, and 40% were from rural areas. Messages created from this campaign generated more than 134 million social media impressions and reached more than 9 million individuals on Facebook and Instagram.

The first MWTM Mental Health Challenge was held in 2024 in response to strong mayoral interest. Mayors hosted events to bring their communities together while engaging in physical activity. Final participation numbers are still pending. MWTM Physical Activity Challenges continue each year.

The National Forum is assiduously nonpartisan and grounds all MWTM communications in sound science. Messages are free from political bias. All recommendations are evidence based, drawn from respected sources such as the Community Guide[11] and the County Health Rankings.[12] The National Forum does not exclude mayors from participation on the basis of political beliefs; mayors are free to participate in MWTM how they choose and can opt to share messages they think will most resonate with their constituents. Through these actions, mayors have come to trust MWTM and understand its nonpartisan nature.

Several large nonpartisan mayoral organizations have endorsed the MWTM initiative, such as the US Conference of Mayors and the African American Mayors Association. The US Conference of Mayors, which represents 1400 mayors from across the political spectrum, has unanimously passed resolutions over the past 5 years urging mayors "to engage members of their community to be more physically active to improve mental and physical health and strengthen individual and community resilience using programs such as Move with the Mayor®."[13]

IMPLEMENTATION CHALLENGES

Recruiting mayors is time intensive. It requires rapport building and consistent engagement with mayors and their teams. Face-to-face interaction (at mayoral conferences) is helpful and requires further resources. Mayoral staff turnover adds to recruitment and retention challenges. To mitigate transitions, all communication with cities is tracked through customer relationship management software. Most social media engagements have been positive. However, trolls and negative comments have posed challenges. The National Forum addresses these challenges by moderating comments, linking to trusted resources, and turning off comments when necessary. Some mayors have struggled with low attendance at events or low engagement. Connecting with other mayors to brainstorm solutions or host joint events has often proven helpful.

OUTCOMES AND IMPACT

Evaluation surveys of participating mayors regularly show strong satisfaction with the MWTM program. In 2023, 83% of survey respondents found the resources provided through weekly e-mail updates very or extremely helpful. Similarly, 83% of respondents found ad hoc communication with their community engagement coordinators very or extremely helpful.

When asked about the best part of participating in MWTM, mayors frequently comment on the opportunities it creates, through events, to engage with their community. Mayors are eager to empower their constituents to make healthy choices.

> [MWTM] is a great opportunity to get out and about with our neighbors here in this city, get moving: do our part around wellness, reducing our risk for cardiovascular disease, a great chance to talk with our neighbors about what's going on in their lives, a great way to reduce stress, improve our mental and emotional well-being.
>
> —Mayor Andrew Ginther, Columbus, Ohio

The National Forum has seen numerous policy changes directly tied to MWTM recommendations. Analyzing data from an MWTM self-assessment tool, the National Forum estimates that responding cities (22 in 2023) were implementing an average of nine evidence-based recommendations from the Community Guide.[11] Systematic reviews have shown that these recommendations increase the amount of time people are physically active, reduce body mass index, and increase fruit and vegetable intake, among other benefits.[11]

In Columbia, South Carolina; Edinburg, Texas; and Green Bay, Wisconsin, decisions to build more sidewalks and trails have come about with MWTM participation. Mayor Ruben Pineda in West Chicago, Illinois, added water fountains in schools and parks to reduce sugary beverage consumption, a recommendation from an MWTM self-assessment report. Participating cities have taken steps toward increasing partnerships for health. Mayor Rod Craig of Hanover Park, Illinois, added a social worker to the police force as a means of allowing police officers to refer directly to health and social services. Mayor Will Hill of Louisville, Mississippi, worked closely with the business community to make improvements to playing fields, playgrounds, splash pads, and a multipurpose building, leading to significant economic development in addition to health benefits.

BUILDING COMMON GROUND WITH MOVE WITH THE MAYOR

Participating mayors represent all political parties; rural, urban, and suburban communities; and a range of races and ethnicities, ages, educational levels, and previous professional experiences. MWTM offers diverse communities the opportunity to come together and learn from one another.

Understanding mayors' motivations is a crucial component of building common ground with MWTM. Many mayors have joined the initiative because it resonates with their personal experiences and values. Mayor Steven Sherlin (Athens, Tennessee) is a stroke survivor. Mayor Rachel Proctor (DeSoto, Texas) lost her father to a stroke. Mayors Keith Sydnor (Laurel, Maryland) and Derrick Wood (Dumfries, Virginia) have been engaged in the military and athletics throughout their lives. Investing time in personal relationships—through dedicated community engagement coordinators—to understand these unique motivations has been crucial to the MWTM initiative. Starting from a shared motivation begins the conversation and provides a bridge to other topic areas in which a common understanding does not exist.

Through MWTM, the National Forum found that mayors understand that a healthy community underlies a socially and economically thriving community. Political differences can be overcome if this is recognized as a motivating factor. With MWTM, the National Forum has worked with cities through mayoral administration changes and as they change political parties (including from Democrat to Republican), and support for MWTM activities continues. As shared by one mayor:

> If there's anything that we can rally around, it is the health of our communities. It's not a Republican issue, not a Democratic issue, or an Independent issue. Working towards health helps improve our entire community.
>
> —Mayor Quentin M. Hart, Waterloo, Iowa

Mayors are experts in getting things done. More so than state or federal leaders, residents see their mayor's impact on their lives. Because of this, mayors are pragmatists. When mayors are presented with evidence-based policies, programs, and infrastructure improvements, they listen and act. Mayors who have repeatedly completed an MWTM self-assessment tool—which incorporates evidence-based policies, programs, and infrastructure improvements—have used it to find more opportunities to promote health.

> Completing the [self-assessment] has been a great way for city departments and partners to review our accomplishments over the year and see what we are doing well and see what we can improve. Each additional year

> we complete the [self-assessment] is a chance to see how far we have progressed.
>
> —Mayor Kim Norton, Rochester, Minnesota

HOW MAYORS BUILD COMMON GROUND FOR HEALTH

Mayors are uniquely positioned to be trusted advisors, building common ground in their own communities. In addition, they are skilled at tailoring messages to their communities. To be effective, mayors must have an up-to-date reading of their community's pulse. They must understand how to communicate with residents to serve all segments of the community. Mayors have adeptly changed the framing and wording of MWTM public health messages to resonate with their communities. They have translated materials into other languages to reach specific segments of their population.

MWTM media campaigns featuring mayors have routinely exceeded social media audience engagement benchmarks, demonstrating the value of these tailored campaigns highlighting local champions. When mayors lead by example and are provided tools to do so, people pay attention and norms shift. As Mayor Lori Bagwell (Carson City, Nevada) shared:

> I was super hesitant to do a video on getting your vaccines. But I went ahead and did it and yesterday, I was going through a drive-through at Starbucks and the young man that handed me my drinks said, "You're our mayor and I went and got my flu shot because you told me to." It showed you how a simple statement or a simple thing that you do can have impact.

Mayors have convening power, a crucial tool for creating common ground in the name of health. They can rapidly bring together public, private, and nonprofit stakeholders to discuss, plan, and act on shared objectives. Mayors Sharon Weston Broome (Baton Rouge, Louisiana), Ruben Pineda (West Chicago, Illinois), and Jim Ross (Arlington, Virginia) established multisector wellness councils linking businesses and health. Within these councils, mayors use MWTM resources to inform their programming.

In conservative Findlay, Ohio, Republican Mayor Christina Muryn (one of the authors) collaborates closely with community leaders, local media, hospitals, and the county health department. Through this collaboration, they have successfully generated community support for science-based approaches to population health. The mayor has framed public health messages to help residents recognize that the information aligns with their values and concerns. Mayor Muryn shares personal stories and concerns and directly addresses misinformation that is being circulated locally. Similarly, she has advanced programs for underserved members of the community.

Furthermore, mayors either directly oversee or indirectly influence many of the public sectors that affect the social determinants of health, including schools, parks and recreation, and transportation, among others.[14] In Allentown, Pennsylvania, Mayor Matt Tuerk prioritized health by making the health director a member of his cabinet, literally seating public health at the table when policy and resource decisions are made. His efforts culminated in Allentown's first city-specific community health assessment, which identified residents' priorities, engaged new stakeholders in the health planning process, and will be used to guide decisions across government going forward. As he described:

> All of the decisions we make as city leaders are public health decisions. The way we support our police and fire departments has an impact on public health. The investments we make in our streets or streetscapes are public health decisions.

CONCLUSION

MWTM has shown that there is a large cohort of mayors who are motivated and willing to be advocates for health in their communities. The approach has been successful in engaging mayors in physical activity and more divisive issues such as COVID-19 vaccinations; it could readily be applied to a wide array of public health topics, even those that may be viewed as divisive. Mayors can play valuable roles in long-term, nonpartisan strategies to build community support for public health. They have powerful potential to bridge diverse stakeholders, serve as trusted messengers, and ultimately champion public health at the local level. AJPH

CORRESPONDENCE

Correspondence should be sent to Emma Waugh, MPH, 1150 Connecticut Ave, NW, Suite 300, Washington, DC 20036-4130 (e-mail: emma.waugh.ic@nationalforum.org). Reprints can be ordered at https://www.ajph.org by clicking the "Reprints" link.

PUBLICATION INFORMATION

Full Citation: Waugh E, Childress J, Snyder M, Muryn C, Clymer J. Mobilizing mayors across the political spectrum to promote population health: the move with the mayor initiative. *Am J Public Health*. 2025;115(4):495–499.

Acceptance Date: December 8, 2024.

DOI: https://doi.org/10.2105/AJPH.2024.307978

ORCID iDs:
Emma Waugh https://orcid.org/0000-0001-8248-3859

John Clymer https://orcid.org/0000-0002-2962-8235

CONTRIBUTORS

All of the authors contributed significantly to this article. E. Waugh led the drafting of the article. J. Childress and M. Snyder contributed to sections on program design, challenges, and implementation. C. Muryn provided significant contributions to sections on mayoral involvement. J. Clymer served as the senior author and provided input on the design and overall guidance of the article.

ACKNOWLEDGMENTS

Funding for the Move with the Mayor initiative has been provided by the Centers for Disease Control and Prevention in partnership with the American Public Health Association, the National Association of Chronic Disease Directors, and the National Association of County and City Health Officials.

We acknowledge the mayors from across the country and their staff who have dedicated themselves to promoting health in all that they do. We also thank the many team members who have worked on the program and contributed to its numerous successes. Finally, we thank the funders that have made this work possible.

CONFLICTS OF INTEREST

The authors have no potential conflicts of interest to declare.

REFERENCES

1. Pew Research Center. Political polarization in the American public. Available at: https://www.pewresearch.org/politics/2014/06/12/political-polarization-in-the-american-public. Accessed May 22, 2024.
2. US Department of Health and Human Services. Confronting health misinformation: the U.S. surgeon general's advisory on building a healthy information environment. Available at: https://www.hhs.gov/sites/default/files/surgeon-general-misinformation-advisory.pdf. Accessed May 22, 2024.
3. Kennedy B, Tyson A, Funk C. Americans' trust in scientists, other groups declines. Available at: https://www.pewresearch.org/science/2022/02/15/americans-trust-in-scientists-other-groups-declines. Accessed May 22, 2024.
4. Lupia A, Allison DB, Jamieson KH, Heimberg J, Skipper M, Wolf SM. Trends in U.S. public confidence in science and opportunities for progress. *Proc Natl Acad Sci U S A*. 2024;121(11):e2319488121. https://doi.org/10.1073/pnas.2319488121
5. World Health Organization. Managing the COVID-19 infodemic: promoting healthy behaviours and mitigating the harm from misinformation and disinformation. Available at: https://www.who.int/news/item/23-09-2020-managing-the-covid-19-infodemic-promoting-healthy-behaviours-and-mitigating-the-harm-from-misinformation-and-disinformation. Accessed May 22, 2024.
6. Kirzinger A, Presiado M, Valdes I, Hamel L, Brodie M. The COVID-19 pandemic: insights from three years of KFF polling. Available at: https://www.kff.org/coronavirus-covid-19/poll-finding/the-covid-19-pandemic-insights-from-three-years-of-kff-polling. Accessed May 31, 2024.
7. Kirzinger A, Kearney A, Hamel L, Brodie M. COVID-19 vaccine monitor: the increasing importance of partisanship in predicting COVID-19 vaccination status. Available at: https://www.kff.org/coronavirus-covid-19/poll-finding/importance-of-partisanship-predicting-vaccination-status. Accessed May 22, 2024.
8. Shah A, Seervia S, Schneider E. How can the U.S. catch up with other countries on COVID-19 vaccination? Available at: https://www.commonwealthfund.org/blog/2021/how-can-us-catch-other-countries-covid-19-vaccination. Accessed May 22, 2024.
9. Network for Public Health Law. Proposed limits on public health authority dangerous for public health. Available at: https://www.networkforphl.org/wp-content/uploads/2021/06/Proposed-Limits-on-Public-Health-Authority-Dangerous-for-Public-Health-FINAL.pdf. Accessed May 22, 2024.
10. Ward JA, Stone EM, Mui P, Resnick B. Pandemic-related workplace violence and its impact on public health officials, March 2020–January 2021. *Am J Public Health*. 2022;112(5):736–746. https://doi.org/10.2105/AJPH.2021.306649
11. Centers for Disease Control and Prevention. Community Guide home page. Available at: https://www.thecommunityguide.org/index.html. Accessed May 31, 2024.
12. University of Wisconsin Population Health Institute. County health rankings and roadmaps. Available at: https://www.countyhealthrankings.org. Accessed May 31, 2024.
13. United States Conference of Mayors. Resolutions. Available at: https://www.usmayors.org/the-conference/resolutions/?category=a0F4N00000S4uUZUAZ&meeting=91st%20Annual%20Meeting. Accessed May 31, 2024.
14. Godinez Puig L, Lusk, K, Glick, D, Einstein, K, Palmer, M, Fox, S, Wang ML. Perceptions of public health priorities and accountability among US mayors. *Public Health Rep*. 2021;136(2):161–171. https://doi.org/10.1177/0033354920966050

Exploring Democratic Deliberation in Public Health: Bridging Division and Enhancing Community Engagement

Michelle Bosché, Rachel Krust, MPP, Archon Fung, PhD, and Aditya S. Pawar, MD

ABOUT THE AUTHORS

Michelle Bosché is a third-year medical student at Harvard Medical School, Boston, MA. Rachel Krust and Archon Fung are with the Ash Center for Democratic Governance and Innovation, Harvard Kennedy School, Boston, MA. Aditya S. Pawar is with the Beth Israel Deaconess Medical Center and Harvard Medical School, Boston, MA.

See also Common Ground, pp. 481–518.

Trust between citizens and the institutions that govern them is essential for effective policy, especially in public health. Across the world, higher levels of trust in government are associated with higher uptake of public health guidance, from vaccinations and use of preventive health services to physical distancing recommendations during epidemics.[1,2] However, against a backdrop of escalating political polarization and rising levels of misinformation, there has been a stark decline in public confidence in government and health institutions. In 1966, 73% of people expressed a "great deal of confidence" in those running the medical system. By 2012, only 34% did.[3] In 2024, the Edelman Trust Barometer revealed that 70% of US respondents worried government leaders were purposely trying to mislead them.[4] This trend has a negative impact on health care delivery at almost every level, from patient–doctor relationships to national population health efforts.

Public participation in decision making is one strategy policymakers can use to strengthen trust in health governance. Citizen engagement has historically been used to inform policies across a range of social issues, often to great success, yet it is still largely underused in the health sector.[5] When efforts have been made to engage communities, they have often been through quantitative and nondeliberative frameworks favored by many health economists, such as discrete choice experiments, surveys, and polls.[6] Meaningful public reasoning is essential to address moral and civic questions, especially in areas of scarce resources that necessitate transparent and inclusive decision-making processes.[7]

In an increasingly divided political atmosphere, there is a pressing need for policymakers to explore innovative ways to engage the public, gather diverse perspectives, and build common ground on controversial and complex issues of public health policy. Democratic deliberation offers such a framework. We argue that, by facilitating formal and goal-driven discussion between leaders and the public, deliberation can be used as a tool to build understanding between participants with competing viewpoints and can ultimately improve the quality and responsiveness of public health policy. Here we examine the potential of democratic deliberation to improve health sector governance. We discuss the unique benefits of deliberative approaches, limitations, and how deliberation can be scaled up to influence public health policy.

AN OVERVIEW OF DEMOCRATIC DELIBERATION

Democratic deliberation refers to a method of public engagement in which people from different backgrounds come together in a formal dialogue to learn about, discuss, and ultimately provide recommendations about a social problem.[8] Although the scale and structure of these dialogues can vary, each facilitates a two-way exchange of information between organizers and participants. Core requirements of democratic deliberation include (1) recruitment of participants with diverse and representative opinions, (2) presentation of accurate and neutral evidence as background information, (3) consideration of various solutions and perspectives of other participants, and (4) pursuit of common ground to ultimately offer a recommendation.[8]

Examples of deliberation include citizen juries, citizen panels, and consensus conferences (Box 1). With these principles, democratic deliberation is distinct from other common forms of public engagement such as town halls, focus groups, and opinion polling in which there is typically a one-way solicitation of feedback without explicit efforts to discuss difficult trade-offs or arm

BOX 1— Methods of Deliberation

Method	Stakeholder Inclusion	Transparency	Efficiency	Outcome
Democratic deliberation	Multistakeholder engagement (e.g., patients, providers, and policymakers)	Open discussions and shared rationale	Time-intensive but inclusive processes	Policies aligned with public/stakeholder needs
Online engagement platforms	Broader participation via digital platforms	Moderately transparent; real-time feedback	Flexible, asynchronous participation	Broad accessibility but potential for digital exclusion
Crowdsourcing	Involvement of large groups, including nonexperts	Limited transparency during synthesis	Fast, creative idea generation	Diverse ideas but requires moderation and synthesis
Digital town halls	Broad audience interaction through virtual platforms	High transparency; live interaction	Real time but requires significant logistics	High engagement, although outcomes can be less structured
Citizen panels	Carefully selected representative groups	High transparency; informed decisions	Time-intensive but in-depth deliberations	Recommendations that reflect informed, diverse perspectives
Asynchronous deliberation	Flexible participation by busy stakeholders	Moderately transparent; iterative input	Time-efficient for individuals	Thoughtful input but lacks dynamic interactions
Gamification/simulations	Stakeholders engage actively through interactive tools	Moderate transparency; scenario based	Engaging but resource intensive	Helps in visualizing outcomes but risks oversimplification
Social media engagement	Large-scale, diverse public input	Limited transparency; social media biases	Fast and scalable	Provides a snapshot of public opinion but lacks depth
Deliberative artificial intelligence (AI) tools	Broad input processed via AI algorithms	Low transparency; algorithm dependent	Highly efficient, scalable	Synthesizes large data sets, although nuanced human insights may be missed

AJPH April 2025, Vol. 115, No. 4

participants with balanced evidence.[9] Some proponents of public deliberation argue that it requires random selection of participants. In this article, we use "democratic deliberation" more broadly to encompass processes that create reasoned discussion among a representative sample of participants but do not entail strict random selection.

The goal of deliberation has historically been to find consensus, but definitions of successful outcomes have expanded in contemporary discussions.[10] Dryzek and Niemeyer argued that meta-consensus—agreement about the credibility of opposing beliefs, if not the beliefs themselves—should be considered a successful outcome. Mansbridge formulated four alternative ends to deliberation other than consensus, including expanding the borders of a problem and introducing new perspectives. Morrissey and Boswell argued that the building of common ground, wherein participants "agree on and seek to further build the shared pool of information," should mark the success of deliberation.[11(p153)] Although consensus is a worthy aim, these alternative goals of deliberation show that its benefits reside not in a specific outcome but instead within the process of deliberation itself. Examples such as the Oregon Health Plan and citizen assemblies in Canada highlight how structured dialogue can reduce polarization and illuminate shared values.[12]

We argue that democratic deliberation offers unique benefits to health policy-making that other frameworks lack, particularly with respect to inclusion of diverse, representative populations; knowledge exchange; and building of common ground. These three areas are especially useful in a climate of increasing distrust and political division that threatens the effectiveness of public health policies. Overall, democratic deliberation can improve responsiveness to and strengthen public trust in health policy decisions.

Inclusion of Diverse, Representative Populations

Traditional health policy decisions are made through feedback from a complex interplay of actors, including interest groups, lobbyists, nongovernmental organizations, and the media. This approach often overlooks the nuanced perspectives of minority groups, economically disadvantaged communities, and other underrepresented voices that typically avoid formal political discourse. Although there have been recent efforts to diversify social participation, health professionals, experts, and government cadres still dominate the process.

Democratic deliberation offers methods of systematically including unheard and previously undervalued voices. It focuses on recruiting a representative sample of participants, often through random selection that can also be stratified according to demographics.[13] Participants in the discussion can be selected to represent groups that would otherwise be left out. For example, in a systematic review of the use of citizen juries in health policy, Street et al. found that most studies explicitly stated an aim to recruit juries that represented the community.[12] In deliberative approaches, representation can be an intentional process and allows an opportunity to weave in voices that would otherwise be neglected.

In addition, deliberations include skilled facilitators who aim to ensure that participants have an equal chance to speak, listen carefully to others, and weigh different options and trade-offs.[14] Instead of hearing predominantly from the "loudest voices" who are best equipped to advocate their perspective, facilitators can help policymakers gather a holistic view of participants' perspectives.[15]

Knowledge Exchange

Deliberative frameworks also act to open communication channels between the public and policymakers. Policymakers can more easily share scientific opinions and research findings with members of the public without fear of obscuration by the media or political spin.[8] By providing background materials that showcase the range of evidence-based views and including experts who can explain complex components of an issue, deliberation can be an effective way of sharing accurate information. For example, a study on a deliberation about the allocation of ventilators in a hypothetical influenza outbreak in Maryland showed a substantial increase in participants' understanding of the discussed issues according to surveys conducted before and after the study. After the deliberation, 80% of the study participants said that they understood issues related to deciding who received medical treatment during emergencies "very well or well," as compared with 44% who reported an understanding of these issues before the study.[16]

In return, public participants can share specific and localized community values to aid in prioritization schemes. The New York City Department of Health and Mental Hygiene used deliberative strategies to gather feedback on how to allocate the distribution of COVID-19 vaccines early in the pandemic. The department found that the combination of background information and structured discussion led to more "carefully considered recommendations, allowing health departments to gain a nuanced understanding not only of what participants think but also underlying reasons why."[17(pp93–94)] This allowed for a "rich exploration of community values" that informed policy development.

This "give and receive" framework offered by deliberative platforms allows both policymakers and the public to benefit. The participants can obtain "stimulating and informative" background data on policy issues that affect them, and policymakers can gather detailed information on community priorities and reasons behind them.[8] This process can facilitate information sharing and trust between decision makers and constituents and pave the way for locally resonant policy development.

Common Ground

Despite the vitriolic nature of most political discourse, common ground does exist even on the most hotly debated issues of health policy. In an Association of American Medical Colleges survey of young adults, the authors were "surprised" by areas of consensus among Democrats, Independents, and Republicans: three quarters of Republicans in the survey agreed with Democrats and Independents that access to health care is a basic human right, and more than two thirds of Republicans said that it is the responsibility of the federal government to ensure that everyone has health care coverage.[18] However, these areas of agreement are often elusive in current policy discussions. Deliberative methods allow time and space for civil discussion that can reveal common ground between participants.

The formal structure of democratic deliberation encourages an environment of mutual respect among participants. By explicitly stating common rules and goals at the outset, employing trained facilitators to help navigate the discussion, and providing evidence-based background information, deliberation allows participants to wrestle with alternative opinions in a civil way. For example, more than 400 residents of Washington, DC, participated in a deliberation exercise to prioritize policies designed to address social determinants of health, such as adult education, job placement programs, housing, and public day care. In a postdeliberation survey, 92% of participants said they were treated with respect and 86% said their views were considered by the rest of the group. Moreover, although nearly 40% of participants said their individual prioritization scheme differed considerably from the group's, more than 70% were still willing to abide by the recommendations that the group agreed on.[19] Even if full consensus is not achieved, deliberation fosters an environment where common ground can be found.

Another measurable proxy for building common ground is participants' willingness to change their mind after deliberation. Many studies on deliberative methods show that participants do change their opinions after discussion. A Canadian citizens' dialogue exploring public opinion on public health system priorities revealed that participants' attitudes underwent "substantial change" as a result of deliberations: the share of participants supporting increased public funding for the Canadian public health care system rose from 48% to 61%, and the percentage supporting systemic reform of the primary care system rose from 56% to 79%.[20] Democratic deliberation can open participants' minds to the validity of other perspectives and help identify areas of agreement.

LIMITATIONS OF DELIBERATIVE METHODS

Although democratic deliberation is a promising and underused tool for public engagement in health policy, there are several limitations of its use. First, even with a focus on random selection, democratic deliberation cannot claim perfect representativeness. The small sample sizes of 10 to 20 people necessary for a successful discussion preclude the ability to represent all perspectives present in a population. Some have argued that this can increase bias in decision-making processes by creating too narrow of a representative body.[21]

Beyond issues of sample size, achieving a representative cross section of the population is often challenging, even when doing so is a stated aim. In the 1980s, Oregon set out to gather broad public feedback about health services included in Medicare's basic plan. Representation was a major criticism of the effort, as 50% of the participants were health professionals, college educated, or White.[22] Part of this difficulty may be participation bias. Deliberative methods require buy-in from participants and a commitment to accepting the norms of a democratic process. Recruiting participants who lack trust in governmental leadership or democratic principles can be difficult.

Deliberations also require extensive time commitments of varying length, from several hours to several days. Even when best efforts are made to reduce barriers to participation (e.g., providing additional reimbursement for child-care expenses, travel, and accommodation), nonparticipation bias still exists and can skew the composition of participants toward those with more flexible schedules.[23] Deliberation is also costly: the Organisation for Economic Co-operation and Development estimates that the cost of deliberative methods can vary widely depending on the model and the number of participants, ranging anywhere from 13 000 to 1.8 million euros.[5] This creates challenges in scaling democratic deliberation and reinforces the importance of better understanding the types of decisions for which it can most effectively be used.[24]

MOVING FORWARD

Given these challenges, what are the best ways to operationalize democratic deliberation to improve public health? We suggest that there are significant opportunities to use deliberative methods to improve health policy development, particularly in areas in which there are multiple ethical and evidence-based options and there is a direct impact on citizens' everyday lives. Community engagement is especially important health policy decisions with multiple ethical options, such as how to prioritize the use of scarce health resources (e.g., organ transplants and pandemic response measures). Deliberative approaches can help decision makers adopt policies that reflect the values of the community and potentially increase the acceptance and quality of public health interventions.[5] Evidence also shows that engaging citizens on issues that affect their daily lives (e.g., mental health service programs and reproductive health services) can strengthen their sense of political efficacy.[25] By reinforcing that citizens played a role in decisions that are important to them, policymakers can build trust in the democratic process.

Although there are many potential opportunities for deliberative approaches in health policy, there are still gaps in research. Critical questions requiring further research and pilots include the following:

1. What issues and contexts are most appropriate for deliberation? For

example, deliberation is often appropriate for ethical questions but has not been used as often for technical or expert questions.

2. What methods of democratic deliberation are most effective at building common ground and trust in governmental processes? How can we better evaluate these endpoints?
3. How can deliberation be optimized for the unique challenges in public health? For example, current methodologies are difficult (although not impossible) to employ in settings where time-sensitive decision making is necessary, such as during health emergencies. Also, some health policy issues may require extensive knowledge for informed deliberation. These questions are particularly important given the resource-intensive nature of deliberation.
4. How can democratic deliberation be scaled or institutionalized to improve its cost-effectiveness?
5. To what extent should processes seek to use random selection over curation of representatives (e.g., patients and advocates)?

CONCLUSION

Amid rising political tensions, the erosion of trust in governing institutions, and worsening health outcomes, we need innovative methods of engaging the public in decision making. Although questions of public health policy are often complex and can generate divergent viewpoints, finding common ground is possible, even in the most nuanced and controversial issues.[18] Democratic deliberation is an underused tool in these efforts. Moving forward, we should use its principles to foster a deeper understanding among health professionals and policymakers, build trust in institutions, and lay a foundation where everyone can find common ground. AJPH

CORRESPONDENCE

Correspondence should be sent to Aditya S. Pawar, MD, 110 Francis St, Lowry, Floor 7, Beth Israel Deaconess Medical Center, Boston, MA 02215 (e-mail: aspawar@bidmc.harvard.edu). Reprints can be ordered at https://www.ajph.org by clicking the "Reprints" link.

PUBLICATION INFORMATION

Full Citation: Bosché M, Krust R, Fung A, Pawar AS. Exploring democratic deliberation in public health: bridging division and enhancing community engagement. *Am J Public Health*. 2025;115(4):500–505.

Acceptance Date: December 18, 2024.

DOI: https://doi.org/10.2105/AJPH.2024.307998

ORCID iDs:
Michelle Bosché https://orcid.org/0009-0001-3568-6634

Archon Fung https://orcid.org/0009-0003-0629-6762

Aditya S. Pawar https://orcid.org/0000-0002-9178-4386

CONTRIBUTORS

M. Bosché and A. S. Pawar conceptualized and designed the work. M. Bosché drafted the article. R. Krust, A. Fung, and A. S. Pawar revised the article for important intellectual content.

CONFLICTS OF INTEREST

The authors report no conflicts of interest.

REFERENCES

1. Bargain O, Aminjonov U. Trust and compliance to public health policies in times of COVID-19. *J Public Econ*. 2020;192:104316. https://doi.org/10.1016/j.jpubeco.2020.104316
2. Darden ME, Macis M. Trust and health care-seeking behavior. Available at: https://www.nber.org/system/files/working_papers/w32028/w32028.pdf. Accessed May 28, 2024.
3. Taylor LA, Solomon MZ, Kaebnick GE. Trust in health care and science: toward common ground on key concepts. *Hastings Cent Rep*. 2023;53(suppl 2):S2–S8. https://doi.org/10.1002/hast.1517
4. Edelman Trust Institute. 2024 Edelman Trust Barometer. Available at: https://www.edelman.com/sites/g/files/aatuss191/files/2024-05/2024%20Edelman%20Trust%20Barometer_U.S.%20Report.pdf. Accessed May 28, 2024.
5. Organisation for Economic Co-operation and Development. Innovative citizen participation and new democratic institutions: catching the deliberative wave. Available at: https://www.oecd.org/content/dam/oecd/en/publications/reports/2020/06/innovative-citizen-participation-and-new-democratic-institutions_11aa2baf/339306da-en.pdf. Accessed May 28, 2024.
6. Schoon R, Chi C. Integrating citizens juries and discrete choice experiments: methodological issues in the measurement of public values in healthcare priority setting. *Soc Sci Med*. 2022;309:115223. https://doi.org/10.1016/j.socscimed.2022.115223
7. Daniels N. Accountability for reasonableness. *BMJ*. 2000;321(7272):1300–1301. https://doi.org/10.1136/bmj.321.7272.1300
8. Safaei J. Deliberative democracy in health care: current challenges and future prospects. *J Healthc Leadersh*. 2015;7:123–136. https://doi.org/10.2147/JHL.S70021
9. Westminster Foundation for Democracy. An introduction to deliberative democracy for members of parliament. Available at: https://www.wfd.org/sites/default/files/2021-11/WFD_newDemocracy_An-introduction-to-deliberative-democracy-for-members-of-parliament_2021.pdf. Accessed May 28, 2024.
10. Dryzek JS, Niemeyer S. Reconciling pluralism and consensus as political ideals. *Am J Pol Sci*. 2006;50(3):634–649. https://doi.org/10.1111/j.1540-5907.2006.00206.x
11. Morrissey L, Boswell J. Finding common ground. *Eur J Polit Theory*. 2023;22(1):141–160. https://doi.org/10.1177/1474885120969920
12. Street J, Duszynski K, Krawczyk S, Braunack-Mayer A. The use of citizens' juries in health policy decision-making: a systematic review. *Soc Sci Med*. 2014;109:1–9. https://doi.org/10.1016/j.socscimed.2014.03.005
13. Steel D, Bolduc N, Jenei K, Burgess M. Rethinking representation and diversity in deliberative mini-publics. *J Deliberative Democracy*. 2020;16(1):46–57. https://doi.org/10.16997/jdd.398
14. Organisation for Economic Co-operation and Development. Good practice principles for deliberative processes for public decision making. Available at: https://www.oecd.org/content/dam/oecd/en/topics/policy-issue-focus/innovative-citizen-participation/good-practice-principles-for-deliberative-processes-for-public-decision-making.pdf. Accessed May 28, 2024.
15. Redman K. Association of Australian Medical Research Institutes deliberative panel. Available at: https://www.newdemocracy.com.au/2023/07/12/association-of-australian-medical-research-institutes-deliberative-panel. Accessed May 28, 2024.
16. Daugherty Biddison EL, Gwon H, Schoch-Spana M, et al. The community speaks: understanding ethical values in allocation of scarce lifesaving resources during disasters. *Ann Am Thorac Soc*. 2014;11(5):777–783. https://doi.org/10.1513/AnnalsATS.201310-379OC

17. Scherer M, Kamler A, Weiss L, Blacksher E, Jeavons J, Gold MR. Using public deliberation to set priorities: the case of COVID-19 vaccine access in New York City. *J Public Health Manag Pract.* 2022;28(1):86–94. https://doi.org/10.1097/PHH.0000000000001471
18. Alberti PM, Orgera K, Alvarado CS. Generation Z challenges partisan divides for health equity. *Am J Public Health.* 2023;113(10):1114–1115. https://doi.org/10.2105/AJPH.2023.307391
19. Pesce JE, Kpaduwa CS, Danis M. Deliberation to enhance awareness of and prioritize socioeconomic interventions for health. *Soc Sci Med.* 2011;72(5):789–797. https://doi.org/10.1016/j.socscimed.2011.01.002
20. Participedia. Citizens' dialogues during the Royal Commission on the Future of Health Care in Canada. Available at: https://participedia.net/case/609. Accessed May 28, 2024.
21. Sandman L, Hofmann B, Bognar G. Rethinking patient involvement in healthcare priority setting. *Bioethics.* 2020;34(4):403–411. https://doi.org/10.1111/bioe.12730
22. Daniels N. Is the Oregon rationing plan fair? *JAMA.* 1991;265(17):2232–2235. https://doi.org/10.1001/jama.1991.03460170086039
23. Biddison ELD, Gwon HS, Schoch-Spana M, et al. Scarce resource allocation during disasters: a mixed-method community engagement study. *Chest.* 2018;153(1):187–195. https://doi.org/10.1016/j.chest.2017.08.001
24. Baker R, Mason H, McHugh N, Donaldson C. Public values and plurality in health priority setting: what to do when people disagree and why we should care about reasons as well as choices. *Soc Sci Med.* 2021;277:113892. https://doi.org/10.1016/j.socscimed.2021.113892
25. Knobloch KR, Barthel ML, Gastil J. Emanating effects: the impact of the Oregon citizens' initiative review on voters' political efficacy. *Polit Stud.* 2020;68(2):426–445. https://doi.org/10.1177/0032321719852254

A "Civity" Approach Helps Build the Civic Muscle That Underlies Healthy Communities

Palma Joy Strand, JD, LLM, and Malka Ranjana Kopell, MPP

ABOUT THE AUTHORS

Palma Joy Strand is with the nonprofit organization Civity, San Francisco, CA, emerita professor at Creighton University, Omaha, NE, and visiting professor at Marquette University School of Law, Milwaukee, WI. Malka Ranjana Kopell is with the nonprofit organization Civity, San Francisco, CA, and California State University, Sacramento, CA.

See also Common Ground, pp. 481–518.

Research from various academic disciplines, including sociology and public health, has established that communities with bridging relationships that link disparate social groups have lower levels of violence,[1] greater capacity to collaborate to address community needs,[2,3] and better health.[4] Although there is strong consensus among researchers that cross-cutting civic networks are powerful positives, there has been little focus on how to create or strengthen relationships across social difference in actual community settings.

Civity is a national nonprofit organization with the mission of operationalizing these findings by creating "civity," which we define as "a culture of deliberately engaging in relationships of respect and empathy with others who are different."[5] Civity's work thus centers on creating positive relationships across social differences.

Increasing the quantity and quality of "weak-tie" bridging connections builds civic capacity for a community to pull together as a whole.[5,6] This civic capacity—also referred to as "relational infrastructure" or "civic muscle"—enables cooperation to strengthen collective supports for all community members. Civic muscle lies at the core of the vital conditions for health and well-being that enable individual and community thriving.[7] Robust communities with strong and flexible civic muscle support the well-being of all members; ensuring that all members of a community are "seen" and valued is a key contributor to that community's health.[8(pp383–387)]

Civity's theory of change recognizes that community members themselves have the ability to strengthen their communities by initiating and engaging in cross-cutting relationships. Our key strategies are to (1) make the "other" visible, particularly to people with more privilege, and (2) strengthen relationships across difference, which together (3) support and increase the effectiveness of existing community-based work, which advances public health. (See Figure 1 for the Civity Theory of Change.) Civity partners with local leaders to help them engage in and facilitate other community members' participation in relationship-building that increases social trust and decreases social distance—acting as a catalyst to transform existing social networks and civic infrastructure.[9,10] Civity's work thus offers a practical example of a relational "civity" approach to building civic muscle.

PERSONAL STORIES STRENGTHEN RELATIONAL INFRASTRUCTURE

The authors of this article, who cofounded Civity, came to this work in similar ways. Both authors are grounded in "head" disciplines (M. R. K. in public health policy and P. J. S. in law) that emphasize the technical and analytical aspects of community problems and opportunities. Yet both of us, through being involved ourselves in decision-making processes at the community level, noticed that relationships—especially those connecting members of disparate social groups—are the essential basis for productive collaborations. Without such relationships, discussions break down, communities get stuck, and people get left out. Bringing this necessary "heart" element to the fore to make progress on intractable yet essential current issues spurred us to focus on relationships in civic life.

In conversations with activists and civic leaders seeking to improve their communities, we heard time and time again that lack of social trust is a barrier and that relationships, particularly relationships across difference, are necessary for community thriving, yet are often lacking. With philanthropic support from The Whitman Institute, Civity developed a protocol for providing people with positive relational experiences with "others" who are socially different from them. We drew from research in psychology, sociology, network theory, and complex adaptive systems to develop a strategy for cultivating the

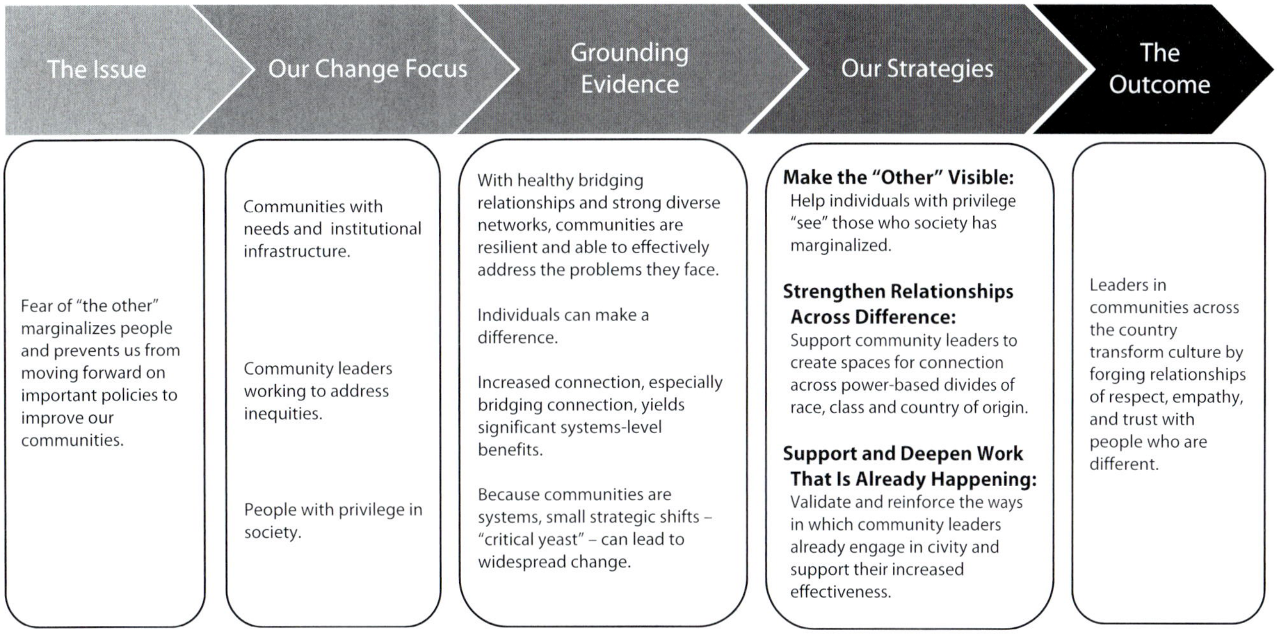

FIGURE 1— Civity Theory of Change

essential personal interactions these on-the-ground leaders identified as necessary.[11]

Combining insights from practice and theory, Civity designed an experiential workshop that we conduct both in person and virtually. This workshop centers structured one-on-one conversations in which participants exchange personal stories, which effectively bring them into authentic relationship in a surprisingly short time (10 minutes). Personal stories that are heart- rather than head-based connect participants with their own nonsurface selves and give them a glimpse into the complexity of someone else. With this approach, participants identify disparate social identities and create genuine connection across and through difference.[5]

Personal stories offer a way for people to begin to engage with social differences. Many people know that these differences are important and potentially divisive but avoid them through anxiety and fear. Telling one's own story and listening to another person's may feel a bit risky because we are often unaccustomed to sharing parts of our authentic selves with people other than friends and family. Through civity experiences, however, people find that relational story-sharing is not just possible but enjoyable. And naming and connecting through difference taps into our natural curiosity and desire for connection.

Many, though not all, of the social differences that keep people apart involve power differentials. Although "civity conversations" do not fully eliminate power differentials, they bring into the mix horizontal relational experiences (i.e., person-to-person conversational interactions centered on people's own stories) that tend to mitigate negative power dynamics. Sharing personal stories creates human-to-human connections that provide an entry point for engagement and erode stereotypes and other power-based "us versus them" mindsets. Our ultimate goal is twofold: to provide people with a positive experience of engaging with someone they regard as "other" and to create a space in which everyone feels that they "matter"—especially people who have been silenced or marginalized.

The story-sharing conversations that Civity workshop participants engage in operate on several levels. Most immediately, these conversations provide the experience of connecting relationally with someone who is not a friend or family member—in fact, with someone who may be unknown to them. Story-sharing also gives participants a structured way to talk to people they perceive as different. Overall, participants leave a Civity workshop with the fundamentals of "practicing civity"—that is, engaging relationally on their own with people who are different, which contributes to building civity in their community.

Civity conversations do not themselves resolve community conflicts; rather, they are the "conversation before the conversation." The relationships that civity conversations create are a necessary precondition for community members to work together productively to address stressors and challenges. Only when diverse parties affected by a problem see each other as "mattering" can they collaborate to develop ways forward that address the full range of interests involved. These relationships need not be close or deep, but they do need to be characterized by respect ("I see you") and empathy ("I hear you"). Civity relationships are a kind of "secret sauce" that enables community norms to move from "us versus them" to "we all belong."

PARTNERING BRINGS A CIVITY APPROACH TO SCALE

The local leaders with whom Civity partners are deeply embedded in their communities' civic infrastructure: in relationships, organizations, and formal and informal institutions and practices. These leaders are government officials, nonprofit heads, civic activists, and community-minded businesspeople. Civity's systems frame recognizes that a small but transformative shift in how people interact—in the places in which they are already interacting—spreads out through existing networks and pathways to grow civity culture.

This work with community leaders serves multiple purposes. It affirms the value of relationships in addressing community challenges. It provides leaders with a frame and language for intentionally engaging in relationship-building themselves, especially bridging relationships. And it supplies them with tools and strategies for creating spaces in their work for other community members to connect relationally. Designated as "seeding civity," this strategy of working with and through existing civic infrastructure is our systems-based strategy for bringing relationship-building to scale.[5]

With support from the William & Flora Hewlett Foundation, we field-tested our partnering model. Over more than a decade, we worked with hundreds of individuals in several dozen organizations in various communities across the country. We supported local leaders in reaching across different social divides such as race, economics, geography, religion, and politics. We assisted them in integrating relationship-building into work on issues ranging from affordable housing to immigration policy to climate change and more. We offer here several examples from Civity initiatives across the United States.

In Louisville, Kentucky, Civity partnered with Compassionate Louisville[12] to support concrete actions to bring the city's declared commitment to compassion to life. Civity reached deeply into Louisville's civic infrastructure, bringing civity language and strategies to business, government, and community organizations—from leadership programs to meditation centers—to provide relationship-building skills and strategies for Louisville residents.

In Nebraska, Civity partnered with the Center for Rural Affairs,[13] cofacilitating community workshop events centered on local leadership development and eventually training the Center's staff to integrate civity relationship-building into their own community-strengthening initiatives. Civity train-the-trainer work is a powerful multiplier for scaling.

In Montana, Civity partnered with Braver Angels[14] and Citizens' Climate Lobby[15] to work with community leaders on how to talk about climate change with people of differing perspectives. Integrating relationality into tough issue-based conversations paves the way for understanding—even when agreement is not forthcoming.

Working with the Welcoming America[16] national network, Civity partnered with local members who saw the value of intentional relationality in creating welcoming environments. From government agencies to long-standing community nonprofits such as the YMCA to community gardens, these local leaders brought civity to their diversified spheres of influence.

We saw, in these and other communities, a hunger for simply being human in interactions with fellow community members. Too often, we were told, the pressure to get things done gets in the way of taking time and creating space for making sure relationships are tended to. Local leaders told us that Civity gave them "permission" to follow their intuitions that relationships are key to community flourishing—the nourishment that civic muscles need to grow and stay strong and flexible.

FOUR KEY ASPECTS OF A CIVITY APPROACH

To scale the civity approach to building civic muscle, we bring the tools of connection via story-sharing to people who can use and spread them: emerging and established community leaders. These leaders hail from various sectors and are working on a wide range of issues and challenges. The common thread is their recognition of the need for and value of relationships in moving forward. Practicing and seeding civity provide local leaders and community members tangible doable actions that they as individuals can take to help build community-level relational infrastructure, the genesis of cooperative initiatives that enhance community well-being. Civity supports this civic muscle-building in four key ways.

First, we provide a name—"civity"—that describes the positive relationship-based culture that is our vision. "Civity" is akin to the word "community" but has the important distinction of focusing on difference rather than similarity. A unique word focuses attention, which is important for creating intention and making the sought-after goal more concrete.[17] "Civity" the word reminds people that being relational, especially across difference, matters; it also provides language for fellow-member-of-my-community relationships without the political charge of "citizenship."

Second, although Civity's relational strategies are powerful, they are also compact, designed to fit easily into what leaders and other community members are already doing. Civity transforms *how* people do their work rather than being an additional to-do. Indeed, an entire set of do-it-yourself activities provides myriad entry points into civity practice. Our DIYcivity web page affirms Civity's overarching "You can do this!!!" message.[5]

Third, seeding civity identifies and defines for local leaders the importance of civic relationships among community members—above and beyond engagement with officials and government.[18] Civic capacity grows when communities are internally interconnected, when a civic web is created. Civity—a "we all belong" culture—is decentered and self-organizing and arises when actions of various individuals in their spheres of influence provide the impetus for change.

Fourth, Civity gives local leaders concrete and specific tools and strategies for integrating civity conversations—relational interactions across difference—into their communities. In addition to our workshops, we provide one-on-one and group coaching that reinforces practice and offers opportunities for mutual support. Building civic muscle and belonging is a shared effort that benefits from mutual support and encouragement.[7]

MEGASTUDY AFFIRMED CIVITY'S PERSONAL STORIES APPROACH

Our primary evaluation methods have been comments collected on-site and postworkshop questionnaires. We review these to continually refine the workshop experience. Because workshop participants often start out with anxiety about connecting across social differences, ensuring that the experience is enjoyable is an important aspect of inviting people into civity practice, which is key to our scaling and sustainability strategies. The questionnaire is thus designed to elicit overall impressions as well as to focus participants' attention on taking the workshop vocabulary and strategies into their outside lives.

In 2021 and 2022, the Stanford University–based Strengthening Democracy Challenge, a megastudy designed to identify effective ways to reduce political division and strengthen US democracy, provided the opportunity to have academic evaluators assess Civity Storytelling: Expanding the Pool of People Who Matter, an eight-minute, one-way online intervention designed to give viewers an experience similar to the two-way person-to-person conversations our workshops provide.[19] The Challenge's outside reviewers assessed the effects of this video form of the Civity workshop intervention, which featured a diverse group of individuals briefly sharing their own stories—described by the researchers as "sympathetic personal narratives."[20(p4)]

The researchers' data affirmed the effectiveness of Civity's personal stories approach.[21] Of the 25 interventions tested in the megastudy (selected from 252 submitted), Civity Storytelling ranked #4 in effectiveness at reducing animosity across political party identity, the specific social difference that was the focus of the study.[20(p6)] Most important from our point of view, Civity Storytelling tested #1 in effectiveness at increasing social trust, a more generalized characteristic that the study also measured.[20(Supp.Mat.90)] Social trust is a foundational quality for constructive collective action.[22] Civity Storytelling also ranked #2 in effectiveness at decreasing social distance,[20(Supp.Mat.91)] a lessening of an "us versus them" dynamic between social groups.

A CIVITY APPROACH AND BUILDING CIVIC MUSCLE

Civity's emphasis on relationships across social differences and strategy for scaling and sustainability are grounded in the recognition that communities are complex adaptive social systems of many individuals interacting in ways that have profound system-level effects. We have previously observed, "Personal relationships lie at the heart and are the drivers of complex adaptive social systems."[23] In particular, bridging relationships across social differences "create enough communication and trust to defuse destructive conflict between distinct groups and to spark creative and collective responses to community, system-level stressors."[23]

Overall, a civity approach moves from understanding communities as systems to operationalizing systems-based change. Civity interventions offer a research-based, workable, and proven strategy to intentionally engage in the enterprise of cultivating the authentic bridging relationships that underlie public health. Bridging relationships that connect different populations with each other tap into disparate perspectives and experiences that can serve as valuable community resources.[24] Civity connections also build social trust, nurture cooperative and collaborative collection action, and grow an overarching sense of belonging—belonging to a larger community of which all members are a part.

Similarly, systems-based approaches to public health highlight that "at the heart of a systems orientation is an emphasis on relationships."[25(p403)] When systems are systems of people, "understanding the nature of the system and its dynamics requires an understanding of people—such as how we interact with each other in social networks."[25(p403)] With people, interactions are relationships. AJPH

CORRESPONDENCE

Correspondence should be sent to Palma Joy Strand, 2601 24th St N, Arlington, VA 22207 (e-mail: palma@civity.org). Reprints can be ordered at https://www.ajph.org by clicking the "Reprints" link.

PUBLICATION INFORMATION

Full Citation: Strand PJ, Kopell MR. A "Civity" approach helps build the civic muscle that underlies healthy communities. *Am J Public Health*. 2025;115(4):506–510.

Acceptance Date: January 7, 2025.

DOI: https://doi.org/10.2105/AJPH.2025.308025

ORCID iDs:

Palma Joy Strand https://orcid.org/0000-0003-0508-6483

Malka Ranjana Kopell https://orcid.org/0009-0003-1355-0685

CONTRIBUTORS

Both authors contributed equally to the work described in this article, with M. R. Kopell taking the lead in the field work and P. J. Strand taking the lead in writing.

ACKNOWLEDGMENTS

Funding support in the form of grants was provided by The Whitman Institute and the William & Flora Hewlett Foundation.

We thank Gina Baleria, EdD, who contributed substantially to the development of the Civity Storytelling intervention.

CONFLICTS OF INTEREST

The authors have no conflicts of interest to report.

REFERENCES

1. Varshney A. *Ethnic Conflict and Civic Life: Hindus and Muslims in India*. New Haven, CT: Yale University Press; 2002.
2. Putnam R. *Making Democracy Work: Civic Traditions in Modern Italy*. Princeton, NJ: Princeton University Press; 1993.
3. Safford S. *Why the Garden Club Couldn't Save Youngstown: The Transformation of the Rust Belt*. Boston, MA: Harvard University Press; 2009.
4. Kawachi I, Berkman L. Social cohesion, social capital, and health. In: Berkman L, Kawachi I, Glymour M, eds. *Social Epidemiology*. 2nd ed. New York, NY: Oxford University Press; 2014:174–189.
5. Kopell M, Strand P. Civity. Available at: https://www.civity.org. Accessed July 3, 2024.
6. Strand P. Cultivating "Civity": enhancing city resilience with bridging relationships and increased trust. *Ida Law Rev*. 2014;50(2):153–191.
7. Milstein B, Payne B, Kelleher C, et al. Organizing around vital conditions moves the social determinants agenda into wider action. Health Affairs Forefront. 2023. Available at: https://www.healthaffairs.org/content/forefront/organizing-around-vital-conditions-moves-social-determinants-agenda-into-wider-action. Accessed November 19, 2024.
8. National Academies of Sciences, Engineering, and Medicine. *Federal Policy to Advance Racial, Ethnic, and Tribal Health Equity*. Washington, DC: National Academies Press, 2023.
9. Christakis N, Fowler J. *Connected: The Surprising Power of Our Social Networks and How They Shape Our Lives*. New York, NY: Little, Brown and Company; 2009.
10. Centola D. *Change: How to Make Big Things Happen*. New York, NY: Little, Brown and Company; 2021.
11. Civity. Civity touchstones and resources. Available at: https://www.civity.org/wp-content/uploads/2023/07/Civity-Touchstones-and-Resources-7.10.23-.pdf. Accessed August 11, 2024.
12. LouisvilleKy.gov. Compassionate cities mission statement. Available at: https://louisvilleky.gov/government/compassionate-cities-mission-statement. Accessed August 11, 2024.
13. Center for Rural Affairs. Available at: https://www.cfra.org. Accessed August 11, 2024.
14. Braver Angels. Available at: https://braverangels.org. Accessed August 11, 2024.
15. Citizens' Climate Lobby. Available at: https://citizensclimatelobby.org. Accessed August 11, 2024.
16. Welcoming America. Available at: https://welcomingamerica.org. Accessed August 11, 2024.
17. Strand P. "Civity" by any other name. . . Civity. December 10, 2018. Available at: https://www.civity.org/civity-by-any-other-name. Accessed July 3, 2024.
18. Strand P. Civity and civic engagement. Civity. January 29, 2020. Available at: https://www.civity.org/civity-and-civic-engagement. Accessed August 11, 2024.
19. Kopell M, Strand P, Baleria G, Fiorina M. Civity storytelling intervention: expanding the pool of people who matter. Civity. Available at: https://sshs.qualtrics.com/jfe/form/SV_88PAor84VsO3X5Y?Condition=Civity_Storytelling, also available at www.civity.org/civity-storytelling-intervention. Accessed August 11, 2024.
20. Voelkel J, Stagnaro MN, Chu JY, et al. Megastudy testing 25 treatments to reduce antidemocratic attitudes and partisan animosity. *Science*. 2024;386(6719):eadh4764. https://doi.org/10.1126/science.adh4764
21. Strand P. A path out of polarization: the strengthening democracy challenge and the Civity storytelling intervention. Beyond intractability. June 8, 2023. Available at: https://www.beyondintractability.org/newsletter-123. Accessed July 3, 2024.
22. Kahan D. The logic of reciprocity: trust, collective action, and law. *Mich Law Rev*. 2003;102(1):71–103. https://doi.org/10.2307/3595400
23. Esterle J, Kopell M, Strand P. It's all about relationships: systems-based changemaking. Medium. November 22, 2020. Available at: https://medium.com/office-of-citizen/its-all-about-relationships-systems-based-changemaking-470207584bf4. Accessed July 10, 2024.
24. Strand P. Our differences are magic. Fulcrum. March 28, 2024. Available at: https://thefulcrum.us/bridging-common-ground/civity-bridge-building. Accessed July 3, 2024.
25. Leischow S, Milstein B. Systems thinking and modeling for public health practice. *Am J Public Health*. 2006;96(3):403–405. https://doi.org/10.2105/AJPH.2005.082842

Public Health Communication Approaches for Building Common Ground

Wen-Ying Sylvia Chou, PhD, MPH, Irina A. Iles, PhD, MPH, Anna Gaysynsky, MPH, and William M. P. Klein, PhD

See also Common Ground, pp. 481–510.

Changes in the information landscape and increasing polarization in society over recent decades have made it more difficult to establish common ground, which poses a profound challenge to effective health communication and public health in general.

We highlight the importance of assessing health communication approaches for their potential to bring people together and reduce polarization. We outline several communication approaches that use existing common ground (e.g., appeals to shared values, shared identity, common goals, social norms) or cultivate common ground (e.g., dialogue to bridge divides, trust-focused communication, efforts to humanize scientists), positing that by furthering common ground, these approaches can serve to increase a shared understanding of contentious health topics and foster greater trust in science and evidence-based health information.

We end by cautioning against the use of approaches that may be shown to be effective on some measures but may also inadvertently create further polarization, such as the use of certain fear appeals, disparaging humor, or stigmatizing language. (*Am J Public Health*. 2025;115(4):511–518. https://doi.org/10.2105/AJPH.2024.308003)

AJPH April 2025, Vol. 115, No. 4

A central function of public health is to effectively communicate with audiences about a diverse range of topics to help individuals take actions to protect their health and well-being. For this communication to be effective in facilitating informed decision-making, the existence of common ground (a shared understanding and alignment of goals between the source and recipient) is often vital. However, our current information landscape, characterized by heightened emotions, increasing amounts of misinformation, and societal polarization, can make establishing common ground difficult, posing a profound challenge to health communication. Consequently, fundamental assumptions long held in public health need to be reconsidered. For example, we can no longer presume that evidence-based information from scientific and health experts will be accepted or that traditional health institutions are necessarily the main sources of information on which people rely.

Structural changes in the media environment since the 1970s, including the rise of cable television, the Internet, social media, and mobile technologies, have contributed to increased polarization by enabling users to self-curate their media diets and exposing them to increasingly divisive content.[1] For instance, social media platform algorithms often reinforce echo chambers in which users exclusively encounter information confirming their existing views and may also lead users further down rabbit holes of more extreme content.[1] Moreover, the spread of poor-quality and false health information may be both driven by and contribute to polarization.[2] These changes in the communication environment are happening against a larger backdrop of rising social divisions, greater mistrust in institutions, and rejection of evidence-based health recommendations by certain segments of the population. Several factors may explain distrust and rejection of science, including identity politics, misinformation, and lived experience (e.g., perceived discrimination).[1]

This confluence of factors makes it critical to carefully assess health communication approaches for their potential to bring people together rather than drive them apart. We outline communication approaches that can help foster and build common ground to ameliorate the effects of polarization, build resiliency against disinformation efforts, and support public health moving forward. We operationally define "communication approaches to build common ground" as communication efforts that have the potential to reduce polarization, increase shared understanding of a health topic, and foster mutual trust. In this essay, we highlight communication strategies that (1) use existing points of commonality, (2) can help to proactively build a foundation for common ground in situations in which common ground is currently lacking, or (3) may be useful for promoting certain public health goals but may also inadvertently create further division and polarization, thereby potentially undermining long-term efforts.

We acknowledge that, in itself, effective communication is insufficient. For example, when cost is a major barrier for a particular behavior (e.g., cancer screening), policies to alleviate financial burden may be better suited than a communication campaign. However, when communication approaches are used in public health, it is important to ensure that they do not also have unintended consequences, such as reducing trust or increasing polarization. Additionally, although finding common ground may be difficult, relationship building remains an important goal that will likely benefit public health practice in the long run.

HEALTH COMMUNICATION APPROACHES THAT USE COMMON GROUND

There remain untapped opportunities for public health communication efforts to use existing areas of common ground. We summarize such strategies, including those that emphasize shared values, shared identity, common goals, and social norms.

Appeal to Shared Values

The values people hold play a prominent role in how they process scientific information and form views on related topics.[3] Several psychological and communication theories emphasize the importance of appealing to people's values to minimize reactance. Although much of value-based communication has focused on targeting messages to the specific values endorsed by specific audiences,[4] in the present polarized environment it may be more useful to explore the impact of identifying and appealing to shared values rather than distinct values. For example, in communicating about a polarized topic such as climate change, broader support for mitigation measures may be garnered with communication frames that use shared values (e.g., protecting personal health and the health of loved ones), instead of environmental protection frames that may resonate with only certain individuals.[5,6] Notably, studies suggest that exposure to moral frames that do not match an individual's values can result in further commitment to one's existing stance and greater animosity toward those on the other side.[7] Therefore, messages focusing on a set of values endorsed by a particular group may have an unintended polarizing effect if they are seen by those outside that group, a likely occurrence in the online environment. Emphasizing common values may be more effective in efforts addressing diverse audiences across ideological and political orientations. Moreover, research suggests substantial similarity in values across cultural groups: Shalom Schwartz's summary of values across 82 countries, for example, showed that, on average, values such as benevolence, universalism, and self-direction were similarly prioritized across different groups.[8] However, more formative work will be needed to identify and use shared values in various health contexts.

Another strategy to appeal to values and build common ground is self-affirmation (i.e., engaging in a reflection on one's cherished values before encountering threatening information, a process that serves to reduce the perceived threat to self-integrity posed by such information, thereby reducing rejection[9]). Meta-analytic evidence shows self-affirmation to increase message acceptance, behavioral intention, and actual behavior change across various health topics.[10] Self-affirmation can also foster prosocial behavior (e.g., helping others) by increasing feelings of self-compassion,[11] suggesting its potential to help build common ground. Self-affirmation strategies could be incorporated into communication contexts that support 2-way engagement (e.g., providers may ask patients about values that are important to them before counseling them on lifestyle changes).

Highlight Shared Identity

Identifying and highlighting shared identity could also help reduce polarization. Political science research suggests that cooperative, positive interactions between members of different groups can lead to reduced out-group prejudice because out-group members are subsequently reconceptualized as belonging to a larger, more inclusive in-group with a shared identity (e.g., "fellow citizens" rather than the "opposing political party").[12,13] A similar effect can be achieved through messages priming with unifying themes or shared characteristics.[12,13] For example, experimental research has shown that messages highlighting a shared national identity can lower political animosity, potentially because they lead members of the opposing political group to be seen as a liked national in-group, rather than a disliked partisan out-group.[13,14]

It may also be beneficial to highlight shared identities between researchers or practitioners and their target audience or between the group being asked to take action and the group that may benefit from this action (e.g., healthy individuals being asked to practice social distancing even though they are at lower risk and those who are immunocompromised and at higher risk). For example, a health department spokesperson trying to promote childhood vaccinations could highlight a shared identity as a parent. Similarly, messages encouraging low-risk individuals to protect others in their community might emphasize a shared identity based on residence (e.g., "protect your fellow Wisconsinites").

Emphasize Shared Goals

Messages that emphasize common goals may serve to unify people around recommended actions. An example is the Congressional Families Cancer Prevention Program, a long-standing effort in which congressional spouses from both sides of the aisle unite to tackle cancer prevention, citing shared personal experiences with cancer and mutual interest in improving the health of Americans.[15] Furthermore, research on intergroup conflict suggests that hostility can be overcome when people from different groups work toward a common goal: the Robbers Cave Experiment conducted by Sherif et al. showed that prejudice and conflict are reduced when previously competing groups have to pursue common superordinate goals.[16] Similarly, creating the opportunity for people who might disagree on specific public health actions (e.g., needle exchange programs) to focus on a shared goal (e.g., protecting their community) may decrease polarization and also set the stage for cooperation on other goals in the future. Messages framing recommended actions in terms of common goals (e.g., "We all want our kids to be safe") could also help increase message acceptability although this hypothesis would need to be validated through additional research.

Communicate Social Norms

Emphasizing social norms is another way to build common ground, particularly when dealing with controversial health topics, as norms communicate what most individuals do or think (descriptive norms) and what is socially acceptable (injunctive norms); consequently, people tend to conform with norms.[17] Social norm messages have been found to positively increase public support even in the context of polarized health topics.[18] Such messaging is a potentially promising avenue for increasing receptivity toward health messages that may not match an individual's preexisting views. Highlighting certain social norms also has the potential to decrease polarization. For example, a political communication study showed that appealing to civic norms rooted in obligation to others reduced affective polarization toward out-party individuals among US military service members.[19] Identifying and using social norms in practice is complex, however, and formative work before disseminating social norm-based messages is needed.

LAYING A FOUNDATION TO FOSTER COMMON GROUND

When relevant shared values, identities, or goals are not immediately available, communication approaches that lay a foundation for building common ground may be required. Traditionally, efforts to actively bridge opposing viewpoints and stimulate constructive dialogue have not been in the purview of public health; however, they could yield sustained impact by enabling different groups to listen to each other and work toward finding points of understanding. These strategies may not directly lead to the attainment of a specific public health goal, but they serve as perennial approaches that build conditions in which people might be more willing to listen and discuss health topics with an open mind.

Create Mutual Understanding Through Dialogue

Social science research suggests that bringing people together for dialogue is a potentially effective way to establish common ground. For example, in an experiment focused on people's willingness to engage with those who hold opposing views on polarizing topics, researchers found that emphasizing common ground with those who think differently (i.e., fundamental human rights and behavioral etiquette) before listening to different views reduced opinion polarization on controversial topics, including abortion, guns, and immigration.[20] Such evidence indicates that creating opportunities for dialogue between individuals with different viewpoints and experiences can meaningfully help people inch closer to shared understanding. Efforts by groups such as Starts With Us to bridge the political and cultural divide on contentious issues offer a possible blueprint for such initiatives.[21] Public health experts could explore opportunities to stimulate dialogue on health topics that have become contentious and among people from different backgrounds to increase understanding of different perspectives.

Bringing people together in person or online is admittedly resource intensive and may be difficult to implement at scale, but similar success might be achieved through mediated experiences such as using chat apps or viewing videos of others having these types of interactions. For example, findings from a recent megastudy showed that one of the most effective strategies for reducing partisan animosity is a "positive contact video" that depicted interactions between pairs of people with different political orientations who connected with one another and found mutual respect.[14] Other research has shown that similar vicarious contact interventions can improve intergroup attitudes toward individuals from different ethnic groups[22] and those with different sexual orientations.[23]

Foster Trusting Relationships

Establishing trusting relationships between public health scientists and practitioners and the populations they serve can lay an important foundation that facilitates the building of common ground. Developing such relationships requires deliberate, long-term, and continuous engagement with communities; endeavoring to understand and meet the needs of those being served (as opposed to focusing narrowly on achieving the goals of an intervention or campaign)[1]; and communicating with empathy, openness, and honesty.[24] As part of relationship-centered communication, it may help to explain the rationale behind a particular recommendation, as well as to acknowledge when circumstances are changing or information is uncertain, as any perception that information is being withheld diminishes trust and can lead people to turn to other sources of information.[24]

Scientists and communicators should also strive to convey empathy and genuine concern: if the public feels that scientists are sincerely concerned for their well-being they are more likely to accept the scientists' recommendations.[24] Displaying empathy may be challenging, especially when addressing concerns that have no scientific basis (e.g., vaccines cause autism). Yet it is especially in those situations that acknowledging people's concerns and ensuring that they feel heard and respected becomes paramount. Recent research finds that empathetic communication in which health care providers sequentially elicit patients' vaccination concerns, affirm patients' values, and then address misperceptions with empathetic language (e.g., "I can see why you would worry about this"; "It's normal to have questions") are significantly more compelling and likely to nurture trust toward the provider than directly delivering the facts (e.g., using phrases such as "that's not true"; "that's the wrong way to look at it").[25]

Humanize Scientists and Health Experts

To maintain and bolster trust in scientists and public health experts, there is also a need to reduce perceptions of experts as elitist and science as exclusionary.[26] Emphasizing the humanity of scientists and the fact that they are not that different from members of the public could help counter these perceptions. Perceived similarity between people has been found to increase openness to differing points of view.[12] For example, a study found that nonpolitical similarities between paired strangers lead to increased feelings of closeness, and such feelings predicted openness toward an opposing view on a political issue expressed by the other person, reducing opinion polarization overall.[12] This suggests that highlighting similarities between the message source (e.g., a health official, a scientist) and the recipient could make recipients more open to the message even when it contradicts their existing views and even when the similarities are not directly relevant to the topic of the message.

Additionally, humanizing experts by sharing relatable details of their personal lives (e.g., pet ownership, sports interest, parental status) could serve not just to deter demonization but also to increase perceived similarity with those they wish to reach. For example, former National Institutes of Health director Francis Collins talked publicly about his faith,[27] and this personal reference could serve to demonstrate to people with shared religious beliefs that they have something in common, making them potentially more open to his views on health and science. He has disclosed a personal cancer diagnosis in an effort to decrease associated stigma, raise awareness, and highlight the importance of the research and medical advances that are now benefiting him. These types of personal disclosures humanize the scientist and highlight the humanity behind the work they champion. An experiment conducted with nearly 4000 students across 36 undergraduate institutions found that including humanizing information about scientists from underrepresented backgrounds in a science activity (i.e., interviews with them about their hobbies and experiences) increased the extent to which students related to those scientists, and this in turn led to higher engagement with the materials.[28] This is not to suggest that scientists should always disclose personal details, but highlighting areas of commonality may help reduce stereotypes, increase trust, and help humanize science and the people who practice it.

SPURRING DIVISION AND DIMINISHING COMMON GROUND

In addition to employing approaches that can build common ground, we also encourage public health communicators to be cautious about the use of communication approaches that may be divisive, thus undermining efforts to build common ground. We briefly describe such approaches based on available evidence and recommend that future communication research routinely assess the polarization potential of messaging strategies in addition to other metrics. Although the strategies referenced may be effective in promoting intended health behaviors among some target audiences in some contexts, it is important to carefully consider the potential unintended consequences of these approaches, such as increasing animosity toward certain groups.

Stigmatizing Language and Imagery

Public health messages sometimes include language and imagery that contrast normative and nonnormative behavior. Such strategies, although grounded in evidence and designed to deter risky behaviors such as tobacco use, may inadvertently contribute to the stigmatization of either the individuals targeted by the campaign or the groups that engage in the behavior or have the condition portrayed in the message more generally. For example, language and imagery in antiobesity campaigns (e.g., language that attributes obesity to poor personal choices, images of overweight individuals) may be viewed as stigmatizing those struggling with weight management.[29]

Furthermore, the common use of certain stigmatizing labels to describe individuals who do not conform to specific public health recommendations can be divisive. For example, labeling vaccine-hesitant individuals "antivaxxers" risks othering them, pushing them further away from information sources and exchanges in which such stigmatizing language might be experienced[30] and may lead to further polarization based on vaccine-related attitudes.

Disparaging Humor

Overall, humorous approaches in public health show mixed effects.[31] Some disparaging or dismissive humor has been found to backfire and increase polarization when used to communicate about partisan topics such as climate change.[32] Sensitivity is particularly important when considering humor appeals that belittle others and when addressing sensationalized and culturally charged issues. Disparaging jokes, in particular, can have negative social consequences, as they increase acceptability of prejudice toward the group being disparaged.[33]

During the height of COVID-19, humor was occasionally deployed in public health communication efforts. For example, the US Food and Drug Administration posted a humorous message mocking the use of ivermectin as a COVID-19 treatment ("You are not a horse. You are not a cow. Seriously, y'all. Stop it.").[34] Although it received a lot of attention, the sarcastic and dismissive tone may have had the unintended consequence of fostering distrust in the message source (the US Food and Drug Administration) among those who were using or considering using ivermectin and inducing prejudice against this group. Additionally, a study exploring prepandemic provaccine memes on Reddit found that these memes mocked vaccine skeptical mothers, suggesting a lack of intelligence and willful ignorance.[35] Although these memes may have been humorous and engaging to those with provaccine attitudes, they presented vaccine attitudes in moralistic and reductive terms and sought to shame those with antivaccine views, which likely did little to help address vaccine hesitancy and may have pushed individuals with these views further away.[35] In short, humor appeals that rely on in-group praise or out-group derogation can not only undermine the effectiveness of communication efforts but also increase polarization—giving one side a sense of superiority and the other side the sense of being attacked.

Fear-Arousing Language

Fear appeals have been used in various public health communication efforts. According to the extended parallel process model and other theories, fear appeals increase perceived risk and susceptibility of the health threat and, when coupled with recommendations for action and self-efficacy, can be successful in promoting protective (or healthy) behaviors.[36] However, the right balance between increased risk perception and self-efficacy is difficult to achieve in a single message. Consequently, high fear-arousing appeals have also been associated with several negative outcomes, such as stigmatization and psychological reactance.[37] Such defensive responses can be detrimental to building common ground because they remove an opportunity for shared understanding (i.e., through rejection of information that would make understanding the other side possible) and may also hinder the credibility of the source disseminating the fear-appeal message (via source derogation), although additional research is needed to investigate these conjectures.

Using fear-based approaches in certain contexts may also limit the range of possible solutions that the public might accept or that might be politically feasible—hindering efforts to reach common ground on policies and programs to address certain issues based on consideration of their effectiveness. For example, fear-based messaging on drug use could lead people to favor criminalization as a solution (given the perceived intensity of the threat) and make them less likely to consider less punitive solutions.[38] Fear also typically leads to a focus on achieving safety when being confronted with a threat and leads people to respond more punitively toward outgroups and to become less tolerant.[39] An experimental study from Austria looking at news media portrayals of terrorism found that articles portraying the threat of terrorism as severe and uncontrollable elicited fear, and fear increased support for anti-Muslim policies (e.g., immigration bans).[39]

CAVEATS, GAPS, AND FUTURE DIRECTIONS

There are important considerations regarding the approaches we have outlined. First, common ground building does not mean false equivalency in contexts in which equipoise does not exist. An illustration can be found in vaccine misinformation, whereby concerted efforts have created an engineered debate on safety issues, despite overwhelming scientific evidence demonstrating the life-saving benefits of vaccination relative to rare side effects. Although we advocate engaging in respectful listening and dialogue, we do not suggest that false assertions should be given equal consideration or acceptance in public health discourse. Established facts (e.g., that the earth is round) are not up for debate. In fact, giving non–evidence-based opinions the same weight as scientific evidence could further destabilize common ground by undermining our shared understanding of reality. However, meeting such opinions with empathy may better serve public health goals,[25] with the understanding that empathy does not equate to endorsement.

Second, the communication approaches we have outlined will need to be tested empirically to elucidate their effect on relevant constructs (e.g., reducing polarization, increasing shared understanding of a health issue, fostering mutual trust). These strategies also need to be evaluated for effectiveness under real-world conditions, not just in laboratory settings or online experiments. Including target audiences in message development and leaning on their experiences in devising outcome measures could also be helpful to ensure that these measures have external validity.

Third, we recommend that relational outcomes (e.g., polarization) be routinely assessed in communication efforts more generally in addition to standard effectiveness measures. We also recommend that researchers and practitioners give careful consideration to the effect of their messages on groups that may not be the primary intended audiences but may be exposed to or affected by them. Assessing for intended and unintended effects on common ground or its antecedents will allow a more holistic understanding of the impact of public health communication efforts in the community. The optimal messaging choice may be one that maximizes intended effects, while also protecting and building common ground.

Finally, it is important to acknowledge that neither effective communication nor finding common ground is always necessary or sufficient to promote behavior change. There are factors shaped by the social determinants of health (e.g., lack of access to health care) that cannot realistically be addressed via messaging alone, and how individuals access, engage with, and respond to health information is also shaped by structural factors.[40]

CONCLUSIONS

Public health is currently challenged by an increasingly siloed online ecosystem, more polarization and politicization, increased skepticism and distrust of public health recommendations among certain populations, and mounting attacks on science (e.g., false accusations of censorship leveled against misinformation research). This complex informational and sociopolitical environment necessitates a reassessment of how we communicate health information to different audiences. Given that effective public health practice depends on effective communication, we are challenged with not only delivering evidence-based information to the public and combating misinformation but also going beyond day-to-day communication practices and Band-Aid solutions to misinformation (e.g., correcting individual falsehoods) to build conditions in which evidence-based information and public health recommendations will be endorsed and acted on by members of the public. It is our assertion that we must take a long-term perspective by testing and deploying approaches that use and help establish common ground and foster trust. AJPH

ABOUT THE AUTHORS

All authors are with the Behavior Research Program, National Cancer Institute, Rockville, MD. Anna Gaysynsky is also with ICF Next, Rockville, MD.

Note. The opinions expressed by the authors are their own, and this material should not be interpreted as representing the official viewpoint of the US Department of Health and Human Services, the National Institutes of Health, or the National Cancer Institute.

CORRESPONDENCE

Correspondence should be sent to Wen-Ying Sylvia Chou, Program Director, Behavioral Research Program, National Cancer Institute, 9609 Medical Center Dr, Rockville, MD 20850 (e-mail: chouws@mail.nih.gov). Reprints can be ordered at https://www.ajph.org by clicking the "Reprints" link.

PUBLICATION INFORMATION

Full Citation: Chou W-YS, Iles IA, Gaysynsky A, Klein WMP. Public health communication approaches for building common ground. *Am J Public Health.* 2025;115(4):511–518.

Acceptance Date: December 18, 2024.

DOI: https://doi.org/10.2105/AJPH.2024.308003

ORCID iDs:

Wen-Ying Sylvia Chou https://orcid.org/0000-0002-9140-6094

Irina A. Iles https://orcid.org/0000-0002-9348-1012

Anna Gaysynsky https://orcid.org/0000-0001-5612-5572

William M. P. Klein https://orcid.org/0000-0002-8847-8193

CONTRIBUTORS

W.-Y. S. Chou, I. A. Iles, and A. Gaysynsky wrote the original draft of the essay. W. M. Klein reviewed subsequent drafts. All authors conceptualized and edited the essay.

CONFLICTS OF INTEREST

The authors have no conflicts of interest to disclose.

HUMAN PARTICIPANT PROTECTION

No protocol approval was necessary because no human participants were involved in this study.

REFERENCES

1. Chou W-YS, Gaysynsky A. A relationship-centered approach to addressing mistrust. *J Commun Healthc.* 2023;16(4):320–323. https://doi.org/10.1080/17538068.2023.2258683
2. Au CH, Ho KKW, Chiu DKW. The role of online misinformation and fake news in ideological polarization: barriers, catalysts, and implications. *Inf Syst Front.* 2022;24:1331–1354. https://doi.org/10.1007/s10796-021-10133-9
3. Kahan DM, Jenkins-Smith H, Braman D. Cultural cognition of scientific consensus. *J Risk Res.* 2011;14(2):147–174. https://doi.org/10.1080/13669877.2010.511246
4. Kaplan JT, Vaccaro A, Henning M, Christov-Moore L. Moral reframing of messages about mask-wearing during the COVID-19 pandemic. *Sci Rep.* 2023;13(1):10140. https://doi.org/10.1038/s41598-023-37075-3
5. Kotcher J, Maibach E, Montoro M, Hassol SJ. How Americans respond to information about global warming's health impacts: evidence from a national survey experiment. *Geohealth.* 2018;2(9):262–275. https://doi.org/10.1029/2018GH000154
6. Rossa-Roccor V, Giang A, Kershaw P. Framing climate change as a human health issue: enough to tip the scale in climate policy? *Lancet Planet Health.* 2021;5(8):e553–e559. https://doi.org/10.1016/S2542-5196(21)00113-3
7. Feinberg M, Willer R. Moral reframing: a technique for effective and persuasive communication across political divides. *Soc Personal Psychol Compass.* 2019;13(12):e12501. https://doi.org/10.1111/spc3.12501
8. Schwartz SH. An overview of the Schwartz theory of basic values. *Online Read Psychol Cult.* 2012;2(1):11. https://doi.org/10.9707/2307-0919.1116
9. Harris PR, Epton T. The impact of self-affirmation on health cognition, health behaviour and other health-related responses: a narrative review. *Soc Personal Psychol Compass.* 2009;3(6):962–978. https://doi.org/10.1111/j.1751-9004.2009.00233.x
10. Epton T, Harris PR, Kane R, van Koningsbruggen GM, Sheeran P. The impact of self-affirmation on health-behavior change: a meta-analysis. *Health Psychol.* 2015;34(3):187–196. https://doi.org/10.1037/hea0000116
11. Lindsay EK, Creswell JD. Helping the self help others: self-affirmation increases self-compassion and pro-social behaviors. *Front Psychol.* 2014;5:82369. https://doi.org/10.3389/fpsyg.2014.00421
12. Balietti S, Getoor L, Goldstein DG, Watts DJ. Reducing opinion polarization: effects of exposure to similar people with differing political views. *Proc Natl Acad Sci USA.* 2021;118(52):e2112552118. https://doi.org/10.1073/pnas.2112552118
13. Levendusky MS. Americans, not partisans: can priming American national identity reduce affective polarization? *J Polit.* 2018;80(1):59–70. https://doi.org/10.1086/693987
14. Voelkel JG, Stagnaro M, Chu J, et al. Megastudy identifying effective interventions to strengthen Americans' democratic attitudes. 2023. Available at: https://www.ipr.northwestern.edu/our-work/working-papers/2022/wp-22-38.html. Accessed January 15, 2025.
15. Walsh D. Bipartisan congressional spouses tackle cancer prevention, and leave politics out. *NPR.* 2024. Available at: https://www.npr.org/2024/05/08/1248795509/congress-spouses-cancer. Accessed January 15, 2025.
16. Onyango VC. Reflections on the Robbers Cave Experiment: finding lessons on political conflict, racism, xenophobia, and business environments. *Am J Hum Psychol.* 2023;1(1):34–38. https://doi.org/10.54536/ajhp.v1i1.2092
17. Cialdini RB. Crafting normative messages to protect the environment. *Curr Dir Psychol Sci.* 2003;12(4):105–109. https://doi.org/10.1111/1467-8721.01242
18. Sabherwal A, Pearson AR, Sparkman G. Anger consensus messaging can enhance expectations for collective action and support for climate mitigation. *J Environ Psychol.* 2021;76:101640. https://doi.org/10.1016/j.jenvp.2021.101640
19. Mullinix KJ, Lythgoe T. Priming norms to combat affective polarization. *Polit Res Q.* 2023;76(1):186–199. https://doi.org/10.1177/10659129211073319
20. Belot M, Briscese G. Reducing polarization on abortion, guns and immigration: an experimental study [preprint]. arXiv:2206.136522022.
21. Silver M. Abortion can be difficult to talk about. These 14 strangers took it on anyway. NPR. 2024. Available at: https://www.npr.org/2024/05/24/nx-s1-4962560/abortion-law-weeks-policy-wisconsin. Accessed January 15, 2025.
22. Vezzali L, Di Bernardo GA, Stathi S, Visintin EP, Hewstone M. Using intercultural videos of direct contact to implement vicarious contact: a school-based intervention that improves intergroup attitudes. *Group Process Intergroup Relat.* 2019;22(7):1059–1076. https://doi.org/10.1177/1368430218809885
23. Preuss S, Steffens MC. A video intervention for every straight man: the role of preattitudes and emotions in vicarious-contact effects. *Group Process Intergroup Relat.* 2021;24(6):921–944. https://doi.org/10.1177/1368430220910462
24. Hyland-Wood B, Gardner J, Leask J, Ecker UK. Toward effective government communication strategies in the era of COVID-19. *Humanit Soc Sci Commun.* 2021;8(1):1–11. https://doi.org/10.1057/s41599-020-00701-w
25. Holford D, Schmid P, Fasce A, Lewandowsky S. The empathetic refutational interview to tackle vaccine misconceptions: four randomized experiments. *Health Psychol.* 2024;43(6):426–437. https://doi.org/10.1037/hea0001354
26. Merkley E, Loewen PJ. Anti-intellectualism and the mass public's response to the COVID-19 pandemic. *Nat Hum Behav.* 2021;5(6):706–715. https://doi.org/10.1038/s41562-021-01112-w

27. Khullar D. Faith, science, and Francis Collins. *The New Yorker*. April 7, 2022. Available at: https://www.newyorker.com/news/persons-of-interest/faith-science-and-francis-collins. Accessed January 15, 2025.
28. Costello RA, Driessen EP, Kjelvik MK, et al. More than a token photo: humanizing scientists enhances student engagement [preprint January 31, 2024]. *bioRxiv*2024. https://doi.org/10.1101/2024.01.29.577791
29. Turner MM, Ford L, Somerville V, Javellana D, Day KR, Lapinski MK. The use of stigmatizing messaging in anti-obesity communications campaigns: quantification of obesity stigmatization. *Commun Rep*. 2020;33(3):107–120. https://doi.org/10.1080/08934215.2020.1793375
30. Mendonça J, Hilário AP. Touching the cornerstone: an illustrative example of the effects of stigma and discrimination on vaccine-hesitant parents. *Public Health Pract (Oxf)*. 2023;6:100438. https://doi.org/10.1016/j.puhip.2023.100438
31. Walter N, Cody MJ, Xu LZ, Murphy ST. A priest, a rabbi, and a minister walk into a bar: a meta-analysis of humor effects on persuasion. *Hum Commun Res*. 2018;44(4):343–373. https://doi.org/10.1093/hcr/hqy005
32. Clarke EJ, Klas A, Stevenson J, Kothe EJ. The role of late-night infotainment comedy in communicating climate change consensus. *Environ Commun*. 2022;16(3):289–295. https://doi.org/10.1080/17524032.2022.2032244
33. Ford TE, Ferguson MA. Social consequences of disparagement humor: a prejudiced norm theory. *Pers Soc Psychol Rev*. 2004;8(1):79–94. https://doi.org/10.1207/S15327957PSPR0801_4
34. Pengelly M. "You are not a horse": FDA tells Americans stop taking dewormer for COVID. *The Guardian*. 2021. Available at: https://www.theguardian.com/us-news/2021/aug/23/fda-horse-message-ivermectin-covid-coronavirus. Accessed January 15, 2025.
35. Brady MJ, Christiansen E, Hiltz E. Good Karen, bad Karen: visual culture and the anti-vaxx mom on Reddit. *J Gend Stud*. 2023;32(6):616–631. https://doi.org/10.1080/09589236.2022.2069088
36. Witte K, Allen M. A meta-analysis of fear appeals: implications for effective public health campaigns. *Health Educ Behav*. 2000;27(5):591–615. https://doi.org/10.1177/109019810002700506
37. Stolow JA, Moses LM, Lederer AM, Carter R. How fear appeal approaches in COVID-19 health communication may be harming the global community. *Health Educ Behav*. 2020;47(4):531–535. https://doi.org/10.1177/1090198120935073
38. Scott T. Repercussions of the crack baby epidemic: why a message of care rather than punishment is needed for pregnant drug-users. *Nat'l Black LJ*. 2005;19:203.
39. Matthes J, Schmuck D, von Sikorski C. Terror, terror everywhere? How terrorism news shape support for anti-Muslim policies as a function of perceived threat severity and controllability. *Polit Psychol*. 2019;40(5):935–951. https://doi.org/10.1111/pops.12576
40. Viswanath K, Ramanadhan S, Kontos E. Macrosocial determinants of population health. In: Galea S, ed. *Mass Media and Population Health: A Macrosocial View*. New York, NY: Springer; 2007:275–294.

Observed Mask Wearing and Presence of SARS-CoV-2 in School Wastewater, San Diego County, CA, 2022

Rebecca Fielding-Miller, PhD, Tommi Gaines, DrPH, Ashkan Hassani, BA, Tina Le, MPH, Vinton Omaleki, MPH, Marlene Flores, MA, Araz Majnoonian, BA, F. Carrissa Wijaya, MPH, Rob Knight, PhD, Smruthi Karthikeyan, PhD, and Richard S. Garfein, PhD

See also Teasdale and Fleary, p. 451.

Objectives. To test the association between directly observed school masking behaviors and the presence of severe acute respiratory syndrome coronavirus 2 (SARS-CoV-2) in school wastewater.

Methods. We randomly sampled a subset of schools participating in a translational study on the effectiveness of passive wastewater surveillance in nonresidential K–12 settings in San Diego County. Trained observers conducted biweekly systematic observations of masking behaviors between March 2 and May 27, 2022.

Results. The proportion of individuals observed masking was a significant predictor of detecting SARS-CoV-2 in school wastewater (adjusted odds ratio = 0.91; 95% confidence interval = 0.85, 0.99; $P = .034$). For every 10% increase in the percentage of observed individuals who were fully masked, the odds of detecting SARS-CoV-2 in school wastewater decreased by nearly 10%.

Conclusions. Masking does not need to be perfect to be effective. Mask mandates are unlikely to be reimplemented in US schools, but interventions that encourage moderate increases in masking may have an important role to play in improving children's health and decreasing the spread of COVID-19 and other respiratory diseases. (*Am J Public Health*. 2025;115(4):519–527. https://doi.org/10.2105/AJPH.2024.307925)

AJPH April 2025, Vol. 115, No. 4

In-person K–12 education is not a major driver of COVID-19 community spread,[1] particularly when compared with spaces frequented by adults such as restaurants and bars.[2] Unlike bars, however, school is mandatory for all children in the United States aged younger than 16 years.[3] As of 2022, roughly 75% of US children aged younger than 12 years had contracted COVID-19,[4] with higher rates of morbidity and mortality among racialized minorities.[5] Although COVID-19 is less severe for children than for adults, up to 25% of children who acquire COVID-19 may experience persistent symptoms for 3 to 6 months after infection, and 15% may experience symptoms for longer than 12 months,[6] and the risk climbs with repeated infections.[7]

Even transient pediatric infections can have serious repercussions via missed school and learning loss.[8] Because women do the bulk of unpaid care work, female caregivers are more likely to lose out on paid work when a sick child must stay home.[9] In addition, young children cannot completely isolate and require a caregiver, which is likely why women have a higher risk of infection from a child index case,[10] resulting in loss of paid work both to provide unpaid care and from their own subsequent illness.[11] Missed work and burnout from COVID-19–related care work has driven systematic professional setbacks for female caregivers across multiple fields.[12] These are especially magnified for women of color, women with less formal education, and people who have a disability.[12,13]

Vaccines reduce the risk of initial infection and reduce long-term symptoms, but pediatric uptake is low: as of May 2024, 13.3% of US children aged 5 to 11 years had received the 2023–2024 COVID-19 vaccine.[14] Children living below the poverty line were less likely to have received a vaccine than their more affluent peers.[14]

Evidence-based infection control measures can significantly mitigate COVID-19 spread in school settings.[1] Masking is an important tool for source control and personal protection,[15] and parents in communities that are more vulnerable to COVID-19 view masking as an acceptable precaution.[16] A growing literature has documented the effectiveness of mask mandates in school settings,[17–19] but there is less evidence on the impact of actual masking behaviors (i.e., compliance with mandates).

Measuring COVID-19 infection as a primary outcome presents a methodological challenge: survey self-report is subject to social desirability and recall bias; clinical data are biased by structural barriers to health care access; and public health case surveillance data are a less reliable indicator since the introduction of at-home antigen tests. Wastewater epidemiology has become a core component of the COVID-19 response because it circumvents these biases while providing a leading indicator for pandemic trends.[20] Severe acute respiratory syndrome coronavirus 2 (SARS-CoV-2) can be detected in wastewater up to 24 hours before an individual is symptomatic or would test positive using a diagnostic reverse-transcriptase polymerase chain reaction test.[21]

The objective of this study was to assess the effectiveness of masking to reduce the spread of COVID-19 in school settings by comparing systematic observations of masking in school settings with the detection of SARS-CoV-2 in school wastewater.

METHODS

The County of San Diego Health and Human Services Agency (SDHHSA) partnered with the University of California, San Diego, between August 2020 and June 2022 to pilot the Safer at School Early Alert (SASEA) program, a SARS-CoV-2 passive wastewater surveillance system for low-income and historically marginalized public schools.

Schools were enrolled based on health equity considerations. All schools in each partner district were assigned a score based on

1. percentage of children eligible for free and reduced-price meals,
2. current COVID-19 vaccine uptake in the census tract in which the school was located,
3. current cases of COVID-19 per 100 000 residents in the school's zip code, and
4. school zip code health equity score, based on California's Healthy Place Index.[22]

We provided district leadership a list of schools with the highest (i.e., most vulnerable) scores, and together selected schools to invite to participate in SASEA based on risk score, district priorities, and school administrator willingness to participate in a wastewater monitoring program.

Twenty-six elementary schools in 4 districts enrolled in SASEA in the 2021–2022 academic year. Indoor masking was mandatory in California for all individuals aged 2 years and older from March 20, 2020, to February 16, 2022. Mask mandates remained in place in schools through February 28, 2022, at which point policies were set by school districts and principals.

Safer at School Early Alert

SASEA was a rapid translation and implementation study to adapt and validate a university-wide wastewater monitoring program called Return to Learn (RTL) for historically marginalized communities in the San Diego region. RTL used Hach autosamplers (Hach, Loveland, CO) for building-level real time SARS-CoV-2 surveillance. Student residences were prioritized, with the program eventually expanding to cover most buildings on campus. Analyses of the RTL program found that wastewater monitoring provided early notification for 85% of diagnosed cases, with an approximately 5-hour turnaround time from sample collection to results.[21]

We conducted a community-engaged implementation and validation study to assess the potential utility of this approach in nonresidential public K–12 schools. In our 2020–2021 validation study, we found that 67% of diagnosed COVID-19 cases at SASEA schools were associated with a positive wastewater signal (95% confidence interval [CI] = 57%, 77%).[20] This rose to 95% of identified cases in the final weeks of the project when more than 70% of staff and students were participating in weekly COVID-19 diagnostic tests.[20] Conversely, 53% (95% CI = 44%, 61%) of wastewater signals were associated with a subsequently diagnosed case. Large retrospective analyses of community wastewater surveillance have found that the approach has a relatively low rate of false positives (approximately 7%–8%), suggesting that SASEA's relatively low specificity is likely attributable to a systematic bias in the risk profiles of individuals who elected to participate in weekly diagnostic testing (i.e., individuals who were more likely to test positive may have been less likely to access a test because of data privacy concerns or the potential economic impact of a positive test).[23,24] In other words, while only 53% of wastewater signals were associated with an identified case, this is likely because individuals who were most likely to test positive were least likely to consent to weekly diagnostic testing, and the "true" specificity of school wastewater surveillance is likely much higher than 53%.

Study Objectives

This was a prospective observational study. Our objective was to determine whether there was an association between the number of individuals observed masking at the end of the school day and the presence of detectable SARS-CoV-2 in elementary school wastewater in the 5 days following an observation. We hypothesized that schools with higher masking uptake would be less likely to have detectable SARS-CoV-2 in school wastewater in the 5 days following an observation.

Outcomes

School wastewater. Our primary outcome of interest was detection of SARS-CoV-2 in school wastewater in the 5 days following an observation event. This was treated as a qualitative, binary indicator. We used a 5-day window assuming (1) a 3- to 4-day adult incubation period for the *o* subvariant (dominant at the time of data collection) and (2) a potentially longer incubation period among children.[25] Because wastewater viral load is not a reliable indicator of caseload with very small sample sizes and near-source sampling approaches, we interpreted the presence of SARS-CoV-2 in school wastewater to mean that there was a minimum of 1 COVID-19 case on campus. We used the Swift Normalase Amplicon Panels kit (Integrated DNA Technologies, Coralville, IA) as described elsewhere.[26]

We considered there to be at least 1 case of COVID-19 on campus in the 7 calendar-days preceding an observation if SARS-CoV-2 was detected in school wastewater within that window. While there is some debate regarding the dynamics of viral shedding, viral load, and infectiousness, we judged that 7 days would conservatively capture the time frame during which a case would most likely be detectable in wastewater and infectious, even if asymptomatic.[27]

Hach autosamplers were installed at manhole or sewage cleanout sites located immediately upstream of the junction where school wastewater entered the city sewage system. Wastewater was sampled every 15 minutes from 7 AM to 4 PM on school days and aggregated for daily collection.

Masking. Masking was directly measured using systematic observation,[28] conducted by pairs of trained researcher–observers using a standardized tally sheet (Appendix, available as a supplement to the online version of this article at https://ajph.org). Observation periods began 10 minutes before students were released at the end of the school day and ended 25 minutes after the last dismissal. Observers only recorded masking among individuals at least 2 years of age (based on observer judgment). Observers recorded masking status of individuals who were within 6 feet of another person and not in a vehicle.

Individuals were recorded as fully masked if their mask completely covered their nose and mouth. All individuals were counted only once, with the first instance of observation given precedence (i.e., if an individual was first seen fully masked but then removed the mask, they were recorded as fully masked). Researcher–observers completed reflexive and ethnographic notes at the end of each event to ensure consistency. Counts were entered into an Excel spreadsheet (Microsoft, Redmond, WA) and compared with the original tracking sheet for quality control. Masking prevalence for each observation event was calculated by dividing the number of fully masked individuals by the total number of individuals observed.

Covariates. We assumed that masking uptake and the presence of COVID-19 cases on campus would both be associated with mask mandates and background case rates in the school's zip code. We also assumed community vaccine uptake would have an impact on both masking behaviors and community case rates, although we did not expect this effect to be strong as children have lower vaccine uptake than adults and vaccines available at the time did not confer sterilizing immunity.[29]

Background case rates were measured as the 7-day average case rate per 100 000 residents in the school's zip code during the week of observation. Vaccination was measured as the proportion of census tract residents aged 5 years and older who had completed their primary vaccination series during the week of observation. We drew data for both indicators from publicly available data sets provided by SDHHSA. We documented the presence or absence of a school mask mandate at each site throughout the research period.

Sampling

Twenty-six schools in 4 districts enrolled in the 2022–2023 SASEA program. We randomly selected 10 sites for this study using stratified random sampling. Two schools were selected from each district with the largest district, San Diego Unified School District, split into 2 clusters: one serves a community with many military-affiliated families, and the other primarily serves a racially and ethnically diverse urban area with a large refugee community.

We created a list of all in-person instruction dates from March 1, 2022, to May 30, 2022, and randomly selected 2 dates per month per school from this list, for a total of 6 observation dates per site and 60 total observation events (10 sites × 6 events).

Analyses

We first assessed univariate frequencies and distributions for our predictor, outcome, and covariates. We then tested our hypothesis that the proportion of individuals observed masking was associated with the probability of detecting SARS-CoV-2 in school wastewater following an observation. First, we measured the unadjusted associations between our outcome of interest (detecting SARS-CoV-2 in school wastewater following an observation) and covariates using the χ^2 test and the student *t* test. To account for correlated observations within the same school site, we analyzed the data with a generalized estimating equations approach.[30,31] We applied a logistic regression model with a logit link function and a binomial distribution to assess the odds of detecting SARS-CoV-2 in school wastewater given the proportion of individuals observed masking. We conducted the analysis using the XTGEE command in Stata version 16.0 (StataCorp LP, College Station, TX). Because of the small number of clusters (n = 10 sites with 6 observations per site) and the random selection of in-person instruction dates for data collection, we used an independent covariance structure. In addition, we applied a correction to the degrees of freedom to obtain robust standard errors.[32]

The primary covariate of interest was the proportion of individuals observed masking (% masking) with the model specified as follows:

$$\log\left(\frac{P(Y_{ij}=1)}{P(Y_{ij}=0)}\right) = \beta_0+\beta_1X_{1ij} + \sum_{k=2}^{5}\beta_kX_{kij}+\epsilon_{ij} \quad (1)$$

where Y_{ij} is the binary outcome (SARS-CoV-2 detected in school wastewater, yes/no) for the *i*th event in the *j*th cluster (school site), β_0 is the intercept, β_1 is the coefficient for % masking, β_k are the coefficients for the remaining covariates in the model, and ϵ_{ij} is the error term specified with an independent covariance structure. We also fitted a similar model that replaced the primary covariate with the binary covariate assessing whether a school mask mandate was in effect during the data collection period. We compared the 2 logistic regression models using the area under the receiver operating characteristic (ROC) curve.[33]

Ethical Considerations

School administrators were informed that observations would take place throughout the spring and provided consent but were not told the days on which observers would be present. We recorded our observations using analog forms rather than video to protect student privacy.

RESULTS

We conducted 6 observations at each school between March 1 and May 30, 2022, for n = 60 total observation events. Our partner schools primarily serve socioeconomically disadvantaged students (i.e., eligible for free or reduced-price meals or parent or guardian without a high-school diploma). On average, 84% (SD = 11%) of the students at each school were considered socioeconomically disadvantaged, and 41% were English-language learners (SD = 23%). Mean enrollment across all 10 schools was 557 (SD = 131). On average, observers recorded n = 260 (SD = 87) children and n = 100 (SD = 42) adults at each observation event.

Vaccination coverage varied spatially but stayed relatively steady within each census tract over time. The 7-day rolling average of COVID-19 cases per 100 000 residents had significant spatial variation and increased in all zip codes from mid-April to the end of the study period (Figure 1). The state school mask mandate was lifted on March 11; district 1 (n = 2 sites) chose to end their campus mask mandate at that time. District 3 lifted its mandate on April 1 (n = 2 sites), district 2 on April 14 (n = 4 sites), and district 4 on April 20 (n = 2 sites). After state and district mandates were lifted, site-level masking policies were at the discretion of the school principal. The 2 sites we sampled in district 4 continued to heavily promote, though not mandate, masking through the end of our observation period. Districts 3 and 4 were on spring break from March 21 to April 1, and districts 1 and 2 were on spring break from March 21 to April 1. Across all time periods, average masking

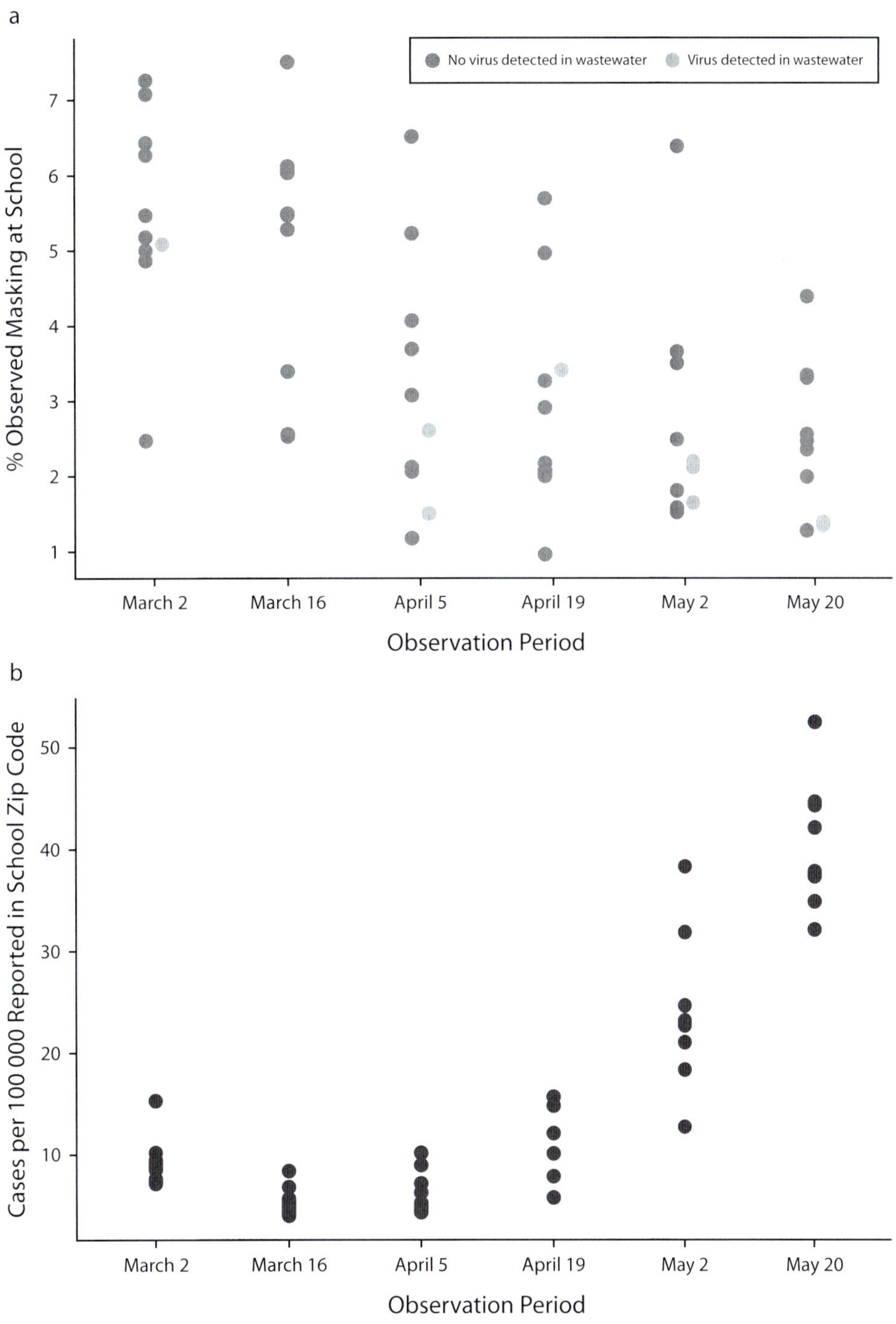

FIGURE 1— Observed Masking Behaviors and Community Case Rates Across the Study Period: San Diego County, CA, 2022

Note. Part a shows the percentage of adults and children directly observed masking at school sites (n = 10) each week of study period and detection of severe acute respiratory syndrome coronavirus 2 (SARS-CoV-2) in wastewater in 5 days following the observation. Part b shows the reported cases of COVID-19 per 100 000 residents in school's zip code during observation week (n = 8; 2 zip codes included 2 school sites; the remainder included just 1).

prevalence was 36% (SD = 19%), with substantial variation by time and place (Figure 1).

SARS-CoV-2 was detected in school wastewater 9 times in the 5 days after an observation. Of our 10 partner school observation sites, 4 had no SARS-CoV-2 detected in school wastewater following an observation, 4 had

TABLE 1— Wastewater SARS-CoV-2 Detections Subsequent to Observation by Site and Week: San Diego County, CA, 2022

	SARS-CoV-2 Detected in Wastewater in 5 Days Following Observation								
Site	D	D	H	E	J	C	H	I	J
Week	1	3	3	4	5	5	5	6	6
Mask mandate in effect	Yes	No	No	No	No	No	No	No	No
% observed masking before detection	50.9	26.0	15.0	34.0	21.9	21.1	16.4	13.5	13.8
Reported cases per 100 000 residents in school zip code	10.2	6.3	9.0	10.1	12.8	21.1	38.3	32.1	32.1
Vaccination coverage in school census tract (% of ages ≥ 5 years)	89.3	93.2	37.8	64.5	71.3	95.8	38.1	69.1	71.3

Note. SARS-CoV-2 = severe acute respiratory syndrome coronavirus 2.

1 detection each, and 2 had SARS-CoV-2 detected in school wastewater twice following an observation day. The 2 sites that had SARS-CoV-2 detected after observation twice had the lowest overall prevalence of masking (18.7%; SD = 9.0, and 23.9%; SD = 13.8), while the 2 sites with no detections had the highest masking prevalence over the 6-week observation period (61.2%; SD = 10.4, and 48.1%; SD = 16.7). A breakdown of each of the 9 postobservation detections is shown in Table 1.

Detecting SARS-CoV-2 in school wastewater 5 days after observation was 2.4 times more likely if virus was also detected in school wastewater preceding the observation (44% vs 18%), although this association was not statistically significant ($P = .07$; Table 2). In unadjusted bivariate tests, detecting SARS-CoV-2 in the 5 days after observation was significantly associated with higher observed masking prevalence (38.6% vs 23.6%; $P = .02$). Neither the number of students enrolled in a school, background community case rate, nor vaccination coverage within the school's census tract were significantly associated with detecting SARS-CoV-2 in school wastewater after an observation.

In model A, the proportion of individuals observed masking was a significant predictor of detecting SARS-CoV-2 in school wastewater (adjusted odds ratio [AOR] = 0.91; 95% confidence interval [CI] = 0.85, 0.99; $P = .034$). Specifically, for every 10% increase in the percentage of observed individuals who were fully masked, the odds of detecting SARS-CoV-2 in school wastewater decreased by nearly 10%. In model B, mask mandates were marginally associated with a lower probability of detecting SARS-CoV-2 in school wastewater, but this association was not significant at the $\alpha = 0.05$ level (AOR = 0.10; 95% CI = 0.10, 1.15;

TABLE 2— Univariate Frequencies and Association With Detectable SARS-CoV-2 in School Wastewater in 5-Day Window Following School Observation: San Diego County, CA, 2022

		SARS-CoV-2 Detected in Wastewater Following Observation		
	All (n = 60), Mean ±SD or No. (%)	No (n = 51), Mean ±SD or No. (%)	Yes (n = 9), Mean ±SD or No. (%)	*P*
% observed masking	36.4 ±18.5	38.6 ±18.6	23.6 ±12.2	.024[a]
School enrollment	557 ±125	557 ±130	562 ±100	.9[a]
Reported cases per 100 000 residents of school zip code	15.9 ±13.1	15.3 ±13.3	19.1 ±12.1	.43[a]
Vaccination coverage in school census tract (% of ages ≥ 5 years)	75.2 ±20.0	76.1 ±19.8	70.0 ±21.4	.4[a]
SARS-CoV-2 detected in school wastewater 7 days before observation	13 (21.7)	9 (17.6)	4 (44.4)	.07[b]
Mask mandate in effect	24 (40)	23 (45.1)	1 (11.1)	.06[b]

Note. SARS-CoV-2 = severe acute respiratory syndrome coronavirus 2.
[a]Student *t* test.
[b]χ^2 test.

$P = .065$). Furthermore, model A, which included the proportion of individuals masking, had better discrimination with ROC = 0.80 compared with model B which included mask mandates, with ROC = 0.77 (Table 3, Appendix Figure A).

DISCUSSION

Using directly observed data, we found that for every 10% increase in masking utilization at school-pickup, the odds of detecting SARS-CoV-2 in school wastewater in the subsequent 5 days decreased by 10% (0.91; 95% CI = 0.85, 0.99). This effect was maintained when holding constant the likely presence of at least 1 case on campus in the week preceding an observation, background case rates, and community vaccination uptake, and accounting for intrasite correlation. There are several possible explanations for this association. Masking might function analogously to herd immunity—a certain threshold of community masking may still protect those who either cannot mask or choose not to do so. Alternatively, individuals who know themselves to be at high risk of transmitting or contracting COVID-19 may have been more likely to choose to mask. The association between the presence of a masking mandate and subsequent infections was not statistically significant. Given the wide confidence interval in our analyses (0.01, 1.15) and the large body of research documenting the effectiveness of school mask mandates,[17,18,34] this finding is likely because of our relatively small sample size (n = 60).

Limitations

While ours is, to our knowledge, the only study to date that has used directly observed and passive measures of SARS-CoV-2 viral presence and school masking behaviors, it must be interpreted with key limitations. First, the SASEA study purposively enrolled elementary schools in neighborhoods that had experienced historic underinvestment and organized abandonment, with the intention of piloting wastewater surveillance as a preferential option for communities that have shouldered the brunt of COVID-19 morbidity and mortality. Our ability to generalize beyond these communities should be considered in that light. Research conducted by our team has found that parents in low-income schools predominantly associate masks with safety, protection, and health and that this effect is more pronounced for parents who predominantly speak Spanish as compared with those who predominantly speak English.[16] It is also likely that schools that choose to enroll in a COVID-19 monitoring project were more likely to not only enforce mask mandates but also to implement additional COVID-19 mitigation procedures including air cleaning and ventilation procedures, accessibility of antigen tests, and symptom-screening stringency.

Second, our team observed masking behaviors after school and outdoors—when masking was not mandatory regardless of current state, district, or school policies—and our data underestimate the true prevalence of masking. In concurrent ethnographic work, we found that most schools had distinct microcultures of COVID-19 prevention attitudes. Schools that continued to mandate masking after the state mandate was lifted may also differ systematically in how they prioritize and implement other mitigation procedures and health communications. The masking behaviors we observed could indicate generally more cautious school-community attitudes toward COVID-19, with higher levels of masking correlated with higher use of other prevention behaviors. Of note, however, masking correlated only with the presence of virus in the wastewater in the days following an observation and not those preceding it, lending credence to our hypothesis that masking is the primary effect driver.

TABLE 3— Adjusted Odds of Detecting SARS-CoV-2 in School Wastewater Subsequent to Observation Event With Proportion Observed Masking: San Diego County, CA, 2022

	AOR (95% CI)
% masking (per 10%)	0.91 (0.85, 0.99)
SARS-CoV-2 detected in wastewater 7 d before observation	6.37 (0.94, 43.33)
Enrollment (per 50 students)	0.94 (0.65, 1.36)
Reported cases per 100 000 residents of school zip code	0.80 (0.43, 1.48)
Vaccination coverage in school census tract (ages ≥ 5 years)	1.29 (0.79, 2.09)
Area under the ROC curve (95% CI of area under the curve)	0.80 (0.67, 0.93)

Note. AOR = adjusted odds ratio; CI = confidence interval; ROC = receiver operating characteristic; SARS-CoV-2 = severe acute respiratory syndrome coronavirus 2.

Public Health Implications

Most children we observed were wearing surgical or reusable cloth masks, and it is extremely unlikely that young children were wearing their masks perfectly throughout a full school day. Our findings suggest that masking in schools does not need to be perfect to be effective. While research in health care settings and controlled laboratory environments has documented the utility of high-quality, well-fitting masks to prevent the spread of COVID-19, we document the real-world effectiveness of predominantly cloth and surgical masks as utilized by children in public school settings. Moreover, a relatively small increase in the proportion of individuals masking was sufficient to significantly reduce risk for the whole campus.

Mask mandates have prompted significant public debate, and it is politically unlikely that they will be implemented again at scale in US elementary schools. However, our findings suggest "softer" interventions designed to increase masking uptake incrementally, rather than unilaterally, may have an important role to play in reducing COVID-19 transmission in schools and beyond. Interventions that encourage masking as a normative behavior, rather than requiring their use through policy mandates, may still have a significant ability to decrease transmission, reducing sick days, learning loss, and potential onward transmission to vulnerable individuals. AJPH

ABOUT THE AUTHORS

Rebecca Fielding-Miller, Ashkan Hassani, Tina Le, Vinton Omaleki, Marlene Flores, F. Carrissa Wijaya, and Richard S. Garfein are with the Herbert Wertheim School of Public Health and Human Longevity Science, University of California, San Diego (UCSD). Tommi Gaines is with the School of Medicine, UCSD. Rob Knight is with the Jacobs School of Engineering and San Diego Center for Microbiome Innovation at UCSD. Smruthi Karthikeyan is with Environmental Sciences and Engineering, California Institute of Technology, Pasadena, CA.

CORRESPONDENCE

Correspondence should be sent to Rebecca Fielding-Miller, 9500 Gilman Dr, San Diego, CA 92123 (e-mail: rfieldingmiller@health.ucsd.edu). Reprints can be ordered at https://www.ajph.org by clicking the "Reprints" link.

PUBLICATION INFORMATION

Full Citation: Fielding-Miller R, Gaines T, Hassani A, et al. Observed mask wearing and presence of SARS-CoV-2 in school wastewater, San Diego County, CA, 2022. *Am J Public Health*. 2025; 115(4):519–527.

Acceptance Date: November 5, 2024.

DOI: https://doi.org/10.2105/AJPH.2024.307925

ORCID iDs:

Rebecca Fielding-Miller https://orcid.org/0000-0002-5099-0589

Ashkan Hassani https://orcid.org/0000-0001-7863-559X

Tina Le https://orcid.org/0000-0002-6097-2130

Vinton Omaleki https://orcid.org/0000-0003-4639-2241

Marlene Flores https://orcid.org/0000-0003-0705-5197

Rob Knight https://orcid.org/0000-0002-0975-9019

Richard S. Garfein https://orcid.org/0000-0003-3663-7153

CONTRIBUTORS

R. Fielding-Miller contributed to conceptualization, methodology, formal analysis, investigation, writing the original draft, visualization, supervision, and funding acquisition. T. Gaines contributed to methodology, formal analysis, and writing the original draft. A. Hassani contributed to methodology, investigation, and data curation. T. Le contributed to the investigation. V. Omaleki, M. Flores, and A. Majnoonian contributed to the investigation and data curation. F. Carrissa Wijaya contributed to supervision and project administration. R. Knight and S. Karthikeyan contributed to methodology, resources, and supervision. R. S. Garfein contributed to methodology and writing the original draft.

ACKNOWLEDGMENTS

This project was funded by the County of San Diego Health and Human Services Agency and the National Institutes of Health grants K01MH112436 and U01HD108787.

We are grateful to the leadership, staff, students, and families at our partner school districts and school sites across San Diego County. This project would not have been possible without their enthusiasm and generosity. We thank our colleagues at the County of San Diego Health and Human Services Agency for their vision and support, particularly John Malone, Sarah Stous, and Rorick Luepton. At UCSD, Isabella Cuturrofo, Jeanessa Mendoza, Kristine Ngo, Jessica Ni, and Elizabeth Frost all provided vital support with project implementation. R. Fielding-Miller thanks Esther J. Krohne for inspiring the project.

CONFLICTS OF INTEREST

The authors have no conflicts of interest to report.

HUMAN PARTICIPANT PROTECTION

This study was approved by the UCSD institutional review board, which provided a waiver of informed consent for observed individuals.

REFERENCES

1. Neil-Sztramko SE, Belita E, Traynor RL, et al. What is the specific role of schools and daycares in COVID-19 transmission? A final report from a living rapid review. *Lancet Child Adolesc Health*. 2024;8(4):290–300. https://doi.org/10.1016/S2352-4642(23)00312-7
2. Liu L, Wang H, Zhang Z, et al. Infectiousness of places—impact of multiscale human activity places in the transmission of COVID-19. *NPJ Urban Sustain*. 2022;2(1):28. https://doi.org/10.1038/s42949-022-00074-w
3. Legislative Analyst's Office. A review of California's Compulsory Education Laws. February 2004. Available at: https://www.lao.ca.gov/2004/compulsory_ed/020304_Compulsory_Education_Laws.htm. Accessed June 7, 2023.
4. Clarke KEN. Seroprevalence of infection-induced SARS-CoV-2 antibodies—United States, September 2021–February 2022. *MMWR Morb Mortal Wkly Rep*. 2022;71(17):606–608. https://doi.org/10.15585/mmwr.mm7117e3
5. Inagaki K, Hobbs CV. COVID-19: a pediatric update in epidemiology, management, prevention, and long-term effects. *Pediatrics*. 2023;44(5):243–254. https://doi.org/10.1542/pir.2022-005686
6. Luo D, Mei B, Wang P, et al. Prevalence and risk factors for persistent symptoms after COVID-19: a systematic review and meta-analysis. *Clin Microbiol Infect*. 2024;30(3):328–335. https://doi.org/10.1016/j.cmi.2023.10.016
7. Morello R, Martino L, Buonsenso D. Diagnosis and management of post-COVID (long COVID) in children: a moving target. *Curr Opin Pediatr*. 2023;35(2):184–192. https://doi.org/10.1097/MOP.0000000000001221
8. Peetoom KKB, Crutzen R, Bohnen JMHA, et al. Optimising decision making on illness absenteeism due to fever and common infections within childcare centres: development of a multicomponent intervention and study protocol of a cluster randomised controlled trial [erratum in *BMC Public Health*. 2017;17(1):736]. *BMC Public Health*. 2017;18(1):61. https://doi.org/10.1186/s12889-017-4602-3
9. Calarco JM, Meanwell E, Anderson EM, Knopf AS. By default: how mothers in different-sex dual-earner couples account for inequalities in pandemic parenting. *Socius*. 2021;7. https://doi.org/10.1177/23780231211038783
10. Tanaka ML, Marentes Ruiz CJ, Malhotra S, et al. SARS-CoV-2 transmission dynamics in households with children, Los Angeles, California. *Front Pediatr*. 2022;9:752993. https://doi.org/10.3389/fped.2021.752993
11. Power K. The COVID-19 pandemic has increased the care burden of women and families. *Sustainability: Science, Practice and Policy*. 2020;16(1):67–73. https://doi.org/10.1080/15487733.2020.1776561
12. Goldin C. *Understanding the Economic Impact of COVID-19 on Women*. Working Paper 29974. Cambridge, MA: National Bureau of Economic Research; 2022:w29974. https://doi.org/10.3386/w29974

13. Streuli S, Garfein RS, Gaines T, Fielding-Miller R. COVID-19 disproportionately impacts access to basic needs among households with disabled members. *Disabil Health J.* 2023;16(2):101443. https://doi.org/10.1016/j.dhjo.2023.101443
14. Centers for Disease Control and Prevention. Child coverage and parental intent for vaccination. COVIDVaxView. March 6, 2024. Available at: https://www.cdc.gov/vaccines/imz-managers/coverage/covidvaxview/interactive/children-coverage-vaccination.html. Accessed August 9, 2024.
15. Li Y, Liang M, Gao L, et al. Face masks to prevent transmission of COVID-19: a systematic review and meta-analysis. *Am J Infect Control.* 2021;49(7):900–906. https://doi.org/10.1016/j.ajic.2020.12.007
16. Omaleki V, Gonzalez AF, Hassani A, et al. "They protect us as if they were our mom." Masking attitudes from freelist survey data and qualitative interviews in San Diego school communities. *J Community Health.* 2023;49(1):17–25. https://doi.org/10.1007/s10900-023-01245-1
17. Hughes AE, Medford RJ, Perl TM, Basit MA, Kapinos KA. District-level universal masking policies and COVID-19 incidence during the first 8 weeks of school in Texas. *Am J Public Health.* 2022;112(6):871–875. https://doi.org/10.2105/AJPH.2022.306769
18. Donovan CV, Rose C, Lewis KN, et al. SARS-CoV-2 incidence in K–12 school districts with mask-required versus mask-optional policies—Arkansas, August–October 2021. *MMWR Morb Mortal Wkly Rep.* 2022;71(10):384–389. https://doi.org/10.15585/mmwr.mm7110e1
19. Cowger TL, Murray EJ, Clarke J, et al. Lifting universal masking in schools—Covid-19 incidence among students and staff. *N Engl J Med.* 2022;387(21):1935–1946. https://doi.org/10.1056/NEJMoa2211029
20. Fielding-Miller R, Karthikeyan S, Gaines T, et al. Safer at School Early Alert: an observational study of wastewater and surface monitoring to detect COVID-19 in elementary schools. *Lancet Reg Health Am.* 2023;19:100449. https://doi.org/10.1016/j.lana.2023.100449
21. Karthikeyan S, Nguyen A, McDonald D, et al. Rapid, large-scale wastewater surveillance and automated reporting system enable early detection of nearly 85% of COVID-19 cases on a university campus. *mSystems.* 2021;6(4):e0079321. https://doi.org/10.1128/msystems.00793-21
22. Maizlish N, Delaney T, Dowling H, et al. California Healthy Places Index: frames matter. *Public Health Rep.* 2019;134(4):354–362. https://doi.org/10.1177/0033354919849882
23. Hassani A, Omaleki V, Erikat J, et al. Overcrowded housing reduces COVID-19 mitigation measures and lowers emotional health among San Diego refugees from September to November of 2020. *PLoS ONE.* 2023;18(6):e0286993. https://doi.org/10.1371/journal.pone.0286993
24. Vo AV, Majnoonian A, Ni J, Garfein RS, Wishard Guerra A, Fielding-Miller R. Challenges of COVID-19 case investigation and contact tracing in school settings: an initial investigation. *J Sch Health.* 2023;93(5):353–359. https://doi.org/10.1111/josh.13308
25. Wu Y, Kang L, Guo Z, Liu J, Liu M, Liang W. Incubation period of COVID-19 caused by unique SARS-CoV-2 strains: a systematic review and meta-analysis. *JAMA Netw Open.* 2022;5(8):e2228008. https://doi.org/10.1001/jamanetworkopen.2022.28008
26. Karthikeyan S, Levy JI, De Hoff P, et al. Wastewater sequencing reveals early cryptic SARS-CoV-2 variant transmission. *Nature.* 2022;609(7925):101–108. https://doi.org/10.1038/s41586-022-05049-6
27. Puhach O, Meyer B, Eckerle I. SARS-CoV-2 viral load and shedding kinetics. *Nat Rev Microbiol.* 2023;21(3):147–161. https://doi.org/10.1038/s41579-022-00822-w
28. Reiss AJ. Systematic observation of natural social phenomena. *Sociol Methodol.* 1971;3:3–33. https://doi.org/10.2307/270816
29. Wahl I, Wardemann H. Sterilizing immunity: understanding COVID-19. *Immunity.* 2022;55(12):2231–2235. https://doi.org/10.1016/j.immuni.2022.10.017
30. Zeger SL, Liang KY. Longitudinal data analysis for discrete and continuous outcomes. *Biometrics.* 1986;42(1):121–130. https://doi.org/10.2307/2531248
31. Hanley JA, Negassa A, deB Edwardes MD, Forrester JE. Statistical analysis of correlated data using generalized estimating equations: an orientation. *Am J Epidemiol.* 2003;157(4):364–375. https://doi.org/10.1093/aje/kwf215
32. Hardin J. Small-sample adjustments to the sandwich estimate of variance. Available at: https://www.stata.com/support/faqs/statistics/sandwich-estimate-of-variance. Accessed July 18, 2024.
33. Hosmer DW, Lemeshow S, Sturdivant RX. *Applied Logistic Regression.* 1st ed. Hoboken, NJ: Wiley; 2013. https://doi.org/10.1002/9781118548387
34. Gurbaxani BM, Hill AN, Patel P. Unpacking Cochrane's update on masks and COVID-19. *Am J Public Health.* 2023;113(10):1074–1078. https://doi.org/10.2105/AJPH.2023.307377

Amplifying Lived Expertise on "Food Is Medicine" in the Mississippi Delta's Legacy of Racism

Vanessa Nicholson-Robinson, DrPH, MPH, Danielle M. Krobath, PhD, Sujata Dixit-Joshi, PhD, Cassandra Hawkins, PhD, Julian Miller, Esq, Daniel J. Schultz, MS, RDN, LD, and Christina Economos, PhD

See also Singleton, p. 463.

For generations, Mississippi Delta residents have been subjected to food inequity and resource deprivation from centuries of racism. The Food Is Medicine (FIM) movement is gaining salience as one solution to address diet-related health conditions in partnership with health care providers, medical systems, and local agriculture groups.

The Delta GREENS (Growing a Resilient, Enriching, Equitable, Nourishing food System) FIM research study conducted focus groups in July and August 2023 to center the perspectives and lived expertise of residents in the Mississippi Delta receiving health care services from the Delta Health Centers.

This analytic essay provides context of the past and present food and farming infrastructure in the Mississippi Delta from the residents of these communities. The goal is to inform equitable and sustainable FIM interventions in the rural South and elsewhere in the country among historically marginalized populations. (*Am J Public Health*. 2025;115(4):528–535. https://doi.org/10.2105/AJPH.2024.307937)

AJPH April 2025, Vol. 115, No. 4

The Food Is Medicine (FIM) movement is gaining traction in the United States as a promising solution for advancing food security and diet quality through partnerships between researchers, clinical providers, and the community.[1,2] However, few FIM published studies have fully integrated diverse partners from different sectors of society into their interventions and programming. The purpose of this analytic essay is to inform nutrition programs that use food as medicine for communities affected by food-related violence caused by racial trauma. Just as important, the primary goal of this study is to improve cardiometabolic health outcomes by creating and testing a produce prescription program delivered through weekly fruit and vegetable boxes grown by local area farmers.

The majority of farmland in Mississippi is used for low-nutrient row crops, such as soybeans (~$1.7 billion), corn (~$643 million), and cotton (~$615 000 000).[3] Furthermore, a segment of the food industry disproportionately markets foods high in sugar, salt, saturated fat, and calories in predominantly Black American and low-income neighborhoods across the United States, threatening their health and well-being.[4]

A driving force behind the lack of healthy food access and availability is the suppression of Black land ownership among centuries of Black Americans in the Delta. Since the end of slavery in the United States, Black Americans have struggled to gain economic capital and self-sustainability. In 1910, about 14% of US farmers were Black and owned more than 16 million acres; since that time, Black land ownership has steadily decreased.[5] In 1967, the US Commission on Civil Rights found that whereas Black farmers received only a total of 129 ownership loans from the US Department of Agriculture (USDA), White farmers received a total of 1380.[6] In 2022, National Public Radio conducted an analysis of USDA data showing that only 36% of Black farmers who applied for direct loans were approved, compared with 72% of White farmers.[7] According to the latest Census of Agriculture, Black farmers now represent just 1% of farmers in the United States and own less than 5 million acres of farmland, translating into a loss of land value of about $326 billion.[8,9] This loss of land ownership compromises the autonomy of Black farmers in deciding the types of food grown in their communities and influences hunger in the Delta.

Food apartheid, as defined by the National Black Food & Justice Alliance, is where systemic racism is used to control one's food, the hypersaturation of destructive food driving out healthier food, and predatory marketing that results in communities of color being disproportionately blocked from healthy food.[10] It represents an ongoing manifestation of the violent history against Black Americans in the US South, causing some of the highest rates of diabetes and heart disease in the country.

Between November 1962 and May 1963, Black American residents of the Delta experienced what is now known as the Greenwood Food Blockade.[11] This blockade by the all-White Leflore County Board of Supervisors was designed to weaponize food to suppress Black American voices and discourage them from registering to vote. The actions of the blockade prevented Black American sharecroppers and their families from accessing a federal food surplus commodities program. In the Delta, administering the federal food surplus program was controlled by county administrators who owned plantations or businessmen who were active members of the White Citizens' Council (WCC). The WCC was a Delta-bred White supremacist organization that controlled the lives of Black people through economic and social resource deprivation; for example, by choosing not to implement the federal food surplus program given that 99.1% of program participants were Black.[12]

The residual impacts of these racist policies and decisions can still be seen in the Delta today: the population has the lowest health ranking in the United States,[13] and USDA data indicate that poverty in the Mississippi Delta is more severe than anywhere else in the nation.[14] In most Delta counties, more than 50% of households live below the federal poverty line.[13,15]

Food deserts are areas without access to grocery stores and supermarkets that sell healthy options, such as fruits and vegetables, whereas food swamps are areas saturated with high-energy, ultra-processed options from convenience stores and fast-food restaurants. Most Delta residents live in food deserts or food swamps, do not have access to fresh and healthy food, and pay unsustainable premiums for fresh fruits and vegetables, when available.[16,17] The majority of residents travel outside their county of residence to acquire fresh produce.[18–20] A recent study assessed the food environment across counties in the lower Mississippi Delta and identified 266 food sources; 45% of these were fast-food restaurants, 32% were convenience stores, and only 4% were grocery stores or supermarkets.[16] Moreover, Feng et al. found that households in the US South, rural locales, and predominantly Black American communities are more likely to utilize dollar stores, which often lack nutrient-dense options, as their primary source of food.[21]

METHODS

The Delta GREENS project is a community-engaged, randomized intervention, a collaboration of Tougaloo College, Ruben V. Anderson Center for Justice, Center for Science in the Public Interest, the Delta Health Center, and Tufts University. It aims to improve health disparities by addressing multiple spheres of influence, bolstering the local food economy, and fostering greater community ownership for long-term implementation and sustainability of FIM interventions to treat chronic conditions. The Delta GREENS FIM Project is a multisectoral, community-engaged intervention in three Mississippi counties: Bolivar, Washington, and Sunflower. The project capitalizes on the long-standing relationship between Tufts University Medical School and the Delta Health Center, along with the prior nutrition work of the Tufts Friedman School of Nutrition at the Delta Health Centers in the Mississippi Delta region.

Recruitment

Prior to launching the Delta GREENS project, the recruitment of three focus groups at Delta Health Center began in July 2023 and ended in August 2023. They were recruited in several ways, including on-site recruitment, phone-assisted screener, and use of a QR code recruitment eligibility screener. These focus groups were held in Bolivar, Washington, and Sunflower counties, where the project is being implemented. The number of people in each focus group ranged from 5 to 11. The purpose of focus groups was to ensure that the voices and perspectives of the affected Delta residents were represented. All participants met the following study criteria: they were (1) aged 21 years or older, (2) patients of the Delta Health Center, and (3) residents of either Bolivar,

Sunflower, or Washington County. Additionally, participants or someone in their household had a diagnosis of diabetes or high blood pressure, or their household experienced food insecurity.

Participants and Procedures for Focus Groups

At the start of focus group sessions, participants were told that they'd talk about everything that affects health and well-being in their respective county, particularly as it related to food. They were also told about our research team's plan to pilot a nutrition program and the participants' insights for developing the program. Focus group sessions were recorded, and each lasted an hour.

Sample questions included the following:

1. What barriers affected their access to fruits and vegetables?
2. Where do they usually buy fruits and vegetables?
3. Have they ever purchased from a local farmer?
4. How interested would they be in participating in a nutrition program offering produce boxes, and how could they have easy access to the produce boxes?

The focus group questions were also designed to assess the perspectives of Delta Health Center patients living in the community, rooted in our understanding of the history of the Mississippi Delta, and present-day challenges with managing chronic diseases in these communities. Focus groups were moderated by members of our research team based at the University of Mississippi and the Reuben V. Anderson Center for Justice.

Data Analysis

We used an inductive approach to coding the qualitative data collected during focus groups. Inductive coding was chosen because our focus group scripts did not explicitly ask about experiences of racism or racialized discrimination, yet these themes were clearly interwoven within numerous responses we received to questions of study logistics, program planning, and household food access. In the following sections, we discuss the themes identified by our team following completion of the focus groups. We transcribed data using NVivo, a software program manufactured by Lumivero (Denver, CO), to assist in the analysis of qualitative and mixed methods data.

RESULTS

In total, 25 participants who received medical care at 1 of 3 Delta Health Center facilities participated in focus groups. The sample almost entirely self-identified as non-Hispanic Black American (Black, n = 24; White, n = 1); 14 identified as women and 11 as men. About one third of the participants directly or indirectly identified aspects of racism and discrimination as central to their perceived access to healthy and nutritious food as well as considerations for implementing Delta GREENS.

We identified 3 themes:

1. food equity assessment,
2. trust level of public health programs and FIM interventions in the Delta, and
3. food access, gentrification, and unhealthy environments.

Theme 1

> The Delta is one of the poorest regions in the country. You're aware of that. Don't confuse poorness with uneducated and ignorance. What I mean clearly about that is for some reason people up north and other places, they want to make a contribution to the Delta in the way of fruit and vegetables. They send these little apples about this size here [participant signals with hands to indicate fruit roughly the size of a golf ball] and they get them. Don't do that. Let us have decent [sized] fruit and vegetables. Don't give us something nobody else wants.

This quote indicates that residents of the Delta are not new to being participants in research studies, often by teams who do not belong to the local community. In addition, this participant indicates that presumably misunderstood bias may translate into low-quality produce delivered via weekly produce boxes.

Theme 2

> Altruistic public programs don't typically last in Mississippi without a proper motive. I'm just curious as to how long should I expect to receive this charity program.

> If this is a successful program, are y'all in talks of expanding it? I don't see a lot of farmers so gung-ho just to, 'Here you go,' as much as I would love them to.

> I don't recall anybody in this community of farmers growing apples, oranges, bananas. I don't recall any of them growing most of this stuff is on the list. Where exactly are we going to get fresh fruit and vegetables, because we don't have farmers that's actually growing this stuff?

These participants expressed hesitancy about trusting the sustainability and long-term impact of the Delta GREENS project. Interactions such as these provide opportunities for researchers to respond in a way in which trust is not mishandled nor information misrepresented, but is rather nurtured by properly addressing such valid concerns over time.

Theme 3

> Basically the concept of your local produce is oftentimes far from where your residency is. Say what we know as Southside, they have various little convenience stores, but it's not fresh produce. They have processed food and stuff like that, and that's a lack of accessibility, and there's no means to get access there. There is a project for community gardens in a local area but these are just pet projects right now.
>
> There's not a systematic push to alleviate poverty and the SNAP program [Supplemental Nutrition Assistance Program] didn't get extended. That's half the issue.
>
> It's barely open. It's kind of gate kept for some more privileged people at the farmer's market. You can tell by the prices. [crosstalk] It's only open 2 days out of the week at 4 hours out of the day and I've been to every farmer's market in the Delta when I sold a bunch of tomatoes at Beaverdam and Cleveland's farmer market, far better. Greenwood's far better. Greenville is just behind the times. It's definitely gatekeeping access to just more affordable foods.
>
> All the food is basically on one side of town. All the food and access to food is on one side of town and it's part of the town that's getting as close to the overpass as possible, for fear of becoming irrelevant. Where they call the town dying. There's next to no access to food.

The lack of access to healthy, fresh produce was a resounding theme. Although we learned about various local farmer's markets, the feasibility of accessing such resources was limited by geography, prices, and operating hours.

DISCUSSION

This section provides interpretation and discussion of the previously mentioned themes.

Theme 1

Food equity[22] is the concept that all people have the ability and opportunity to grow and consume healthful, affordable, and culturally significant foods. Participants within our focus groups, however, discussed experiences incompatible with this definition. Based on their feedback, there is a misalignment between the nutritional options that have been offered to them in the past and the food options they truly desire.

There's been a long-standing and complex relationship between the Black American community and hunger, food access, and quality. Enslaved people in all regions and time periods often lacked enough to eat and, under desperate circumstances, some slaves would steal food from the master.[23] House slaves would slip food from leftovers in the kitchen but had to be very careful not to get caught by their White masters as, oftentimes, punishment was harsh.

Recent literature highlights the impact of food labels (expiration and processing dates) on perceived quality. There remains an ongoing debate as to whether food acquired past the labeled expiration date is ethical to distribute or fit for consumption. Furthermore, there remains a need to determine if Black Americans perceive food that they are given through FIM programs as "leftovers," expired, or of low quality. Rectifying these perceptions may improve the likelihood of Black Americans participating in FIM programs, thus supporting their healthy long-term nutritional behavior.[24] Some academic–industry partnerships have attempted to close gaps in food inequity by creating bargain retail stores in low-income communities, such as the Daily Table model in Boston, Massachusetts. However, additional research, in partnership with communities, is needed to ensure widespread scale and sustainability while maintaining dignity and basic human rights.[25]

Over the course of history, the practice of using leftover food as a means of survival has transitioned into a stigmatized assumption that Black Americans are satisfied with and even deserve food that is poorer in quality and nutrients. This sentiment was reflected during formative work with participants. There remains a long-standing need for quality food on a consistent basis. Citizens of the Mississippi Delta have been forced to deal with many inadequacies apparent in the food economy made available to them. To resolve these inadequacies, it is necessary to provide multilevel solutions. Nutrition programs should listen to the desires of their populations of interest and apply what they've learned in their programs. Our study creates produce boxes based on the fruits and vegetables the participants desire to eat. We assess their perspective on how best to make these foods available and how often they'd want to receive the boxes. Furthermore, policies should advocate for making more nutritious food available for all, including marginalized communities; such communities, including the Mississippi Delta, deserve respect and autonomy. The policies should be created to sustain and support the local food economy for local community members.

Theme 2

Although several attempts have been made to include Black Americans in research study and design, they are still often less likely to participate than Whites, partially through mistrust.[26] There is some uncertainty about whether public health programs and FIM interventions will be sustained in the Delta. Historical events in research, including the Tuskegee Syphilis Study and the "Mississippi Appendectomy," are examples of how prior scientific mistreatment involving Black Americans has had a profoundly negative impact on community experience and perception of scientific research. The Tuskegee Syphilis Study was a nearly 40-year experiment to observe the impact of untreated syphilis on poor Black male sharecroppers while withholding the treatment, penicillin.[27] Although there were several ethical boundaries that were ignored in the study, perhaps the most impactful was that information was intentionally withheld from participants regarding their positive syphilis status and instead were told they were being treated for "bad blood." Therefore, many of these men unknowingly passed the disease on to their wives and children, resulting in a legacy of pain, harm, and trauma.

The "Mississippi Appendectomy," coined by the civil rights martyr Fannie Lou Hamer, was just as heinous by directly compromising the reproductive health of Black American women in Mississippi. The process involved the forced sterilization via a complete hysterectomy of Black American women without their consent and, oftentimes, knowledge.[28,29] Hamer found that from the 1920s to the 1970s, 3 out of 5 Black American women from her Sunflower County Mississippi Delta community underwent unwanted sterilization.[30] The researchers behind the forced sterilization of poor Black American women claimed that the practice was intended for the greater good of society by preventing a poverty increase in the Black American population. However, the practice deepened mistrust among Black American women when they were unknowingly left without their uteruses, and "appendectomies" were highly observed in areas of intense civil rights actions and movements.[29] It is unknown exactly how many Black American women were directly affected; however, it has been suggested that the number is in the hundreds of thousands—these "appendectomies" spanned the 1920s through the 1980s.

Through institutional review boards, modern-day studies, including our FIM study, maintain more ethical standards of research. Refinement of public health programs is ongoing and necessary to ensure health equity for all. Therefore, to improve the participation of Black Americans in FIM programs, programs must be grounded in community mobilization and appropriate cultural frameworks, and must gain the support of legislatures. Legislators need to have a vested interest in FIM programs and be in positions to establish policies that advocate against prejudices of marginalized groups, including Black farmers and their local communities. For example, legislatures can work in partnership with nutritional health experts and famers to create a special commission and coalitions that specifically target legal barriers of accessing healthy food.

Theme 3

The Mississippi Delta has one of the highest obesity rates in the United States. One study showed that 22.9% of participants were overweight and 62.1% were obese.[31] Another study showed that the prevalence of childhood overweight and obesity in the Mississippi Delta was 47.1% (18.3% overweight and 28.8% obese).[32] Mississippi Delta communities are particularly at risk for obesity because they are most likely to reside in a food desert or food swamp. The lower cost and convenience of these options aid the consumption of unhealthy foods and diets lower in nutrient quality.[33] However, the Mississippi Delta is particularly unique in that despite its suboptimal food environment, it is a highly profitable agricultural community; the food, however, does not make its way onto the tables of residents—a sentiment captured during focus groups.

Conclusion

Next steps to improve racial equity within FIM programs. FIM programs were a key component under the Biden–Harris administration National Strategy on Hunger, Nutrition and Health. FIM includes medically tailored meals, medically tailored groceries, and produce prescriptions like the Delta GREENS project.[34] FIM must aim to improve not just the physiological needs of marginalized communities but also to apply culturally based methodologies that support the growth and sustainability of food economies for communities. These methods should be inclusive of lived experiences provided by those whom FIM is designed to serve.

Although some research has been completed to assess the experiences of Black Americans on antihunger and nutrition interventions, this research is limited. For example, in a scoping review published by the Nutrition Research Reviews, the authors noted that Black Americans were dissatisfied with nutrition education interventions. This information, however, was only uncovered when qualitative methods were used to examine interventions providing education alone versus programs with policy, systems, and environmental change interventions.[35] The scoping review summarized Black Americans' perceptions of and experiences with participating in nutrition interventions. Two findings emerged:

1. Nutrition educators working with Black Americans should consider evaluating future FIM interventions using qualitative methods in addition to a quantitative assessment, allowing for a more holistic understanding of solutions that align the features of FIM supporting the short- and long-term needs of the community.
2. FIM provides an avenue to address historical mistrust via interventions that are codesigned with eligible participants and appropriate community stakeholders. More attention is necessary to understand the full context required to achieve nutrition equity.

Recommendations for future FIMs in communities historically exposed to racism.

1. Researchers should acknowledge and address medical maltreatment when designing, implementing, and evaluating FIM interventions.[36–38] Medical maltreatment causes mistrust and is a significant barrier to health and health care utilization across populations. Because of racism and racist abuse in research and clinical encounters, Black Americans may be the least likely to participate in and benefit from FIM interventions and programming because of stress-inducing situations across entire sectors of health care systems, which are critical partners in ensuring lasting FIM success.

Researchers should consider the sustainability and feasibility of establishing local food economies prior to program implementation. This allows for space and time for thinking through local farmer infrastructure that is inclusive of factors such as transportation, food storage, quality food availability, and delivery. Funding agencies, such as the National Institutes of Health, must be equipped and willing to invest in sustaining the local agriculture economy when soliciting research to improve FIM interventions.

2. Researchers and participants should work alongside each other, with the population of interest involved in the cocreation of study procedures and decision-making on produce availability with food acting as medicine. This approach could not only support the elevation of Black American voice by listening to the preferences of participants, but also support the healing of Black Americans from chronic illness and disease resulting from the history of systemic racism.
3. The federal, state, and local governments must invest major resources for Black Americans harmed by slavery, particularly in the American South. The details on what the investments would look like must be informed by the input of those with lived experiences to ensure justice and equity.
4. Participant input on study design and data collection should be solicited to assess the community of interest's satisfaction with what they are presently receiving. This method not only helps to facilitate participation in the future, but it also tells researchers if and when they may need to change their method for the duration of the project, which may be especially beneficial in longitudinal studies.
5. Funding agencies must be equipped and willing to invest in sustaining the local agriculture economy when soliciting research to improve FIM interventions.
6. Researchers should be included who are not only racially similar to our study population but are also from the Mississippi and Delta areas. As our study is ongoing, we practice and suggest additional practices for future FIMs, including frequent training regarding data collection, inclusion of student community members of the local area, and cultural history training of the area being served. AJPH

ABOUT THE AUTHORS

Vanessa Nicholson-Robinson is with the School of Medicine, Tufts University, Boston MA. Danielle M. Krobath is with the Arnold School of Public Health, University of South Carolina, Columbia. Sujata Dixit-Joshi, Daniel J. Schultz, and Christina Economos are with the Tufts Friedman School of Nutrition, Tufts University, Boston, MA. Cassandra Hawkins is with the Department of Social Sciences, Mississippi Valley State University, Itta Bena, MS. Julian Miller is with the Reuben V. Anderson Institute for Social Justice, Tougaloo College, Jackson, MS.

CORRESPONDENCE

Correspondence should be sent to Vanessa Nicholson-Robinson, DrPH, MPH, 136 Harrison Ave, Boston, MA 02111 (e-mail: Vanessa.nicholson@tufts.edu). Reprints can be ordered at https://www.ajph.org by clicking the "Reprints" link.

PUBLICATION INFORMATION

Full Citation: Nicholson-Robinson V, Krobath DM, Dixit-Joshi S, et al. Amplifying lived expertise on "Food Is Medicine" in the Mississippi Delta's legacy of racism. *Am J Public Health*. 2025;115(4):528–535.

Acceptance Date: November 11, 2024.

DOI: https://doi.org/10.2105/AJPH.2024.307937

ORCID iDs:

Vanessa Nicholson-Robinson https://orcid.org/0000-0002-4320-1895

Danielle M. Krobath https://orcid.org/0000-0003-2607-5302

Sujata Dixit-Joshi https://orcid.org/0000-0002-2458-7948

Cassandra Hawkins https://orcid.org/0000-0003-4360-0164

Daniel J. Schultz https://orcid.org/0000-0001-7330-8370

Christina Economos https://orcid.org/0000-0002-0410-5294

CONTRIBUTORS

V. Nicholson-Robinson led the conceptualization of the manuscript, interpretation, and thematic analysis of the qualitative data, drafting, and the revising of the manuscript. D. Krobath contributed to the interpretation and thematic analysis of the qualitative data and the conceptualization, drafting, and revising of the article. S. Dixit-Joshi contributed to the development of data collection instruments, data collection, and reviewing the manuscript. C. Hawkins and D. J. Schultz contributed to the manuscript by assisting with data collection and supporting the manuscript review process. J. Miller and C. Economos contributed to the manuscript by assisting with the manuscript review process.

ACKNOWLEDGMENTS

We thank the National Institutes of Health for funding our research to inform on future nutrition programs including Food is Medicine programs.

We acknowledge Bobby J. Smith II of the University of Illinois Urbana-Champaign, who initiated the discussion on the role of food power politics and experiences of food trauma in the Mississippi Delta. We thank the late Fannie Lou Hamer, a native daughter of the Delta, whose past work of investigating unwanted hysterectomies among local Black Mississippi residents help to guide the thought process of needing to preserve the trust of future public health programs. We acknowledge the late H. Jack Geiger, professor emeritus of Tufts School of Medicine, and the late Count Gibson (professor emeritus of health research and policy) for laying the foundation of our work when in the 1960s they partnered with Tufts to help establish the country's first community health centers including the Delta Health Center. Finally, we thank the citizens of the Mississippi Delta. It is through their willingness to engage and provide us with their experiences that we can share their stories for a better and brighter future.

CONFLICTS OF INTEREST

The authors declare no conflicts of interest.

HUMAN PARTICIPANT PROTECTION

Participants were required to provide informed consent prior to study participation. Participants were also told by researchers that their identities would remain confidential.

REFERENCES

1. Bleich SN, Dupuis R, Seligman HK. Food Is Medicine movement—key actions inside and outside the government. *JAMA Health Forum*. 2023;4(8):e233149. https://doi.org/10.1001/jamahealthforum.2023.3149
2. Food as medicine: translating the evidence. *Nat Med*. 2023;29(4):753–754. https://doi.org/10.1038/s41591-023-02330-7
3. US Dept of Agriculture, National Agriculture Statistics Services. 2023 state agriculture overview for Mississippi. Available at: https://www.nass.usda.gov/Quick_Stats/Ag_Overview/stateOverview.php?state=MIS SISSIPPI. Accessed April 5, 2024.
4. Breen T. New study shows unhealthy food advertising continues to disproportionately target consumers of color. UConn Today. November 16, 2022. Available at: https://uconnruddcenter.org/wp-content/uploads/sites/2909/2022/12/Rudd-Targeted-Marketing-PR.pdf. Accessed April 5, 2024.
5. "Gaining Ground" highlights black American farmers' efforts to reclaim lost land. PBS News Weekend. Available at: https://www.pbs.org/newshour/show/gaining-ground-highlights-black-farmers-efforts-to-reclaim-lost-land. Accessed April 5, 2024.
6. Grant G, Wood S, Wright W. Black farmers united: the struggle against power and principalities. *J Pan Afr Stud*. 2012;5(1):1–22. Available at: https://www.jpanafrican.org/docs/vol5no1/5.1BlackFarmers.pdf. Accessed April 5, 2024.
7. Bustillo X. In 2022, black farmers were persistently left behind from the USDA's loan system. 2023. Available at: https://www.npr.org/2023/02/19/1156851675/in-2022-black-farmers-were-persistently-left-behind-from-the-usdas-loan-system. Accessed January 2025.
8. Meredith E. A brief history of America's Black farmers, from the past to present. Feeding America. Available at: https://www.feedingamerica.org/hunger-blog/americas-black-farmers. Accessed April 5, 2024.
9. Gilbert J, Wood S, Sharp G. Who owns the land? Agricultural land ownership by race/ethnicity. Available at: https://ageconsearch.umn.edu/record/289693?v=pdf. Accessed April 5, 2024.
10. Colson-Fearon B, Versey HS. Urban agriculture as a means to food sovereignty? A case study of Baltimore City residents. *Int J Environ Res Public Health*. 2022;19(19):12752. https://doi.org/10.3390/ijerph191912752
11. Smith B II. Food and the Mississippi Civil Rights Movement: re-reading the 1962–1963 Greenwood Food Blockade. *Food Cult Soc*. 2020;23(3):382–298. https://doi.org/10.1080/15528014.2020.1741066
12. Martin Luther King, Jr. Research and Education Institute. White Citizens' Councils (WCC). Available at: https://kinginstitute.stanford.edu/white-citizens-councils-wcc. Accessed April 5, 2024.
13. Wang SC, Crook L, Connell C, Yadrick K. "We need help in the Delta": barriers to health promotion among older Black American men in the Mississippi Delta. *Am J Mens Health*. 2017;11(2):414–425. https://doi.org/10.1177/1557988316684472
14. US Dept of Agriculture, Economic Research Service. Rural poverty & well-being. Available at: https://www.ers.usda.gov/topics/rural-economy-population/rural-poverty-well-being#geography. Accessed April 5, 2024.
15. US Commission on Civil Rights. Chapter 1: equality of economic opportunity. Available at: https://www.usccr.gov/files/pubs/msdelta/ch1.htm. Accessed April 5, 2024.
16. Goodman M, Thomson J, Landry A. Food environment in the lower Mississippi Delta: food deserts, food swamps and hot spots. *Int J Environ Res Public Health*. 2020;17(10):3354. https://doi.org/10.3390/ijerph17103354
17. Canales E. A market basket assessment: prices and availability of healthy foods across SNAP-authorized food outlets in counties with high obesity rates in Mississippi. *Prev Chronic Dis*. 2021;18:210173. https://doi.org/10.5888/pcd18.210173
18. Liese AD, Weis KE, Pluto D, Smith E, Lawson A. Food store types, availability, and cost of foods in a rural environment. *J Am Diet Assoc*. 2007;107(11):1916–1923. https://doi.org/10.1016/j.jada.2007.08.012
19. McCabe-Sellers BJ, Bowman S, Stuff JE, Champagne CM, Simpson PM, Bogle ML. Assessment of the diet quality of US adults in the lower Mississippi Delta. *Am J Clin Nutr*. 2007;86(3):697–706. https://doi.org/10.1093/ajcn/86.3.697
20. Hossfeld LH, Rico Mendez G. Looking for food: food access, food insecurity, and the food environment in rural Mississippi. *Fam Community Health*. 2018;41(suppl 2):S7–S14. https://doi.org/10.1097/FCH.0000000000000182
21. Feng W, Page ET, Cash SB. Dollar stores and food access for rural households in the United States, 2008–2020. *Am J Public Health*. 2023;113(3):331–336. https://doi.org/10.2105/AJPH.2022.307193
22. Raja S. Cultivating Food Equity. University at Buffalo, Global Health Equity. Available at: https://www.buffalo.edu/globalhealthequity/global-projects/foodequity.html. Accessed January 2025.
23. Slavery and the making of America. The slave experience: living conditions. PBS. Available at: https://www.thirteen.org/wnet/slavery/experience/living/history2.html. Accessed April 5, 2024.
24. Palakshappa D, Daftary G, Feudtner C. An ethically appropriate strategy to combat obesity and food insecurity: the urban food initiative. *JAMA Pediatr*. 2014;168(10):881–882. https://doi.org/10.1001/jamapediatrics.2014.1154

25. Jurkowski J. An interview with social entrepreneur Doug Rauch on his solution to food insecurity. *J Public Aff.* 2019;19(3):e1997. https://doi.org/10.1002/pa.1997
26. Scharff DP, Mathews KJ, Jackson P, Hoffsuemmer J, Martin E, Edwards D. More than Tuskegee: understanding mistrust about research participation. *J Health Care Poor Underserved.* 2010;21(3):879–897. https://doi.org/10.1353/hpu.0.0323
27. Tobin MJ. Fiftieth anniversary of uncovering the Tuskegee Syphilis Study: the story and timeless lessons. *Am J Respir Crit Care Med.* 2022;205(10):1145–1158. https://doi.org/10.1164/rccm.202201-0136SO
28. Averbach S, Ha D, Meadows A, Brubaker L, Gyamfi-Bannerman C. Failure to progress: structural racism in women's healthcare. *EClinicalMedicine.* 2023;57:101861. https://doi.org/10.1016/j.eclinm.2023.101861
29. Kluchin R. How should a physician respond to discovering her patient has been forcibly sterilized? *AMA J Ethics.* 2021;23(1):E18–E25. https://doi.org/10.1001/amajethics.2021.18
30. Larson KC. Mississippi appendectomy. In: Larson KC, ed. *Walk With Me: A Biography of Fannie Lou Hamer.* New York, NY: Oxford University Press; 2021:35–49. https://doi.org/10.1093/oso/9780190096847.003.0004
31. Halfacre K, Buys DR, Holmes ME, King E, Roach J. Barriers to healthy eating and physical activity in the Mississippi Delta. *J Healthy Eat Act Living.* 2022;2(1):32–44. https://doi.org/10.51250/jheal.v2i1.36
32. Gamble A, Waddell D, Ford MA, Bentley JP, Woodyard CD, Hallam JS. Obesity and health risk of children in the Mississippi Delta. *J Sch Health.* 2012;82(10):478–483. https://doi.org/10.1111/j.1746-1561.2012.00725.x
33. US Dept of Agriculture, Economic Research Service. Access to affordable, nutritious food is limited in "food deserts." Available at: https://www.ers.usda.gov/amber-waves/2010/march/access-to-affordable-nutritious-food-is-limited-in-food-deserts. Accessed April 5, 2024.
34. Downer S, Berkowitz SA, Harlan TS, Olstad DL, Mozaffarian D. Food is medicine: actions to integrate food and nutrition into healthcare. *BMJ.* 2020;369:m2482. https://doi.org/10.1136/bmj.m2482
35. Greene M, Houghtaling B, Sadeghzadeh C, et al. African Americans' perceptions of nutrition interventions: a scoping review. *Nutr Res Rev.* 2023;36(2):320–339. https://doi.org/10.1017/S0954422422000099
36. Cuevas AG, O'Brien K, Saha S. African American experiences in healthcare: "I always feel like I'm getting skipped over. *Health Psychol.* 2016;35(9):987–995. https://doi.org/10.1037/hea0000368
37. Benkert R, Cuevas A, Thompson HS, Dove-Medows E, Knuckles D. Ubiquitous yet unclear: a systematic review of medical mistrust. *Behav Med.* 2019;45(2):86–101. https://doi.org/10.1080/08964289.2019.1588220
38. Lewis TE, Van Dyke ME. Discrimination and the health of Black Americans: the potential importance of intersectionalities. *Curr Dir Psychol Sci.* 2018;27(3):176–182.

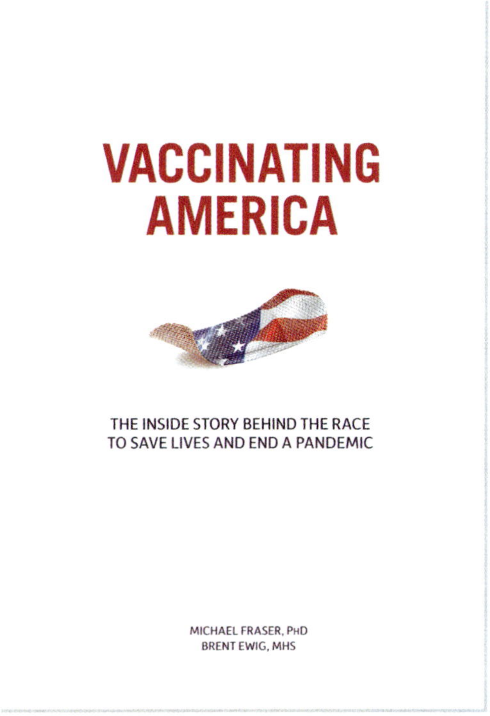

Distribution and Specialties of Broadly Versus Narrowly Defined Public Health Nurses Working in Government Settings in the United States, 2022

Betty Bekemeier, RN, PhD, MPH, Paula M. Kett, RN, PhD, MPH, Greg Whitman, BA, Kelly Chadwick, MPH, and Joyce K. Edmonds, RN, PhD, MPH

See also Kneipp, p. 460.

AJPH April 2025, Vol. 115, No. 4

Objectives. To estimate the size of the US governmental public health nurse (PHN) workforce by setting and specialty, including those working outside of health departments.

Methods. We used 2022 data from the National Council of State Boards of Nursing, representing 2846 registered nurses (RNs) in almost all states, with weights applied. We examined "setting" and "specialty" of PHNs according to broad and more restricted definitions.

Results. Using a broad definition, PHNs in government settings made up 3.7% of the RN workforce, and 1.8% when specialty areas were narrowly defined. These percentages varied by state. PHNs working in public health, school health, and correctional health settings largely indicated their specialty practice areas as public health, school health, and "unspecified" rather than more narrow specialty areas.

Conclusions. PHNs are a small proportion of the RN workforce. They consider themselves generalists and can be identified by specialty and when working in governmental settings outside of health departments.

Public Health Implications. States with few PHNs may be underserving their communities. Better data are needed to understand specific functions and activities of the PHN workforce. (*Am J Public Health*. 2025;115(4):536–545. https://doi.org/10.2105/AJPH.2024.307950)

The public health systems and services research agenda published in December 2023 is rich with practical research questions pertaining to the public health workforce.[1] The COVID-19 pandemic brought the issue of an inadequately sized and prepared public health workforce into sharp focus.[2] Since 2020, there has been an influx of unprecedented federal funding directed to public health workforce research,[3] workforce development,[4] and public health–related educational scholarship initiatives.[5] Yet we have had limited research evidence with which to guide these efforts.

Public health nurses (PHNs), who play a vital role in promoting and protecting population health, are the largest segment of the public health workforce.[6,7] Yet, over the past decade, the number of PHNs has dwindled more dramatically than any other type of governmental public health worker, with PHNs declining "approximately 36% from an estimated 33,200 in 2008 to 21,200 in 2019."[8(p2)] This decline comes despite research showing that PHNs in health departments bring unique, critical skills to public health emergencies and played a primary role in the COVID-19 response, compared with their non-nurse counterparts.[7] More broadly, researchers have highlighted the ways PHNs in leadership positions tend to excel at maintaining relationships with key partners and emphasizing activities focused on root causes, such as facilitating healthy policy change and supporting community-driven decision-making.[9–11] Workforce development and related research are essential to ensure an adequate supply and distribution of PHNs in governmental public health to meet ongoing and emergent health needs. However, such efforts lack basic information needed to succeed—namely, an understanding of how many PHNs currently serve in governmental public health settings, how they are distributed and utilized, and how many are required to meet local needs.

In 2008, a national minimum standard of a public health nurse-to-population ratio of 1:5000 was recommended.[12] Yet, confirming or updating this 2008 recommendation with field evidence, including the numbers and distribution of PHNs along with what is needed to meet existing population health needs, has been neglected.[13] The establishment of nurse-to-patient ratios in health care delivery settings has influenced patient outcomes—most markedly in reducing hospital mortality when the ratio decreases.[14] Without a means to identify PHNs in practice, we are unable to move forward with defining the number of PHNs that might be necessary for a given state or community. This further leaves us without a means to monitor, assess, and advocate for an adequate supply of PHNs for public health systems, both during and aside from crises.

The necessary supply of PHNs working in governmental public health settings may be considered dependent upon the extent to which clinical services are provided by an agency, as nurses are generally educated with a focus on clinical skills and competencies.[15,16] With the conceptual development and spread of Public Health 3.0 among US health departments within the last decade, many state and local governmental public health agencies examined their services and made system changes to shift focus toward population-level prevention activities and reduce (or eliminate) direct service delivery.[17] As such, some agencies may have considered PHNs as less critical to their Public Health 3.0 efforts, despite recent studies indicating that PHNs have unique skills related to emergency response and other areas of practice, and nurse leaders of local health departments (LHDs) appear to have a significantly positive influence on the competencies of their whole staff and the health of the communities they serve.[7,18]

LHDs also vary relative to the characteristics of their jurisdictions and by state and region in terms of the range and type of services they provide.[19] As a result, some LHDs may necessarily offer some clinical services, work very closely with local health care providers and systems, provide jail health services, supply school nurses, or provide school health services. PHNs working in government settings, therefore, may work in settings that sit within or outside of a health department, just by the nature of how public health services are organized in their community, state, or region.

Public health nursing practice is not defined by work setting but instead by activities that involve "promoting and protecting the health of populations using knowledge from nursing, social, and public health sciences."[20(p54)] However, research about PHNs and the overall public health workforce has been largely restricted to those working in governmental public health agencies.[21] Similarly, enumerations of the public health nursing workforce and the overall public health workforce have typically used data drawn from governmental public health agencies, categorizing PHNs by their setting rather than roles or functions.[22] In our study, we aimed to expand upon previous work by using national nursing-specific data to estimate the size of the US governmental PHN workforce, categorizing PHNs both by setting and specialty, and identifying those who may be working outside of public health departments.

METHODS

We obtained data from the National Council of State Boards of Nursing's (NCSBN's) 2022 National Nursing Workforce Survey of Registered Nurses. The NCSBN sample survey is fielded every 2 years by NCSBN, in partnership with the National Forum of State Nursing Workforce Centers.[23] The NCSBN's survey instrument follows the recommended survey items for the National Nursing Workforce Minimum Dataset—items that are uniformly defined data elements intended to standardize information collected by each state about the nursing workforce.[24] The data set we obtained consisted of de-identified, individual-level data representing 2846 nurses in 45 states and the District of Columbia with data pertaining to state, license, employment status, primary work setting, primary specialty, position title, gender, race, ethnicity, academic degree for entry into nursing (e.g., Bachelor's degree in nursing), highest education level, and an overall weight that adjusted the distribution across states, age, and gender. The main variables of interest were nurses' reported "primary setting" (e.g., public health, school health) and "primary specialty" (e.g., public health, school health, pediatrics). The NCSBN's survey lists 15 specific settings and 31 specific specialties for respondents to choose from.[25] The 5 states not included were Missouri, North Carolina, New Mexico, Washington, and Wyoming because the conditions of the data agreement between these states and NCSBN did not allow NCSBN to supply their data to us.

Public Health Nursing Definitions

Our study team used NCSBN setting and specialty variables to create 2 groups of PHNs. The groupings were formed from existing literature, including the Public Health Nursing Scope and Standards,[26] which sets the widely accepted scope of practice for PHNs. We also obtained expert consultation from nationally recognized PHN workforce scholars and practice leaders to help refine and confirm the variables from the NCSBN survey that we included. Based on our review of literature and expert review, we did not include settings such as "assisted living facility," "hospital," or "dialysis center" nor specialties such as "palliative care/hospice," "orthopedic," or "urologic" care that were options in the NCSBN survey.

Our approach resulted in the final items illustrated in Figure 1. In this figure, we depict the settings and specialties of 2 groups we consider to be most likely working in government settings and functioning as PHNs: broad government PHNs and restricted government PHNs. The broad government PHN group included nurses working in "public health," "school health," or "correctional health" settings in combination with 19 specialties available from the data set. By contrast, the restricted government PHNs are a subset of broad government PHNs, with specialties limited to public health, community health, maternal and child health, school health, and infectious diseases. We selected these restricted government PHNs specialties as they align most closely with Public Health 3.0 activities.[17] Although PHN practice is defined by activities or functions rather than setting,[20] we first organized our groups by setting, as setting represented the most robust data available, and then by specialty, using it as a proxy for function.

Analysis

We applied population weights provided by NCSBN first at the state level, then aggregated to the national level, to describe the total number of registered nurses (RNs) in each of the 2 groups of PHNs (Figure 1). In addition, we conducted basic descriptive statistics to characterize the nature and distribution of government PHNs at both the state and national levels.

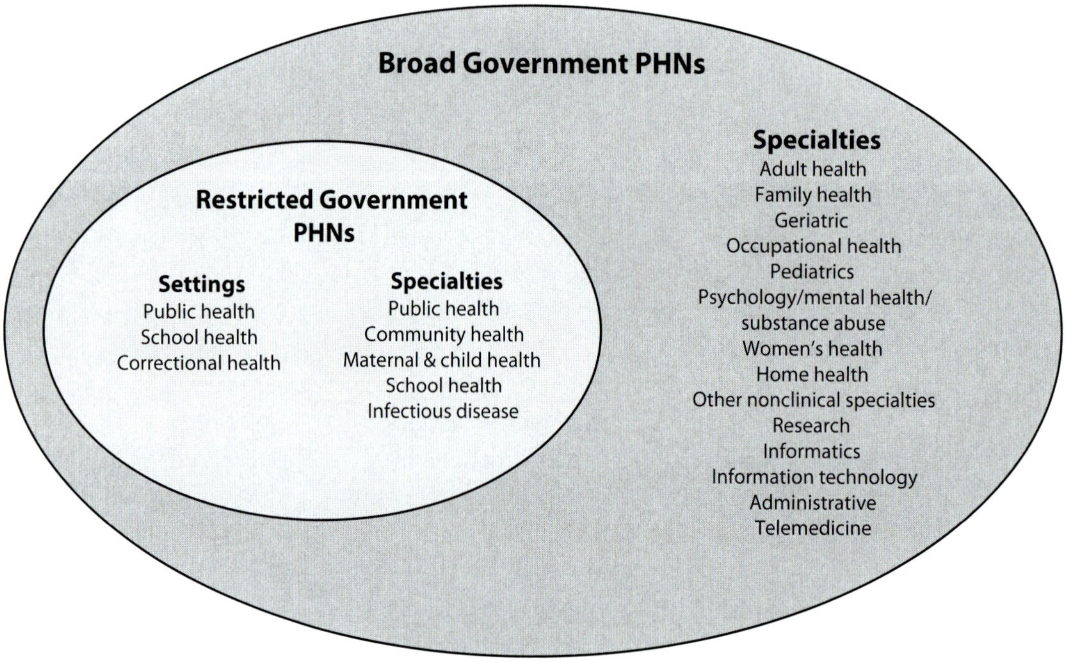

FIGURE 1— Public Health Nurse (PHN) Settings and Specialties Definition Diagram

Note. The broad government PHN group is inclusive of the settings and specialties in the restricted government PHN group, as well as additional specialties specific to the broad government PHN group.

TABLE 1— Distribution of Government Public Health Nurses (PHNs): United States, 2022

	Unweighted No.[a]	Weighted No.[a] (%)
PHN groups		
Restricted government PHNs[b]	536	73 438 (1.8)
Broad government PHNs[b]	1 111	147 957 (3.7)
Restricted government PHNs—specialty distribution by setting		
Public health setting		
Public health specialty	285	35 678 (48.6)
Maternal and child health specialty	16	1 980 (2.7)
Community health specialty	15	2 010 (2.7)
School health specialty	3	156 (0.2)
School health setting		
School health specialty	196	31 340 (42.7)
Community health specialty		327 (0.4)
Public health specialty		110 (0.1)
Correctional health setting		
Community health specialty		1 202 (1.6)
Public health specialty		635 (0.9)
Broad government PHNs—specialty distribution by setting		
Public health setting		
Public health specialty	285	35 678 (24.1)
Unspecified specialty	56	6 405 (4.3)
Pediatrics specialty	12	2 192 (1.5)
Community health specialty	15	2 010 (1.4)
Maternal and child health specialty	16	1 980 (1.3)
Family health specialty	13	1 872 (1.3)
Women's health specialty	6	1 588 (1.1)
Adult health specialty	3	395 (0.3)
Other nonclinical specialty	2	377 (0.3)
Geriatric specialty	3	342 (0.2)
Psychiatric specialty	2	279 (0.2)
Occupational health specialty	2	214 (0.1)
School health specialty	3	156 (0.1)
Informatics specialty	1	207 (0.1)
School health setting		
Unspecified specialty	314	40 880 (27.6)
School health specialty	196	31 340 (21.2)
Pediatrics specialty	58	5 938 (4.0)
Family health specialty	6	891 (0.6)
Community health specialty	4	327 (0.2)
Geriatric specialty	2	306 (0.2)
Adult health specialty	1	178 (0.1)
Psychiatric specialty	2	114 (0.1)
Public health specialty	3	110 (0.1)
Other nonclinical specialty	1	74 (0.1)
Occupational health specialty	1	63 (0.0)

Continued

RESULTS

Our findings indicate that PHNs in our restricted definition represent only 1.8% (n = 73 478) of the total estimated RNs (n = 4 047 872) in the United States. The most common combinations of setting and specialties for restricted government PHNs were those working in public health settings with a public health specialty (n = 35 678; 48.6%) or in school health settings with a school health specialty (n = 31 340; 42.7%; Table 1). When applying the broader definition of primary specialties among nurses working in the government settings, the numbers of PHNs more than doubled, representing 3.7% (n = 147 957) of all RNs in this NCSBN weighted sample. PHNs in the broader group were still largely serving in public health settings with a public health specialty (n = 35 678; 24.1%) or school health settings with a school health specialty (n = 31 340; 21.2%). Many PHNs in the broad government PHN group working in school and correctional health settings, however, did not specify a specialty of practice. In addition, 22.9% (n = 33 856) of nurses in the broad government PHN group reported other combinations of settings and specialties such as correctional health setting with an adult health specialty and school health setting with a pediatrics specialty. These other specialties were relatively small compared with those specialties indicated as public health, school health, and "unspecified" (Table 1).

Whether using our restricted or broad definitions, the PHNs in our sample overwhelmingly identified themselves as female (89% and 91%, respectively), White (81% and 84%, respectively), and most often aged 51 years or older (37% and 44%,

TABLE 1— Continued

	Unweighted No.[a]	Weighted No.[a] (%)
Correctional health setting		
Unspecified specialty	48	6 204 (4.2)
Adult health specialty	23	3 751 (2.5)
Community health specialty	9	1 202 (0.8)
Psychiatric specialty	8	1 006 (0.7)
Public health specialty	5	635 (0.4)
Family health specialty	6	597 (0.4)
Pediatrics specialty	3	478 (0.3)
Informatics specialty	1	153 (0.1)
Women's health specialty	1	16 (0.01)

Note. Data are based on an estimated registered nurse total of 4 047 872.
[a]All numbers are rounded to the nearest whole number.
[b]Restricted government PHNs refers to PHNs working in government settings in public health, community health, maternal and child health, school health, and infectious disease specialty areas. Broad government PHNs refers to PHNs working in government settings, which includes the specialty areas in the restricted group, but also areas such as occupational health, pediatrics, and administration, which are more broadly reflective of PHN practice.

respectively) and had no advanced degree (Table A, available as a supplement to the online version of this article at https://ajph.org). In both groups, PHNs identifying as any racial or ethnic group other than White made up 7% or less of the PHNs in these 2 groups, and those who were aged 40 years or younger made up only about 25% of the PHNs in these 2 groups.

PHN counts, groupings, and setting–specialty combinations varied widely by state. When examining PHNs according to our restricted definition, nurses in Washington, DC (0.3%), Florida (0.5%), Indiana (0.7%), and Maine (0.9%) had the smallest proportions of PHNs in their RN workforce. By contrast, North Dakota (4.5%), Rhode Island (3.4%), Minnesota (3.1%), and New York (3.1%) had the largest proportions of PHNs in their RN workforce (Figure 2). This changed only slightly when we examined PHNs according to our broad government PHN definition—Florida and Washington, DC, remained the lowest proportional group, joined by Ohio and Arizona. The states with the largest proportions of broad government PHNs still included North Dakota and Minnesota, along with Texas and Alaska. Alaska had the largest proportion of broad government PHNs of all states in the data set (n = 925; 5.9%; Figure 3). In almost every state, the count of PHNs was higher when our estimates used public health setting only to define PHNs—at times substantially higher—compared with the count of PHNs when our restricted or broad definitions were applied and, thus, filtered out the specialties where roles and function were not relevant to PHN practice.

DISCUSSION

In 2022, Kneipp et al. decried the limitations of enumeration studies that counted PHNs based on their setting alone.[27] They suggested that, without including the functions and role that define PHNs, "a chasm exists between the roles and functions reflected in them [i.e., definitions of a PHN] and how we identify which segment of the nursing workforce fulfills these roles."[27(pS293)] While we limited our study to PHNs working in what can reasonably be considered government settings, our study expands upon previous enumeration studies by including "specialty" areas of practice and a wider range of what are likely governmental settings beyond health departments.

Our novel approach to enumerating the governmental PHN workforce using NCSBN data demonstrates that the percentage and distribution of PHNs is dependent on how PHNs are defined including the range of specialties nurses may work in. In a recent enumeration of specific occupational groups, focused on settings only and limited to those working in state and local health departments, a national total of 29 387 "public health or community health nurses" were identified.[28] This number (29 387) is relatively close to our finding of 35 678 nurses reporting working in a public health setting with a public health specialty, given that the public health settings in our definition are inclusive of more than state and local health departments alone. However, even as our study captures a wider range of specialties than in previous approaches to counting this workforce,[22,27] our analyses indicate that PHNs nationally, using our restricted government PHN definition, make up only 1.8% of the overall RN workforce, and at the broadest definition, only 3.7% of the same workforce. This underscores the small representation of PHNs within the overall nursing workforce, highlighting the gaps in public health capacity and the need for targeted strategies to bolster this critical segment of health professionals.

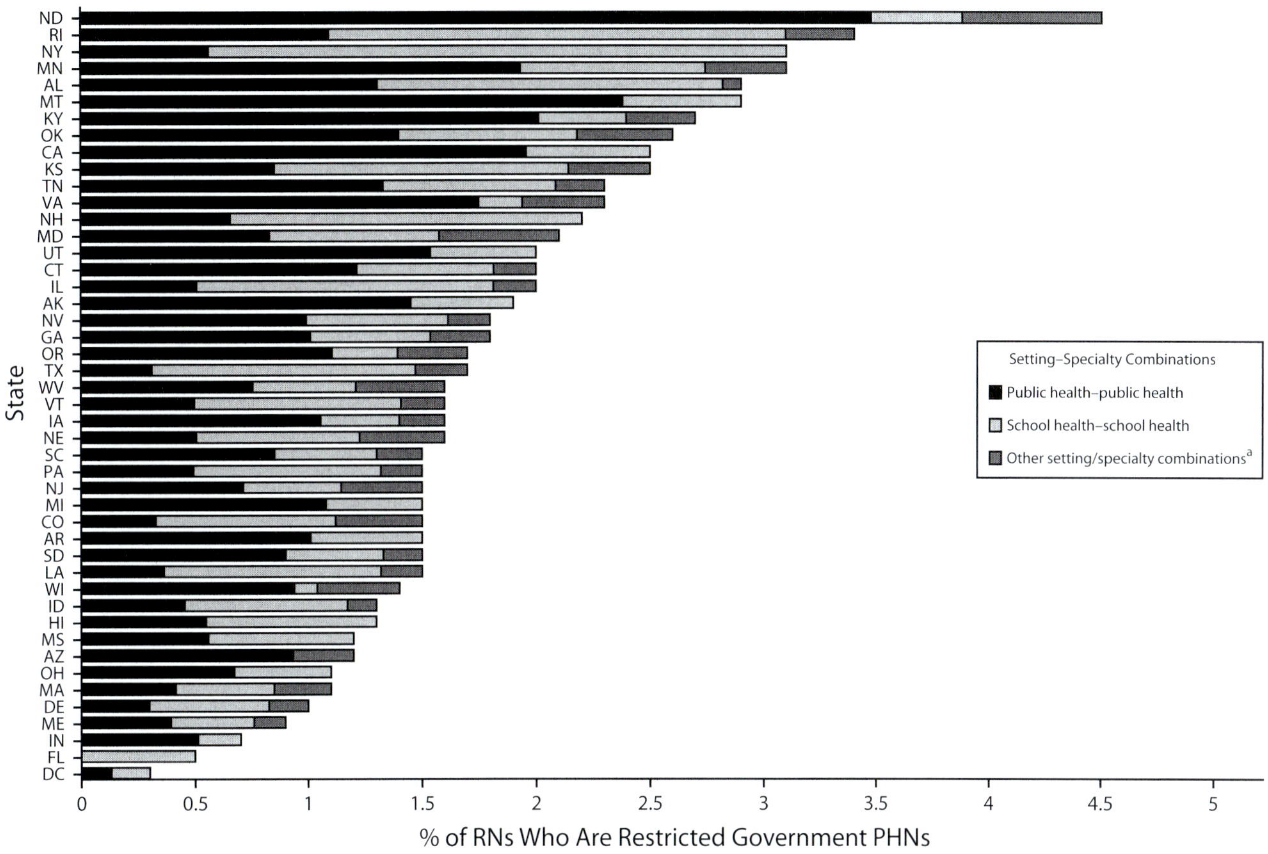

FIGURE 2— State-Level Distribution of Restricted Government Public Health Nurses (PHNs) as a Percentage of Total Registered Nurses (RNs), Broken Down by Major Setting-Specialty Combinations: United States, 2022

[a]This combination includes other combinations depicted in Table 1 such as public health–community health, public health–maternal and child health, and public health–school health.

The nurses surveyed by the NCSBN had 31 specific specialty areas to choose from, with 19 included in our definitions. Despite this variety, a high proportion of nurses working in the government settings that we identified indicated that their primary specialty practice areas were "public health" or "school health." Even in the broad government PHN group, narrower specialty areas such as adult health or geriatrics were less common. This suggests that nurses in these government settings see themselves as working in more comprehensive and population-focused roles rather than clinically focused ones. In addition, many PHNs may have difficulty choosing a primary specialty because of their wide-ranging responsibilities. This can be inferred by the large group of broad governmental PHNs in school and correctional settings where specialty was unspecified in our sample (Table 1). Identifying the comprehensive and population-focused roles these PHNs indicated may also underscore their contributions to the Public Health 3.0 strategies of their agencies.[17]

Governmental health departments in the United States vary widely in the services they provide and may or may not, for example, include correctional or school health among their programs. The "waters become murky,"[27(pS294)] as a result, when trying to identify PHNs doing public health work outside of public health departments. Unlike public health workforce enumerations that use health department data alone, however, our findings capture the substantial proportion of PHNs working in settings such as school or correctional health, regardless of whether a state or local health department oversees these services. Our approach, therefore, identifies more PHNs working in governmental roles than when examining data collected among health departments alone through identifying PHN specialty areas of practice within these non–health department settings, which, to our knowledge, has not been done before.

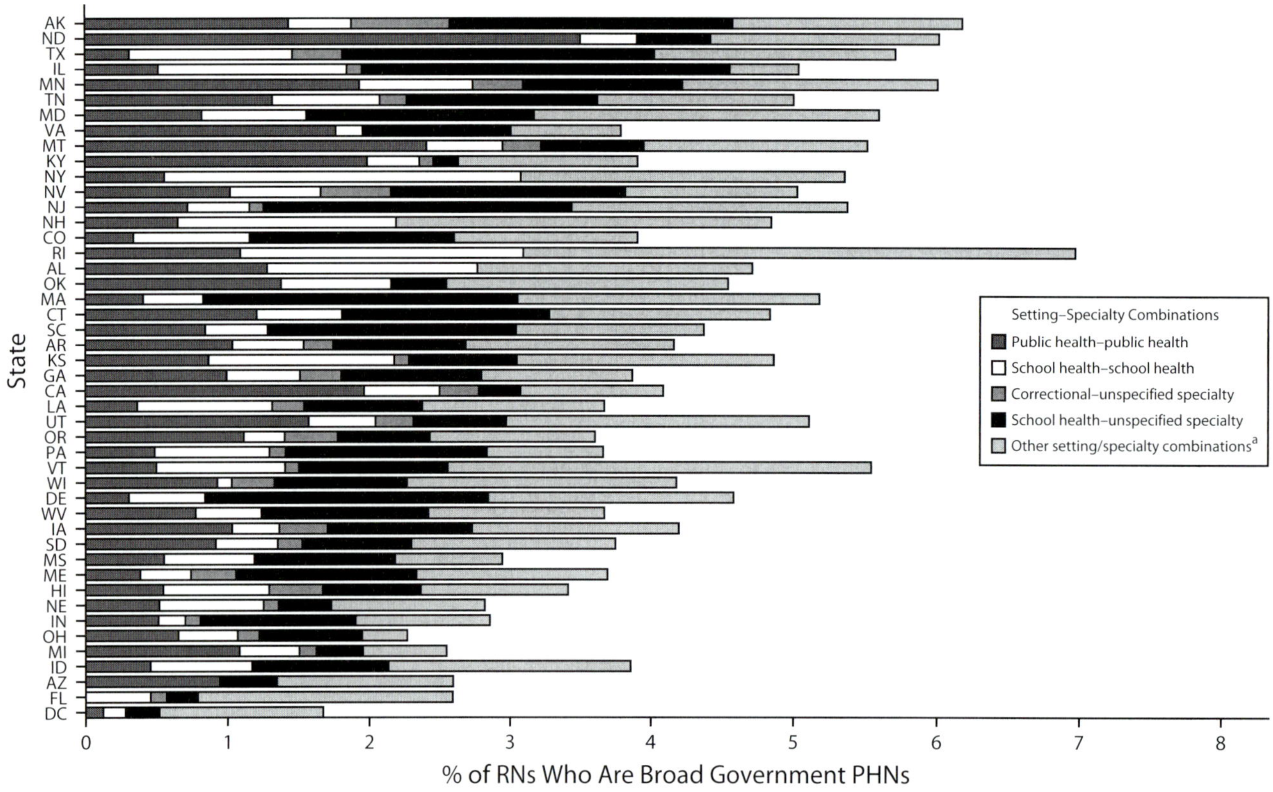

FIGURE 3— State-Level Distribution of Broad Government Public Health Nurses (PHNs) as a Percentage of Total Registered Nurses (RNs), Broken Down by Major Setting–Specialty Combinations: United States, 2022

[a]This combination includes other combinations depicted in Table 1 such as public health–community health, public health–adult health, public health–family health, and public health–geriatric health.

The wide variation in how these PHNs are proportioned by setting and specialty across states also mirrors how widely the public health systems and their services vary by state. Although these NCSBN data are from a sample survey, there is face validity in our findings for certain states. For example, Alaska had a particularly high proportion of the state's nurses working as PHNs, especially within the broad government PHN group. The number of PHNs in Alaska increased considerably from the restricted to the broad group when the "unspecified specialty" was included for PHNs in the broad government PHN group. This suggests that Alaska PHNs may consider themselves in very generalist roles and not identify as often with a particular specialty. This aligns with the comprehensive nature of public health nursing in Alaska.[29] Our findings also have face validity regarding school nurses in terms of states in the US Northeast having more stringent regulations that often necessitate the use of RNs as school nurses (rather than licensed practical nurses, for example).[30] This may account for why we see high proportions of RNs in school health settings and with school health or "unspecified" specialties in many of the northeastern states in our sample (Figures 2 and 3).

Much like the RN population as a whole in the NCSBN's *2022 National Nursing Workforce Survey Report*,[31] PHNs in our sample identified as predominantly White and female regardless of our PHN definition, although this was more prominent in the broad government PHN group compared with the restricted government PHN group (Table A). The high percentage of White-identifying PHNs is similar to other studies of the PHN workforce[7] and school nurse workforce[30] and generally aligns with NCSBN's description of the nursing workforce as a whole.[31] By broadening our restricted sample of PHNs to include those in a wider array of public health–related specialties, it appears that the PHNs included with those in school health and correctional health further increases the proportion of older and of White- and female-identifying PHNs. This highlights an area where greater work is needed—as PHNs are expected to be "promoting and protecting the health of populations"[20(p54)] and with a particular focus on health equity,[11,32,33] studies indicate that the PHN profession and the communities PHNs serve could greatly benefit from having a more diverse workforce.[32]

Public Health Implications

In using NCSBN data to enumerate the governmental PHN workforce, we were able to generate a diverse sample of PHNs working in a variety of government settings, while also excluding those who were arguably serving in specialty areas within these government settings that would not typically be considered fulfilling the roles or functions specific to public health nursing. In our study, we were able to exclude nurses who indicated, for example, that they worked in a public health setting and that their specialty was "nephrology" or other specialties arguably not relevant to PHN practice. Enumerating PHNs solely by setting, as in previous studies, risks including nurses who would not be part of even the broadest definition of public health–related specialties or activities. Our approach via these detailed NCSBN data provides a more accurate picture of the PHN workforce and supports examination into the state distribution of PHNs in terms of their settings and specialties. Because PHNs have a unique influence on local health outcomes[18] and in public health crisis response,[7] a deeper understanding of areas where PHNs are particularly lacking is critical for public health planners, policymakers, educators, and the public.

Limitations

As the NCSBN data represent a national sample survey with weighted estimates, the data may be skewed at the state level, given the relatively small number of NCSBN nurse respondents included in our PHN groups. For example, in South Dakota, there were 52 unweighted respondents in our sample out of 669 total responses (7.7% of South Dakota RN respondents), while in Alaska, the unweighted respondents in our sample represented about 11% of the total NCSBN state survey respondents. This makes it difficult to determine the representativeness of the sample in each state, as public health nursing is a relatively small field, and certain specialties may be overrepresented based on the respondents from a particular state. We are also limited by the lack of information from the 5 states that were not included in our sample. While we consider the overall proportion of PHNs to NCSBN RNs to be accurate, the specific distribution of PHNs by specialty in each state should be interpreted with caution.

We were also limited by the "specialty areas" used by the NCSBN (which included specialties outlined in the National Nursing Workforce Minimum Dataset),[24] for which some items could be considered vague (e.g., "other nonclinical specialties") and none of which were defined for respondents. Because of this limitation, the specialty areas we could draw from in the NCSBN were not necessarily the same as the "roles, functions, and job tasks or activities" called for by Kneipp et al. such as activities more specifically related to emergency preparedness, cross-sector collaboration, care coordination, or policy and advocacy.[27(pS293)] Further research is needed to develop measures that can more effectively capture such PHN work, as our study highlights the need for more detailed and precise data collection. Finally, our study could not answer questions that persist regarding what total number and distribution of PHNs are needed for responding effectively to a public health crisis and for meeting ongoing health promotion and protection needs in communities. Better data collection and related research are needed to examine both the supply of and demand for PHNs to assure prevention needs are adequately met in communities.

Conclusion

Our findings provide a new and critical understanding of the PHN workforce in the United States with respect to its distribution, settings, and specialties. We saw that even at the broadest definition, PHNs encompass only 3.7% of nurses in the United States. In addition, the nurses in our sample saw themselves as predominantly working in public health and school health specialty areas, or perhaps as generalists with an "unspecified," wide scope of responsibilities. Our findings also provide valuable information regarding which states may require giving more attention to building up their PHN workforce and offer a greater understanding of how PHNs perceive their specialty areas of practice. Yet, more precise data are clearly needed to understand the specific functions and activities of the PHN workforce. These data and related research are essential for guiding public health practitioners, policymakers, and educators in meeting PHN workforce needs in support of communities. AJPH

ABOUT THE AUTHORS

Betty Bekemeier is with the University of Washington School of Nursing and the Northwest Center for Public Health Practice in the University of Washington School of Public Health, Seattle. Paula M. Kett is with the University of Washington Center for Health Workforce Studies, Seattle. Greg Whitman and Kelly Chadwick are with the Northwest Center for Public

Health Practice in the University of Washington School of Public Health, Seattle. Joyce K. Edmonds is with the ZHAW Institute for Midwifery and Reproductive Health, Winterthur, Switzerland.

CORRESPONDENCE

Correspondence should be sent to Betty Bekemeier, University of Washington School of Nursing, Child, Family, and Population Health Nursing, Box 357263, Seattle, WA 98195-7263 (e-mail: bettybek@uw.edu). Reprints can be ordered at https://www.ajph.org by clicking the "Reprints" link.

PUBLICATION INFORMATION

Full Citation: Bekemeier B, Kett PM, Whitman G, Chadwick K, Edmonds JK. Distribution and specialties of broadly versus narrowly defined public health nurses working in government settings in the United States, 2022. *Am J Public Health*. 2025;115(4):536–545.

Acceptance Date: November 17, 2024.

DOI: https://doi.org/10.2105/AJPH.2024.307950

ORCID iDs:

Betty Bekemeier https://orcid.org/0000-0002-9034-2746

Paula M. Kett https://orcid.org/0000-0002-8524-6493

Greg Whitman https://orcid.org/0000-0003-3380-2950

Kelly Chadwick https://orcid.org/0000-0003-4901-4895

Joyce K. Edmonds https://orcid.org/0000-0002-0465-9043

CONTRIBUTORS

B. Bekemeier originated this research, interpreted data findings, and took substantial responsibility for writing and final approval of the article. P.M. Kett designed this research, analyzed and interpreted data findings, and contributed substantially to the writing and approval of the article. G. Whitman and K. Chadwick collected and analyzed data and contributed to writing and approval of the article. J.K. Edmonds collected data, helped design this research, interpreted findings, and contributed to writing and approval of the article.

ACKNOWLEDGMENTS

This research was conducted through the Public Health Accreditation Board (PHAB) in partnership with the Consortium for Workforce Research in Public Health. Funds for this study were made available from the Centers for Disease Control and Prevention (CDC) of the US Department of Health and Human Services (HHS), National Center for State, Tribal, Local, and Territorial Public Health Infrastructure and Workforce, through the OE22-2203: Strengthening US Public Health Infrastructure, Workforce, and Data Systems grant.

This study was presented at the 2024 American Public Health Association conference.

Note. The contents are those of the authors and do not necessarily represent the official views of, nor an endorsement, by CDC/HHS, the US government, or PHAB.

CONFLICTS OF INTEREST

The authors have no conflicts of interest to disclose.

HUMAN PARTICIPANT PROTECTION

This study used de-identified secondary data and was determined not to be human participant research according to the University of Washington institutional review board.

REFERENCES

1. *A Research Agenda for an Evolving Public Health System: Directions for the Field of Public Health Services and Systems Research*. AcademyHealth, American Public Health Association. December 2023. Available at: https://academyhealth.org/sites/default/files/publication/%5Bfield_date%3Acustom%3AY%5D-%5Bfield_date%3Acustom%3Am%5D/phssr_final_report.pdf. Accessed August 8, 2024.
2. Brownson RC, Burke TA, Colditz GA, Samet JM. Reimagining public health in the aftermath of a pandemic. *Am J Public Health*. 2020;110(11):1605–1610. https://doi.org/10.2105/AJPH.2020.305861
3. Centers for Disease Control and Prevention. Public Health Workforce Research Center. 2024. Available at: https://www.cdc.gov/workforce/php/about/public-health-workforce-research-center.html. Accessed August 5, 2024.
4. Centers for Disease Control and Prevention. OE22-2203 Strengthening U.S. public health infrastructure, workforce, and data systems. 2022. Available at: https://www.cdc.gov/infrastructure-phig/about/index.html. Accessed August 8, 2024.
5. Health Resources and Services Administration. Public Health Scholarship Program. Available at: https://www.hrsa.gov/grants/find-funding/HRSA-22-122. Accessed August 5, 2024.
6. Leider JP, Balio CP, Hogg-Graham R, et al. *An Enumeration of the Public Health Workforce in 2024*. Consortium for Workforce Research in Public Health. 2024. Available at: https://cworph.umn.edu/sites/cworph.umn.edu/files/2024-08/enumeration-2024.pdf. Accessed November 15, 2024.
7. Kett PM, Shahrir S, Bekemeier B. Public health nurses' proficiencies and training needs in an emergency response: a cross-sectional observational study. *J Public Health Manag Pract*. 2024;30(3):354–366. https://doi.org/10.1097/PHH.0000000000001888
8. Grenadier A. *NACCHO's 2019 Profile Study: Changes in Local Health Department Workforce and Finance Capacity Since 2008*. National Association of County and City Health Officials. May 2020. Available at: https://www.naccho.org/uploads/downloadable-resources/2019-Profile-Workforce-and-Finance-Capacity.pdf. Accessed August 5, 2024.
9. Kett PM, Bekemeier B, Altman MR, Herting JR. "Not everybody approaches it that way": nurse-trained health department directors' leadership strategies and skills in public health. *Nurs Inq*. 2022;29(4):e12487. https://doi.org/10.1111/nin.12487
10. Martsolf GR, Sloan J, Villarruel A, Mason D, Sullivan C. Promoting a culture of health through cross-sector collaborations. *Health Promot Pract*. 2018;19(5):784–791. https://doi.org/10.1177/1524839918772284
11. Blacksin B. Civic engagement: school-based health centers and public health nursing. *Public Health Nurs*. 2021;38(3):357–366. https://doi.org/10.1111/phn.12871
12. Association of State and Territorial Directors of Nursing. Report on a Public Health Nurse to Population Ratio. September 2008. Available at: https://www.cphno.org/wp-content/uploads/2020/08/ASTHOReportPublicHealthNursetoPopRatio2008.pdf. Accessed August 8, 2024.
13. Kub JE, Kulbok PA, Miner S, Merrill JA. Increasing the capacity of public health nursing to strengthen the public health infrastructure and to promote and protect the health of communities and populations. *Nurs Outlook*. 2017;65(5):661–664. https://doi.org/10.1016/j.outlook.2017.08.009
14. Driscoll A, Grant MJ, Carroll D, et al. The effect of nurse-to-patient ratios on nurse-sensitive patient outcomes in acute specialist units: a systematic review and meta-analysis. *Eur J Cardiovasc Nurs*. 2018;17(1):6–22. https://doi.org/10.1177/1474515117721561
15. Wolf A. Adapting nursing programs to competency-based education. *Nursing*. 2022;52(2):12–13. https://doi.org/10.1097/01.NURSE.0000806200.13094.90
16. Bekemeier B, Kuehnert P, Zahner SJ, Johnson KH, Kaneshiro J, Swider SM. A critical gap: advanced practice nurses focused on the public's health. *Nurs Outlook*. 2021;69(5):865–874. https://doi.org/10.1016/j.outlook.2021.03.023
17. DeSalvo KB, Claire Wang Y, Harris A, Auerbach J, Koo D, O'Carroll P. Public Health 3.0: a call to action for public health to meet the challenges of the 21st century. *Prev Chronic Dis*. 2017;14(9):170017. https://doi.org/10.5888/pcd14.170017
18. Kett PM, Bekemeier B, Herting JR, Altman MR. Addressing health disparities: the health department nurse lead executive's relationship to improved community health. *J Public Health Manag Pract*. 2022;28(2):E566–E576. https://doi.org/10.1097/PHH.0000000000001425
19. Bekemeier B, Pantazis A, Dunbar MD, Herting JR. Classifying local health departments on the basis of the constellation of services they provide. *Am J Public Health*. 2014;104(12):e77–e82. https://doi.org/10.2105/AJPH.2014.302281
20. Bekemeier B, Walker Linderman T, Kneipp S, Zahner SJ. Updating the definition and role of public health nursing to advance and guide the specialty. *Public Health Nurs*. 2015;32(1):50–57. https://doi.org/10.1111/phn.12157
21. Castner J, Stanislo K, Castner M, Monsen KA. Public health nursing workforce and learning needs: a national sample survey analysis. *Public Health Nurs*. 2023;40(3):339–352. https://doi.org/10.1111/phn.13171
22. Beck AJ, Boulton ML. The public health nurse workforce in U.S. state and local health departments, 2012. *Public Health Rep*. 2016;131(1):145–152. https://doi.org/10.1177/003335491613100121

23. National Council of State Boards of Nursing. National Nursing Workforce Study. Available at: https://www.ncsbn.org/research/recent-research/workforce.page. Accessed August 5, 2024.
24. National Forum of State Nursing Workforce Centers. Nursing Workforce Minimum Datasets. Available at: https://nursingworkforcecenters.org/dataset. Accessed August 5, 2024.
25. Smiley RA, Allgeyer RL, Shobo Y, et al. The 2022 National Nursing Workforce Survey. *J Nurs Regul.* 2023;14(1):S1–S90. https://doi.org/10.1016/S2155-8256(23)00047-9
26. *Public Health Nursing: Scope and Standards of Practice.* 3rd ed. Silver Spring, MD: American Nurses Association Inc; 2022.
27. Kneipp SM, Edmonds JK, Cooper J, Campbell LA, Little SH, Mix AK. Enumeration of public health nurses in the United States: limits of current standards. *Am J Public Health.* 2022;112(suppl 3):S292–S297. https://doi.org/10.2105/AJPH.2022.306782
28. Leider JP, Balio CP, Hogg-Graham R, et al. Enumeration 2024: what we know and what we wish we knew about the governmental public health workforce in a COVID recovery landscape. *Am J Public Health.* In Press.
29. Alaska Department of Health. Public health nursing services. Available at: https://health.alaska.gov/dph/Nursing/Pages/services.aspx. Accessed August 5, 2024.
30. Willgerodt MA, Tanner A, McCabe E, Jameson B, Brock D. Public school nurses in the United States: National School Nurse Workforce Study 2.0. *J Sch Nurs.* 2024;40(5):468–481. https://doi.org/10.1177/10598405241253565
31. National Council of State Boards of Nursing. Welcome to the FY22 NCSBN Annual Report. 2022. Available at: https://www.ncsbn.org/public-files/2022_NCSBN_Annual_Report.pdf. Accessed August 8, 2024.
32. National Academies of Sciences, Engineering, and Medicine; National Academy of Medicine; Committee on the Future of Nursing 2020–2030; Flaubert JL, Le Menestrel S, Williams DR, Wakefield MK, eds. *The Future of Nursing 2020–2030: Charting a Path to Achieve Health Equity.* Washington, DC: National Academies Press; 2021. https://doi.org/10.17226/25982
33. Baxter C, Schofield R, Currie G, Gauley P. Community health nurses leadership in advancing health equity. *Public Health Nurs.* 2024;41(2):310–317. https://doi.org/10.1111/phn.13286

State-Level Influenza Hospitalization Burden in the United States, 2022–2023

Alexia Couture, MPH, A. Danielle Iuliano, PhD, Howard H. Chang, PhD, Ryan Threlkel, MPH, Matthew Gilmer, MS, Alissa O'Halloran, MSPH, Dawud Ujamaa, MS, Matthew Biggerstaff, ScD, and Carrie Reed, ScD

See also Hochheiser and Kumar, p. 454.

Objectives. To develop a method leveraging hospital-based surveillance to estimate influenza-related hospitalizations by state, age, and month as a means of enhancing current US influenza burden estimation efforts.

Methods. Using data from the Influenza Hospitalization Surveillance Network (FluSurv-NET), we extrapolated monthly FluSurv-NET hospitalization rates after adjusting for testing practices and diagnostic test sensitivities to non-FluSurv-NET states. We used a Poisson zero-inflated model with an overdispersion parameter within the Bayesian hierarchical framework and accounted for uncertainty and variability between states and across time. Model validation included checking the sensitivity of results to input data, as well as model convergence diagnostics and comparing the results with independent data sources.

Results. We estimated 379 300 (90% credible interval [CrI] = 305 400, 479 300) influenza-related hospitalizations in the United States for the 2022–2023 season. Median cumulative state rates ranged widely from 23.2 to 249.0 per 100 000 people.

Conclusions. Our estimates were comparable to national burden estimates incorporating other approaches while accounting for variations in the timing and geography of disease activity and changes in detection and reporting. Our results provide a complementary framework to calculate estimates at finer geographic scales. (*Am J Public Health*. 2025;115(4):546–554. https://doi.org/10.2105/AJPH.2024.307928)

AJPH April 2025, Vol. 115, No. 4

The Centers for Disease Control and Prevention (CDC) has estimated the national influenza disease burden annually in the United States since the 2010–2011 season. Disease burden models help estimate the full impact of the disease, unlike other disease-related indicators that are often affected by care seeking, testing practices, and reporting.[1] Disease burden estimates provide a more complete picture of the true impact of a disease on public health and society, which is often unrecognized through case counting. By understanding the influenza disease burden, public health officials can better assess disease severity and target prevention and control measures to reduce morbidity and mortality. Currently, cumulative deaths, hospitalizations, medically attended illnesses, and symptomatic cases are estimated at the national level each week during and at the end of each season by age group. During the 2022–2023 season, the CDC estimated that 298 700 to 678 200 influenza-related hospitalizations occurred.[2]

Although the CDC has a long-established history of estimating the influenza disease burden at the national level, routine and robust methods to estimate state-level influenza-related hospitalization burdens have been lacking. During the 2009 influenza pandemic, the CDC began reporting timely national disease burden estimates that adjusted for underdetection, and methods have continued developing since; however, there is not yet state-level reporting.[3,4]

Currently, some state health departments report influenza hospitalizations on their Web sites. They often report data on hospitalizations from the Influenza Hospitalization Surveillance Network (FluSurv-NET) or the National Healthcare Safety Network (NHSN), which present unadjusted reported numbers.[5,6] Although these systems and numbers are extremely useful and important, crude or unadjusted reports of surveillance data underestimate the true burden of influenza hospitalizations as a result of multiple underdetection factors.[3,7]

There have been ad hoc efforts to estimate influenza burdens at state levels. One study estimated influenza-related hospitalizations in Utah with adjustment for testing practices, and another study in Washington used the statewide hospitalization system and modeled influenza hospitalization incidence; however, neither investigation accounted for testing practices or diagnostic assay sensitivities.[8,9] Although these studies provide useful information on the burden of disease in specific states, they do not serve as national models accounting for uncertainty and allowing for stratification by state, age, and month. Drawing inspiration from a previous study that estimated the global influenza burden by leveraging country-level reported data, we recognize the inherent variability in the influenza burden among states, as with the variation between countries.[10]

Accurate state-level estimation of influenza-related hospitalizations is important for public health planning, assessments of the impact of preventive measures, and resource allocation. We adapted methods from a project designed to estimate COVID-19 state-level hospitalizations during the pandemic that leveraged available surveillance data and employed a Bayesian hierarchical model.[11] We aimed to provide state-level influenza-related hospitalization estimates modeled with an understanding of spatial and temporal patterns to complement current national hospitalization burden estimates.

Our objective was to calculate monthly state-level influenza-related hospitalization rates by multiple age groups. We applied this new method to the 2022–2023 influenza season.

METHODS

We used hospitalization case count data from the CDC's FluSurv-NET collected during the 2022–2023 season. The network conducts population-based surveillance of hospitalized patients with a positive laboratory influenza test during a hospitalization or within 14 days before a hospitalization. The network includes hospitals in approximately 77 selected counties across 14 participating sites in 13 states: California, Colorado, Connecticut, Georgia, Maryland, Michigan, Minnesota, New Mexico, New York (2 sites; combined for this analysis), Ohio, Oregon, Tennessee, and Utah.

Catchment areas are defined according to patient residence within the selected counties; most data are received from hospitals inside the catchment area. Residents in each catchment area within a state are combined to create the population denominator for calculation of hospitalization rates. The network covers a total catchment population of more than 27 million people, representing about 9% of the US population. The network has been described in detail elsewhere.[12] For our model, the data were aggregated by state, month of hospitalization, and 7 age groups: 0 to 4, 5 to 17, 18 to 49, 50 to 64, 65 to 74, 75 to 84, and 85 years or older. Data are collected from October 1 through April 30 for each influenza season. Therefore, our hospitalization estimates span the period October 2022 through April 2023.

Because not all hospitalized patients undergo influenza testing, we corrected influenza hospitalization rates for underdetection by applying weights based on influenza testing practices and diagnostic test sensitivity using methods described previously.[4] Influenza testing practices were defined as the probability that a person who was hospitalized with a respiratory infection was tested for influenza in participating FluSurv-NET hospitals.[4] Data on testing practices during the 2022–2023 season were unavailable at the time of this study. For the most conservative adjustments, we used the highest observed testing probabilities over 10 influenza seasons (2010–2011 through 2019–2020) by state, month, and age. Ohio was the only FluSurv-NET site without site-specific testing probabilities, so data from all sites were combined by age and month for each season and the highest observed testing probability across seasons was used for the adjustment. Testing probabilities for different states, months, and age groups ranged from 0.1 to 1.0.

In addition, rates were adjusted for diagnostic test sensitivity. The assay sensitivity data were obtained from the literature and ranged from 0.76 to 0.91.[4] We calculated adjusted hospitalization rates using FluSurv-NET catchment populations for each state. Seven distinct models were employed for each age group:

$$\textit{Adjusted Flu Count}_{sm} = \frac{\textit{Raw Flu Count}_{sm}}{\left\{\begin{matrix}\textit{Prob. of Being Tested}_{sm} * \\ \textit{Testing Sensitivity}\end{matrix}\right\}} \quad (1)$$

where $s = 1, \ldots, S$ for each FluSurv-NET state and $m = 1, \ldots, M$ for each month.

Covariates

To extend influenza hospitalization rate estimates beyond FluSurv-NET states to those not included in the network, we incorporated covariates based on state-, month-, and age-specific demographic and epidemiological data. We used various data from multiple sources to address differences between states included and not included in FluSurv-NET (Table A, available as a supplement to the online version of this article at http://www.ajph.org). Including subpopulation-specific covariates allowed us to estimate hospitalizations by age group, month, and state. Covariates were both time-varying and fixed state-level factors.

Time-varying covariates included the percentage of positive influenza tests from commercial and public health laboratories (obtained from the National Respiratory and Enteric Virus Surveillance System), the percentage of all-cause deaths attributed to influenza based on National Center for Health Statistics data from the National Vital Statistics System, the percentage of the population vaccinated against influenza (FluVax), the percentage of outpatient visits to health care providers for an influenza-like illness (from the US Outpatient Influenza-like Illness Surveillance Network), and hospital capacity indicators such as the percentage of influenza patients among all inpatients and the percentage of intensive care unit beds occupied among all available intensive care unit beds (from NHSN).[6,13–16]

To account for the lag between symptom onset and hospitalization, we included the percentage of influenza tests that were positive with a 1-week lag. Likewise, a 1-week lead was added to the percentage of influenza deaths among all deaths to address the gap between hospitalizations and death. In the case of hospital capacity data, if hospitals reported less than 80% of days in a given month, they were excluded from state calculated percentages. Regarding time-invariant covariates, we used the percentages of non-White and Hispanic populations from 2021, state rural-to-urban proportions from 2020, Social Vulnerability Index variables from 2020, and the prevalence of certain comorbid conditions from 2021 (obtained from the Behavioral Risk Factor Surveillance System).[17–20] For age groups younger than 18 years, only asthma and obesity were included as chronic condition or disease covariates because of insufficient evidence that the prevalence of other chronic conditions or diseases affected those groups.

Outliers for each time-varying covariate, such as extreme values, were identified and mitigated through the Winsorization process.[21] We used adjusted influenza hospitalization rates as the outcome variable to guide the selection of covariates, and this procedure was carried out independently for each age group. The method employed for covariate selection was the spike and slab approach within the Bayesian model.[22] This robust method aided in identifying and incorporating the most predictive covariates into the final model for each age group while accounting for model selection uncertainties.

Bayesian Hierarchical Model

Building on previous work, we implemented a Poisson zero-inflated model with an overdispersion parameter within a Bayesian hierarchical framework. Let A_{sm} denote the estimated adjusted influenza hospitalization counts from the FluSurv-NET states during the influenza season starting in October 2022; states are represented as $s=1,\ldots,S$, with $S=13$ states in FluSurv-NET, and months are represented as $m=1,\ldots,M$, with $M=7$ for each month included in the model. A Poisson probability distribution was assumed for the observed hospitalization count. These estimated adjusted influenza hospitalization counts, along with the FluSurv-NET catchment populations and selected covariates, were used in the following Bayesian hierarchical model:

$$\text{Level 1: } A_{sm} \sim Pois(\theta_{sm} * Population_s/100,000) \quad (2)$$

$$\theta_{sm} = \varphi_{sm} * z_{sm}$$

$$z_{sm} \sim Bern(\rho)$$

where $A_{sm} = Adjusted\ FluSurv\text{-}NET\ Count_{sm}$ (the adjusted hospitalization count from FluSurv-NET), $Population_s$ is the catchment population for state s, θ_{sm} *and* φ_{sm} are the unobserved true hospitalization rates, and z_{sm} is an indicator for whether the rate is zero.

$$\text{Level 2: } \varphi_{sm} \sim logNormal\left(\mu + \sum_{j=1}^{k} \gamma_j X_{smj} + \delta_{sm}, \sigma^2\right) \quad (3)$$

$$\delta_{sm} \sim N(0, \tau)$$

where X is the covariate matrix and δ is the overdispersion parameter.

$$\text{Level 3: } \gamma_k \sim N(0, 1000000^{(1-g_k)} * 0.001) \quad (4)$$

$$g_k \sim Bern(0.25)$$

$$\text{Priors: } \mu \sim N(0, 10^{-6})$$

$$\sigma^2 \sim Unif(0, 1000)$$

$$\rho \sim Unif(0, 1)$$

$$\tau \sim Gamma(0.001, 0.001)$$

where $k = 1, \ldots, K$ and K is the number of selected covariates.

We carried out inference calculations using Markov chain Monte Carlo simulations with 110 000 iterations, 10 000 burn-ins, and thinning of 2 with the "rjags" package in R software version 4.1.2 (R Foundation for Statistical Computing, Vienna, Austria), which interfaces between R and JAGS software version 4.3.0 (https://sourceforge.net/projects/mcmc-jags). The model outputted the posterior distribution of influenza-related hospitalizations for each state and month. We calculated medians and 90% credible intervals (CrIs) for hospitalization counts, rounded to hundreds because of Monte Carlo errors, and used 2021 state and age populations to calculate hospitalization rates. Posterior samples were summed to calculate all-age, age by month, age by state, and state by month hospitalizations and rates.

The medians of sums did not equal the sums of medians, which led to slightly different total hospitalizations depending on which grouping was used to sum. Total hospitalizations were calculated from all-age medians, age by month medians, and age by state total medians. We took a Bayesian approach to incorporate multiple levels of variability and have a flexible framework for a hierarchical approach. We chose vague priors for our model's iteration (as defined in the model); as state-level data become more available, however, priors can be adjusted to be more informed. Priors were varied slightly to check the robustness of the results.

Sensitivity and Comparisons

We conducted multiple sensitivity and comparison analyses to assess the performance of the model. First, we compared the model's aggregate national rates by age group to the CDC burden estimates from the 2022–2023 season.[2] Second, to validate the model, we removed each FluSurv-NET state, one at a time, and compared how the model estimated hospitalizations for the removed state with the FluSurv-NET adjusted hospitalization rate.

Third, we compared the model's state estimates with NHSN data.[6] Developed and managed by the CDC, NHSN provides a standardized platform for health care facilities to monitor health care–associated infections and includes state-level hospitalization data for influenza hospitalizations by week. According to Healthdata.gov, NHSN data have reliable counts of new influenza hospitalizations starting on February 2, 2022, as a result of mandatory influenza reporting. However, the NHSN data are derived from reports at the facility level and do not account for nonresponse, nontesting, test sensitivity, or missing data. Finally, we compared the model's state estimates with hospitalizations reported by state health departments. We compiled data publicly posted to each state's health department Web site that provided influenza-related hospitalizations at the end of the 2022–2023 season. Sources and notes on each source are detailed in Table B (available as a supplement to the online version of this article at http://www.ajph.org).

RESULTS

From October 2022 through April 2023, our model estimated 379 300 (90% CrI = 305 400, 479 300) influenza-related hospitalizations in the United States, with a cumulative hospitalization rate of 114.5 (90% CrI = 92.2, 144.7) per 100 000 people. Rates varied by age, state, and month. The highest estimated rate of cumulative hospitalizations for the 2022–2023 season was in New York, with a rate of 249.0 (90% CrI = 205.1, 303.7) per 100 000 people from an estimated count of 49 400 (90% CrI = 40 700, 60 200). The lowest estimated cumulative hospitalization rate was in Alaska, with a rate of 23.2 (90% CrI = 13.8, 38.8) per 100 000 people from an estimated count of 170 (90% CrI = 100, 280). Figure 1 and Figure A (available as a supplement to the online version of this article at http://www.ajph.org) show the cumulative hospitalization rate for each state. In Figure 1, cumulative hospitalization counts by state are presented to show the difference in burden of counts versus rates. FluSurv-NET states were well distributed throughout all state estimates.

Hospitalization rates varied by age group. The highest cumulative rate was observed among those aged 85 years or older, with a rate of 625.2 (90% CrI = 507.4, 768.0) per 100 000 people. The lowest cumulative rate was observed among those aged 18 to 49 years, with a rate of 47.7 (90% CrI = 39.5, 55.0) per 100 000 people (Table 1). Hospitalization rates for all age groups peaked in December 2022 except for those aged 5 to 17 years; the rate for this group peaked in November 2022 (Figure B, available as a supplement to the online version of this article at http://www.ajph.org). Across all ages, the largest peak occurred in December 2022 (51.1 per 100 000), followed by November 2022 (41.7 per 100 000), and the lowest occurred in April 2023 (2.2 per 100 000).

Monthly state-level hospitalization rates varied widely, with different timings and magnitudes of peaks. For example, some states (e.g., Arkansas and Michigan) were estimated to have

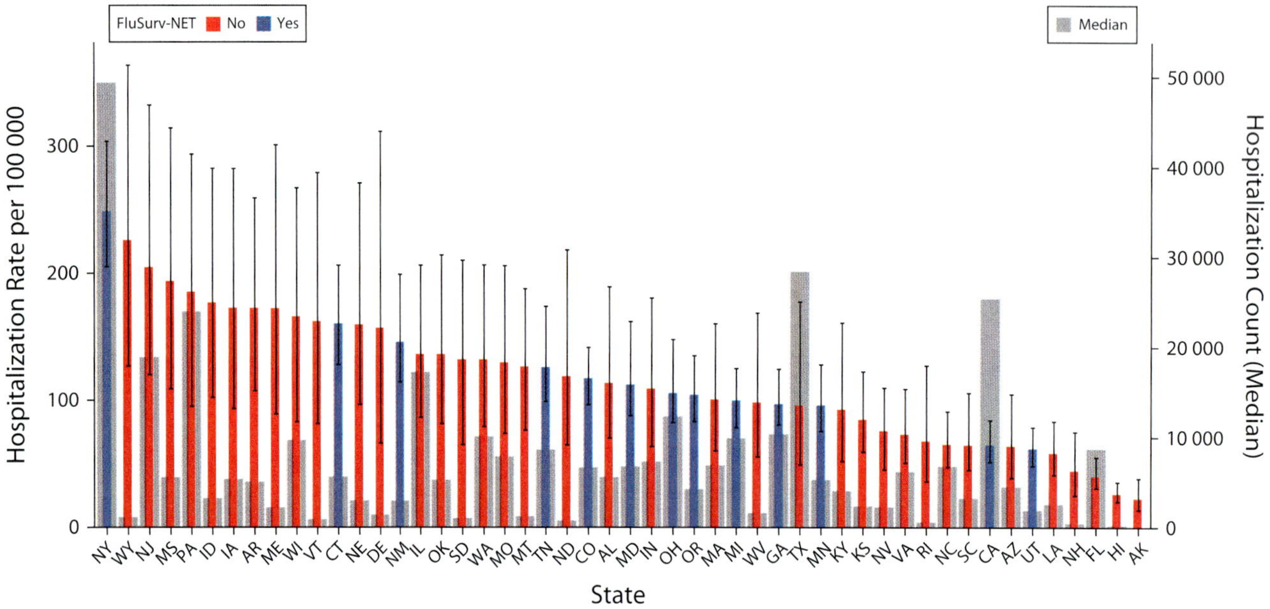

FIGURE 1— Median Cumulative Influenza-Related Hospitalization Rates From Our Bayesian Model, With FluSurv-NET and Non-FluSurv-NET State Rates: United States, October 2022–April 2023

Note. Whiskers indicate 90% credible intervals. The bar graph is ordered by median value for cumulative influenza-related hospitalization, which cannot be interpreted without intervals.

discrete peaks, whereas other states had multiple months with higher hospitalizations (e.g., Connecticut and Illinois). Figure C (available as a supplement to the online version of this article at http://www.ajph.org) shows each state's curve over time, highlighting the variability in the influenza-related hospitalization burden between states and within states by month. Varying model priors had no impact on the results.

According to the comparison analysis, this state-level model produced similar estimates to published national burden estimates by age group (Figure 2). The median hospitalization rate produced by the model falls inside the 95% uncertainty intervals of published burden estimates for all age groups, and the mean hospitalization rate of the published burden falls within the model's 90% credible intervals for all ages. For the sensitivity analysis in which FluSurv-NET states were dropped one at a time, model estimates were mostly consistent whether inputted to build the model or extrapolated (i.e., dropped from the model). Most of the FluSurv-NET states' extrapolated estimates had overlapping credible intervals (Figure 3). When they did not overlap, extrapolated estimates were lower except for Ohio's and Oregon's peak months, which were higher when extrapolated.

When making comparisons at the state level, we found a wide range of similarities with and discrepancies from our model estimates, NHSN, unadjusted FluSurv-NET rates, and hospitalizations reported by state health departments. Figure C shows states where all sources agreed, but we also

TABLE 1— Cumulative Influenza-Related Hospitalization Count and Rate by Age: United States, October 2022–April 2023

Age Group, y	Hospitalization Count, Median (90% CrI)	Hospitalization Rate per 100 000 (90% CrI)
< 5	15 500 (10 800, 27 800)	82.4 (57.6, 148.2)
5–17	28 300 (19 800, 40 000)	51.9 (36.2, 73.1)
18–49	66 000 (54 600, 80 200)	47.7 (39.5, 58.0)
50–64	73 500 (60 900, 89 800)	115.1 (95.7, 141.2)
65–74	86 400 (69 300, 108 700)	251.0 (206.0, 323.3)
75–84	72 400 (59 700, 87 000)	447.3 (368.7, 537.4)
≥ 85	37 300 (30 300, 45 800)	625.2 (507.4, 768.0)
Total	379 300 (305 400, 479 300)	114.5 (92.2, 144.7)

Note. CrI = credible interval. Data are from our Bayesian model.

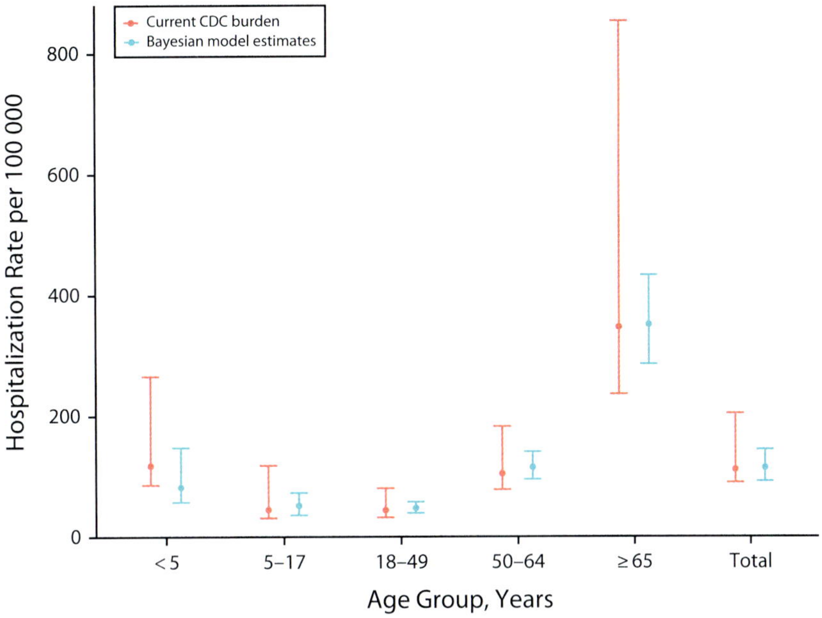

FIGURE 2— Comparison of Influenza-Related Hospitalization Rates From Our Bayesian Model With the Current Centers for Disease Control and Prevention (CDC) Published Burden, Aggregated by Age Groups: United States, October 2022–April 2023

Note. Whiskers indicate 90% credible intervals from our Bayesian model and 95% uncertainty intervals from the CDC published burden.

observed instances in which state-reported rates were higher than our model estimates and NHSN. In general, our model estimates caught overall timing trends and were slightly higher than other sources of reported hospitalizations at the state level, most likely because of our adjustments for testing probability and diagnostic sensitivity.

DISCUSSION

Overall, we estimated that 379 300 cumulative influenza-related hospitalizations occurred in the United States from October 2022 through April 2023. Our model estimated national influenza-related hospitalizations by age group similar to CDC published burden estimates. Our model showed that there was wide variability between states and within states between months with respect to influenza-related hospitalizations during the 2022–2023 season. We found that most states peaked in November and December 2022, following trends observed in influenza surveillance indicators (Figure C).

From our sensitivity analysis, we found that our model was able to reasonably estimate data for states when they were dropped as an input. When there was discordance between estimates, the extrapolated estimates were often more conservative. When comparing our estimates with available outside sources, such as NHSN and figures reported by state health departments, we found that our model was well validated in trends but that there were important differences in magnitude and peak timing. For example, if a state started to peak in November according to our model, it was often not detected in the other sources. This could have been due to early peaking being missed by incorporating the probability of being tested. However, our credible intervals often covered other sources.

Our study introduces a novel approach leveraging state-level information and providing granularity across states, months, and age groups. The absence of such state-level estimates has been a gap in the CDC's efforts to understand the burden of influenza across the country and has limited the understanding of the spatial and temporal dynamics of influenza-related hospitalizations. Our findings underscore the critical role of state-level data in capturing the variable impact of influenza, revealing spatial and temporal patterns that might otherwise be obscured by national-level analyses. Our method aimed to create estimates that account for variation in the timing and geography of disease activity and changes in detection and reporting to produce monthly state-level estimates at the end of the influenza season.

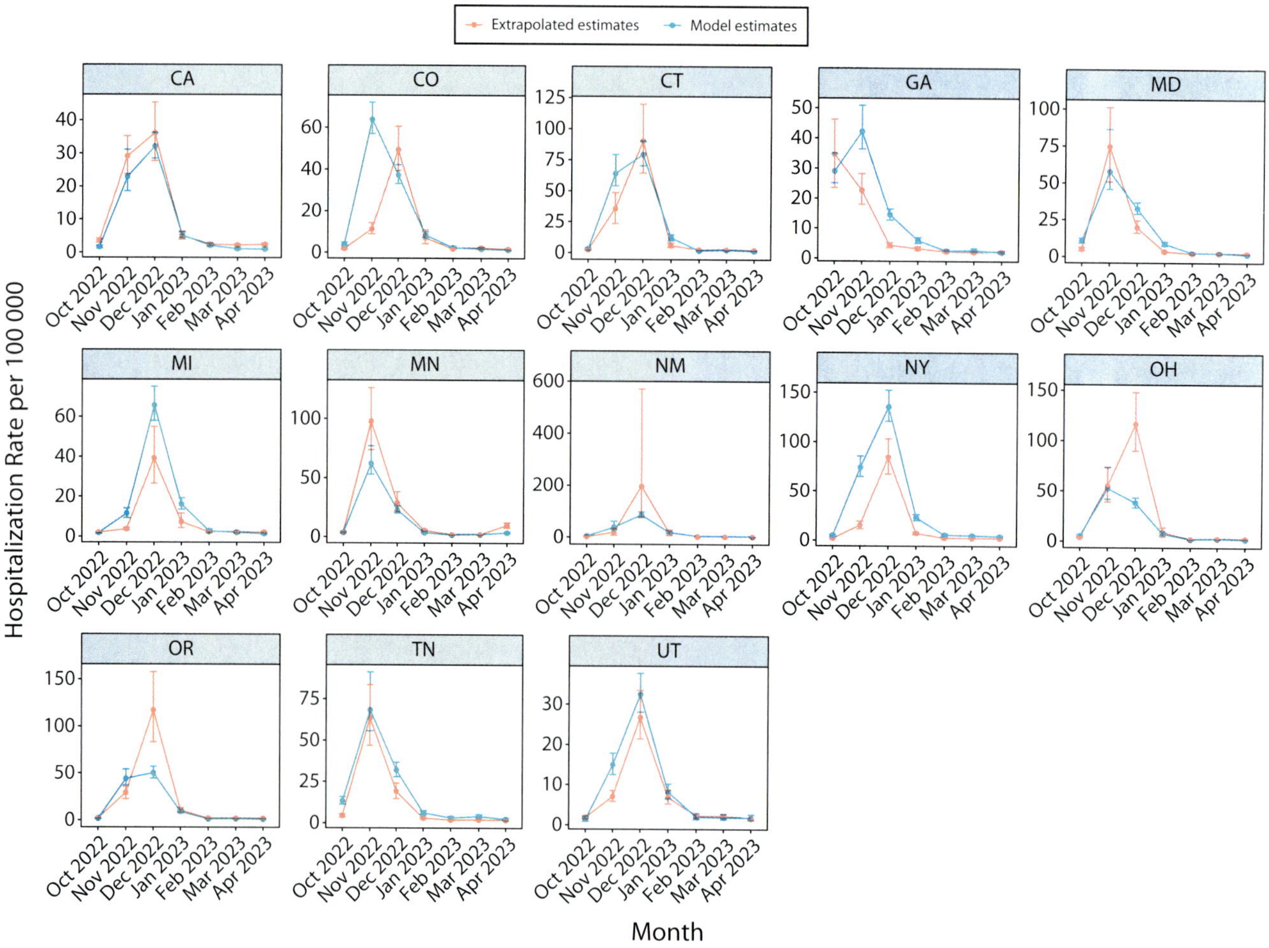

FIGURE 3— **Comparison of Influenza-Related Hospitalization Rates From Our Bayesian Model for Each State in FluSurv-NET Showing the Final Rate From the Model and the Extrapolated Rate When the State Was Not Inputted in the Model: United States, October 2022–April 2023**

Note. Whiskers indicate 90% credible intervals.

This approach provides a framework for monitoring disease burden using surveillance data.

We found that the unadjusted estimates from FluSurv-NET and NHSN aligned well with our results. The difference between our results and NHSN was expected because, unlike our model, the data from the NHSN system did not account for testing practices and sensitivity. This difference limited comparability between our estimates and reporting sources and the ability to know whether our model estimated the true level of the influenza-related hospitalization burden. There is no available true gold standard with which to compare hospitalization burden estimates because sources do not account for reasons hospitalizations may be underascertained, including the propensity to test individuals for influenza and test performance. Therefore, there is still potential for future work in this framework, including refining the model to account for evolving influenza strains or integrating real-time data to improve the timeliness and accuracy of estimates.

The method's adaptability, drawn from experiences during the COVID-19 pandemic, speaks to its potential for creating a framework applicable beyond the current study.[11] Our model is also advantageous in the context of influenza, wherein dynamics exhibit considerable temporal and spatial variability. The Bayesian framework accommodates uncertainty inherent in disease burden estimation, in which factors influencing hospitalization rates may exhibit considerable fluctuations. The ability to quantify uncertainties is crucial when interpreting and using results in public health decision making. Furthermore, the model allows for the incorporation of additional covariates. As new information becomes available or as the landscape of influenza evolves (e.g., availability of large-scale wastewater data for the influenza virus), the model can be updated to reflect these changes so that the estimates remain current and relevant. This adaptability is pertinent in the context of emerging infectious diseases, in which the ability to integrate evolving information enhances the utility and longevity of the methodology.

Limitations

Our study has several limitations. First, our approach relies on the assumption that FluSurv-NET sites are representative of the entire state. The composition of FluSurv-NET sites varies across states; in some states, they encompass most counties, whereas in others they include only a small number of counties. Consequently, our model may involve overestimation or underestimation for FluSurv-NET states depending on the extent to which the catchment area aligns with the influenza activity in the entire state. Despite our efforts to accommodate state-level variability and uncertainty within the model, our ability to accurately capture the full state's reality is constrained by the representativeness of a FluSurv-NET site relative to the entire state and might be biased with respect to the variability of testing practices across the state.

Second, we assume that FluSurv-NET states encompass sufficient diversity to extrapolate data to all states. Although the states within FluSurv-NET exhibit variability across multiple dimensions, we cannot guarantee that they encompass the full spectrum of variations in influenza-related hospitalizations, including adequate rural representation or use of respiratory illness mitigation strategies.

Third, our reliance on covariates to inform extrapolation is constrained by the quality, completeness, and availability of data. Essential information pertaining to influenza-related hospitalization rates, such as underlying risk factors in the population, could be missing. However, our model does incorporate time-varying covariates that describe the seasonal impact in each state, including metrics such as vaccination rates.

Fourth, some states have wide credible intervals, increasing the margin of error in determining actual hospitalization figures and inferring medians. In addition, we did not adjust for test specificity because specificities in hospital settings were high, ranging from 96% to 100% regardless of age group.[23,24] Although adjustment for false-positive test results might decrease our estimates, the impact on the overall rates would be minimal. Finally, our approach involved distinct models for each age group, restricting our ability to interpret hospitalization estimates by month and state, potentially underestimating variability, and failing to capture correlations between age groups.

Conclusion

Our independent approach aligns with the results of published burden methods. Our method helps provide a better understanding of the actual burden of influenza in the United States because observed hospitalization data are likely to underrepresent the true burden of influenza owing to testing practices and test sensitivity. Furthermore, developing a method to estimate postseason, state-level burdens enhances our understanding of the impact of influenza by state and time. Our method offers a way to estimate state-level influenza hospitalization burdens for all states using routinely collected surveillance and demographic data. State-level estimates can also be used for further public health awareness (e.g., vaccine-averted burden). Our method, initially used to estimate the global influenza burden and then the US COVID-19 burden, may be useful as well for other levels of the disease burden pyramid or other diseases. Our estimates can help in better informing the differential burden of influenza by state over time and better understanding the potential impact of factors such as differences in vaccination coverage in future analyses. AJPH

ABOUT THE AUTHORS

Alexia Couture, A. Danielle Iuliano, Ryan Threlkel, Matthew Gilmer, Alissa O'Halloran, Dawud Ujamaa, Matthew Biggerstaff, and Carrie Reed are with the National Center for Immunization and Respiratory Diseases, Centers for Disease Control and Prevention, Atlanta, GA. Howard H. Chang is with the Department of Biostatistics and Bioinformatics, Rollins School of Public Health, Emory University, Atlanta, GA.

CORRESPONDENCE

Correspondence should be sent to Alexia Couture, MPH, 1600 Clifton Rd NE, H24-7, Atlanta, GA 30333 (e-mail: njh6@cdc.gov). Reprints can be ordered at https://www.ajph.org by clicking the "Reprints" link.

PUBLICATION INFORMATION

Full Citation: Couture A, Iuliano AD, Chang HH, et al. State-level influenza hospitalization burden in the United States, 2022–2023. *Am J Public Health*. 2025;115(4):546–554.

Acceptance Date: November 7, 2024.

DOI: https://doi.org/10.2105/AJPH.2024.307928

ORCID iDs:

Alexia Couture https://orcid.org/0000-0002-4257-3697

Matthew Gilmer https://orcid.org/0000-0003-3283-0909

Matthew Biggerstaff https://orcid.org/0000-0001-5108-8311

CONTRIBUTORS

All of the authors were involved in the study conceptualization. A. Couture, A. D. Iuliano, R.

Threlkel, M. Gilmer, M. Biggerstaff, and C. Reed analyzed the primary and input data. A. Couture and H. H. Chang coded the model and A. Couture was responsible for running model analyses. A. Couture, A. D. Iuliano, R. Threlkel, M. Gilmer, A. O'Halloran, and D. Ujamaa validated the data used in the analysis. A. Couture, A. D. Iuliano, M. Biggerstaff, and C. Reed led the initial drafting of the article. All of the authors contributed ideas for analysis and to editing of the article.

ACKNOWLEDGMENTS

This work was supported by the Centers for Disease Control and Prevention (CDC).

Our results relied on data contributed by many health care providers, public health practitioners, and laboratorians, to whom we are grateful for the privilege of working with these data, including FluSurv-NET.

Note. The views expressed in this article are those of the authors and not necessarily those of the CDC.

CONFLICTS OF INTEREST

The authors declare that they have no competing interests.

HUMAN PARTICIPANT PROTECTION

This activity was reviewed by the Centers for Disease Control and Prevention and determined to be consistent with non–human participant research activity. Informed consent was waived as the data were de-identified and aggregated.

REFERENCES

1. Centers for Disease Control and Prevention. Disease burden of flu. Available at: https://www.cdc.gov/flu/about/burden/index.html. Accessed March 11, 2024.
2. Centers for Disease Control and Prevention. Preliminary estimated influenza illnesses, medical visits, hospitalizations, and deaths in the United States—2022–2023 influenza season. Available at: https://www.cdc.gov/flu/about/burden/2022-2023.htm. Accessed March 11, 2024.
3. Reed C, Angulo FJ, Swerdlow DL, et al. Estimates of the prevalence of pandemic (H1N1) 2009, United States, April–July 2009. *Emerg Infect Dis.* 2009;15(12):2004–2007. https://doi.org/10.3201/eid1512.091413
4. Reed C, Chaves SS, Daily Kirley P, et al. Estimating influenza disease burden from population-based surveillance data in the United States. *PLoS One.* 2015;10(3):e0118369. https://doi.org/10.1371/journal.pone.0118369
5. Centers for Disease Control and Prevention. Influenza Hospitalization Surveillance Network (FluSurv-NET). Available at: https://www.cdc.gov/flu/weekly/influenza-hospitalization-surveillance.htm. Accessed March 11, 2024.
6. Centers for Disease Control and Prevention. National Healthcare Safety Network. Available at: https://www.cdc.gov/nhsn/index.html. Accessed March 11, 2024.
7. Shrestha SS, Swerdlow DL, Borse RH, et al. Estimating the burden of 2009 pandemic influenza A (H1N1) in the United States (April 2009–April 2010). *Clin Infect Dis.* 2011;52(suppl 1):S75–S82. https://doi.org/10.1093/cid/ciq012
8. Hughes MM, Carmack AE, McCaffrey K, et al. Estimating the incidence of influenza at the state level—Utah, 2016–17 and 2017–18 influenza seasons. *MMWR Morb Mortal Wkly Rep.* 2019; 68(50):1158–1161. https://doi.org/10.15585/mmwr.mm6850a2
9. Somayaji R, Neradilek MB, Szpiro AA, et al. Effects of air pollution and other environmental exposures on estimates of severe influenza illness, Washington, USA. *Emerg Infect Dis.* 2020;26(5): 920–929. https://doi.org/10.3201/eid2605.190599
10. Iuliano AD, Roguski KM, Chang HH, et al. Estimates of global seasonal influenza-associated respiratory mortality: a modelling study. *Lancet.* 2018;391(10127):1285–1300. https://doi.org/10.1016/S0140-6736(17)33293-2
11. Couture A, Iuliano AD, Chang HH, et al. Estimating COVID-19 hospitalizations in the United States with surveillance data using a Bayesian hierarchical model: modeling study. *JMIR Public Health Surveill.* 2022;8(6):e34296. https://doi.org/10.2196/34296
12. Chaves SS, Lynfield R, Lindegren ML, Bresee J, Finelli L. The US Influenza Hospitalization Surveillance Network. *Emerg Infect Dis.* 2015;21(9): 1543–1550. https://doi.org/10.3201/eid2109.141912
13. Centers for Disease Control and Prevention. National Respiratory and Enteric Virus Surveillance System. Available at: https://www.cdc.gov/surveillance/nrevss/index.html. Accessed March 11, 2024.
14. National Center for Health Statistics. National Vital Statistics System. Available at: https://www.cdc.gov/nchs/nvss/index.htm. Accessed March 11, 2024.
15. Centers for Disease Control and Prevention. FluVaxView. Available at: https://www.cdc.gov/flu/fluvaxview/index.htm. Accessed March 11, 2024.
16. Centers for Disease Control and Prevention. US influenza surveillance: purpose and methods. Available at: https://www.cdc.gov/fluview/overview/index.html. Accessed March 11, 2024.
17. Centers for Disease Control and Prevention. Bridged-race population estimates. Available at: https://wonder.cdc.gov/bridged-race-population.html. Accessed March 11, 2024.
18. US Census Bureau. Urban and rural. Available at: https://www.census.gov/programs-surveys/geography/guidance/geo-areas/urban-rural.html. Accessed March 11, 2024.
19. Agency for Toxic Substances and Disease Registry. CDC/ATSDR Social Vulnerability Index. Available at: https://www.atsdr.cdc.gov/placeandhealth/svi/index.html. Accessed March 11, 2024.
20. Centers for Disease Control and Prevention. Behavioral Risk Factor Surveillance System. Available at: https://www.cdc.gov/brfss/index.html. Accessed March 11, 2024.
21. Ruppert D. Trimming and Winsorization. In: Balakrishnan N, Colton T, Everitt B, Piegorsch W, Ruggeri F, Teugels JL, eds. *Wiley StatsRef: Statistics Reference Online.* Hoboken, NJ: Wiley Blackwell; 2006:8765.
22. Ishwaran H, Rao JS. Spike and slab variable selection: frequentist and Bayesian strategies. *Ann Stat.* 2005;33(2):1. https://doi.org/10.1214/009053604000001147
23. Chartrand C, Leeflang MM, Minion J, et al. Accuracy of rapid influenza diagnostic tests: a meta-analysis. *Ann Intern Med.* 2012;156(7):500–511. https://doi.org/10.7326/0003-4819-156-7-201204030-00403
24. Kumar S, Henrickson KJ. Update on influenza diagnostics: lessons from the novel H1N1 influenza A pandemic. *Clin Microbiol Rev.* 2012;25(2): 344–361. https://doi.org/10.1128/CMR.05016-11

The Fourth Wave of the Opioid Epidemic: Increasing Combination of Fentanyl With Stimulants

Katie Diekhans, MFS, Jihau Yu, MS, Sue Pearring, MS, Robert Almeida, MS, and Luke N. Rodda, PhD

See also Aronowitz and Reed, p. 457.

Objectives. To identify drug prevalence through the analysis of drug material and paraphernalia (DMP) collected from scenes of fentanyl-involved fatal accidental drug overdoses in San Francisco, California, throughout 2022.

Methods. We conducted gas chromatography–mass spectrometry testing on 409 items of DMP (e.g., glass pipes, syringes, aluminum foil, powders) from 137 cases, and we further tested 132 DMP items using liquid chromatography–tandem mass spectrometry in context with decedent information and toxicology findings.

Results. We detected fentanyl in 106 cases (77%); 35 (33%) contained fentanyl either alone or with fentanyl precursors or breakdown products. Of the 106 fentanyl-positive cases, we codetected cocaine in 29 (27%) and methamphetamine in 16 (15%). Overall, we detected methamphetamine in 58 (42%) cases (25 in isolation), cocaine in 68 (50%) cases (18 in isolation), and fentanyl analogs in 33 (24%) cases (4 in isolation). We detected 38 novel fentanyl analogs and precursors of analogs.

Conclusions. We observed fentanyl use in combination with stimulants (a characteristic pattern of the opioid epidemic fourth wave). Smoking fentanyl powder using aluminum foil or snorting were the most inferred. We established polysubstance use and emerging potent novel fentanyl analogs use. (*Am J Public Health*. 2025;115(4):555–565. https://doi.org/10.2105/AJPH.2024.307948)

AJPH April 2025, Vol. 115, No. 4

Throughout the United States, from March 2022 to March 2023, there were more than 100 000 reported drug overdose deaths from predominately synthetic opioids, mainly fentanyl.[1] As the opioid epidemic has progressed, deaths involving fentanyl combined with the stimulants methamphetamine or cocaine have also increased, which has been described as the "fourth wave" of the opioid overdose crisis.[2] In San Francisco, California, fentanyl-related deaths increased from 9 in 2009 to 230 in 2019, an increase of more than 2000%.[3]

In 2022, San Francisco saw 649 deaths from accidental overdoses.[4] Of these, fentanyl was listed as a causal drug in 459 (71%), methamphetamine in 354 (55%), cocaine in 252 (39%), heroin in 64 (10%), and medicinal opioids in 52 (8%). Fentanyl in combination with methamphetamine or cocaine was detected in 258 (40%) and 178 (27%) cases, respectively, and all 3 together were detected in 50 (8%), suggesting significant polysubstance drug use, which is indicative of this fourth wave.[4] Additionally, the region saw the introduction of novel fentanyl analogs (fentalogs), posing further risk because of often increased potency compared with fentanyl, potential synergistic effects, and individuals being unaware of these novel substances in their drug supply.[5]

Drug paraphernalia have been the subject of several studies that examined the prevalence of drugs in certain regions of the United States and Europe.[6–8] It has been reported that the number of adults in the United States who inject drugs has increased from approximately 774 000 in 2011 to nearly 3.7 million in 2018.[9,10] However, in San Francisco and throughout other US regions, the number of injections has decreased in recent years, a positive public health trend, as continuously emerging fentanyl substances are administered through smoking instead.[11,12]

As many illicit drugs require the use of paraphernalia, the analysis of drug material and paraphernalia (DMP) can better characterize drug use, providing objective data regarding the prevalence of drugs available and in use. Such information can aid harm reduction and public health services to better address the ongoing drug overdose epidemic and identify emerging substances. We analyzed DMP collected from scenes of fentanyl-related accidental overdose deaths in 2022 to investigate drug prevalence and polysubstance use in San Francisco.

METHODS

The Office of the Chief Medical Examiner for the City and County of San Francisco determines the cause and manner of death resulting from all homicides, accidents, suicides, undetermined circumstances, and certain natural circumstances. Beyond comprehensive medicolegal death investigations, including thorough toxicology analysis, investigators collect DMP items deemed relevant to the case during scene investigations.

The case inclusion criterion for our study was submission of DMP in 2022 accidental overdose cases in which fentanyl was detected in the decedent's blood. A flowchart presenting these criteria is displayed in Figure A (available as a supplement to the online version of this article at http://www.ajph.org). We did not test clearly unused DMP or pharmaceuticals unless we suspected them to be illicit. Of particular interest were fentanyl, stimulants, emerging substances such as xylazine and fentalogs, and other drugs of abuse such as heroin, ketamine, and THC (tetrahydrocannabinol).

Sample Preparation

Before analysis, we photographed the original DMP container and the DMP inside it and recorded the physical characteristics of the DMP. The general procedure for each type of evidence is displayed in Table A (available as a supplement to the online version of this article at http://www.ajph.org). After extraction, we subjected samples to gas chromatography–mass spectrometry (GC–MS) analysis and, if applicable, liquid chromatography–tandem mass spectrometry (LC–MS/MS).

Drug Analysis

The GC–MS method parameters and spectral libraries we used are displayed in Table B (available as a supplement to the online version of this article at http://www.ajph.org). We confirmed compounds with a spectral library match of 70 or more and a retention time within plus or minus 2% of the standard analyte. We employed 2 quality controls to monitor the response and retention times of certain compounds to ensure proper instrument operation and to compare unknowns using retention time and an MS library search.

Following GC–MS analysis, we subjected selected DMP to a previously published LC–MS/MS method that analyzes more than 250 novel synthetic opioids, including fentalogs, nitazenes, utopioids, other nonfentanyl opioids, and xylazine.[13] We tested cases that were positive for novel synthetic opioids or xylazine using this method, either in DMP with the previously described GC–MS analysis or in blood or urine from a previous study using LC–MS/MS.[5] The sample preparation procedure for LC–MS/MS analysis is displayed in Table C (available as a supplement to the online version of this article at http://www.ajph.org).

RESULTS

We present our results from GC–MS and LC–MS/MS together.

Of the 649 accidental overdose death cases in 2022 in San Franciso, DMP were submitted for 182 (28%) cases. Of these, 137 (75%) were among the 459 fentanyl-related deaths. From these 137 cases, 409 individual DMP items were tested, with 393 (96%) resulting in positive drug findings. In 16 (4%) DMP samples, we detected no drugs or we identified out-of-scope substances such as amino acids, cholesterol, and fatty acids.

Drug Material and Paraphernalia

We combined results for baggies, bindles, and powders (hereafter called "baggies and powders") because of their similarities and composition of primarily powders or powder residue. Overall, baggies and powders (in 121 [30%] samples) were the sample type that we most often encountered, followed by nonbulbous glass pipes (in 86 [21%] samples), which are often used to smoke crack cocaine (Figure 1). There were 38 (9%) samples of aluminum foil, which is typically used to heat the drug material, producing smoke that is then inhaled through a straw. Bulbous glass pipes, often used to smoke methamphetamine, were in 37 DMP samples (9%). There were 32 (8%) syringe samples, 20 (5%) straws, 20 (5%) crystal substances, and 15 (4%) pills. Of the pills, the majority were commercially available benzodiazepines and 3 were illicit. DMP samples that we

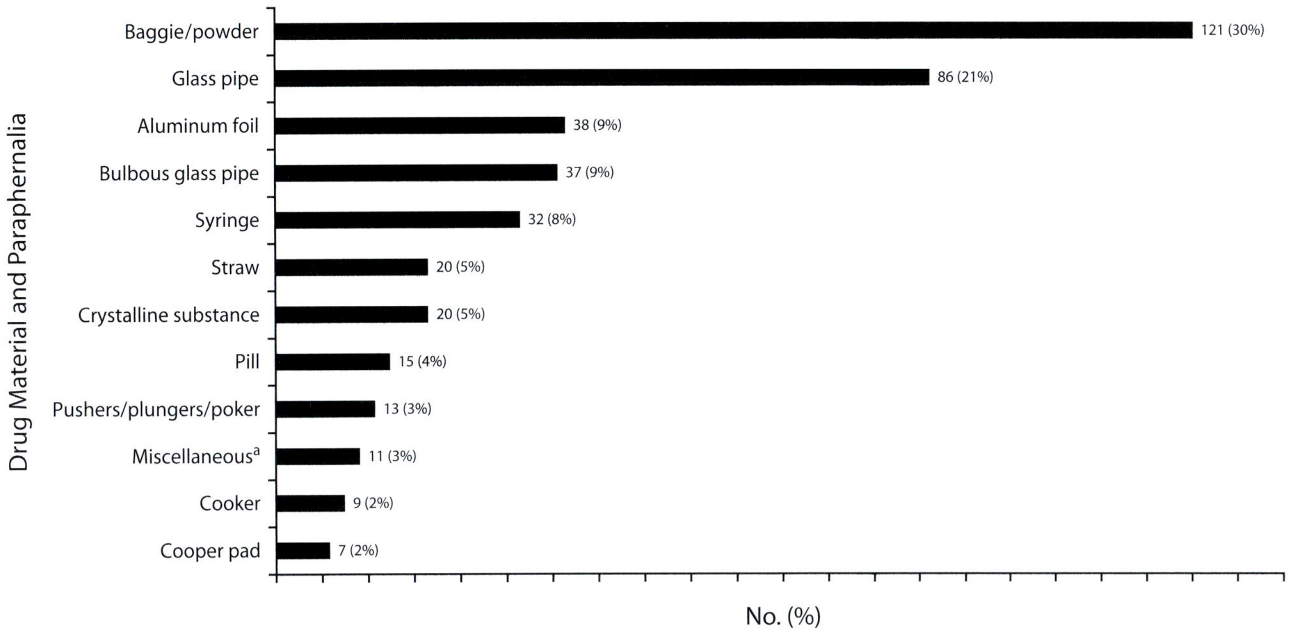

FIGURE 1— Prevalence of Drug Material and Paraphernalia Types Tested Among Fatal Fentanyl Overdose Decedents: San Francisco, CA, 2022

Note. The sample size was n = 409.
[a]Miscellaneous included a bindle with nonpowder (black tarry substance), a baggie of nonpowder (mushrooms), brown substance (n = 3), green vegetable material (n = 2), a joint (n = 2), a razor blade, and a vape pen.

encountered less often are included in Figure 1.

Types of DMP and decedent demographic information are presented in Table 1. Overall, many DMP types corresponded to the sample population in this study (e.g., 79% of baggies and powders and 69% of nonbulbous glass pipes, correlating with 77% of the sample population being male). Notable exceptions were syringes, with 60% contributed by the female population (which made up only 23% of this sample population) and crystalline substances, with 86% being contributed by White individuals although White individuals made up 53% of the sample population. The most common DMP type among males were baggies and powders, glass pipes (bulbous and nonbulbous), and aluminum foil, with glass pipes (bulbous and nonbulbous), syringes, and baggies and powders being most common among females. Additionally, aluminum foil was a common DMP type among those aged 25 to 34 years and syringes and crystalline substances among those aged 35 to 44 years.

As displayed in Table 2, the most common drug detected in baggies and powders was fentanyl alone or with fentanyl precursors or breakdown products (hereafter called "fentanyl alone"; 23% of baggies/powders samples), followed by fentanyl plus cocaine (14%), and then fentanyl plus fentalogs (9%). Bulbous glass pipes had a high instance of methamphetamine alone (51%), whereas nonbulbous glass pipes had a high instance of fentanyl plus cocaine (24%), cocaine alone (17%), or fentanyl combined with fentalogs and cocaine (17%). Among crystalline substances and syringes, methamphetamine alone was detected in 60% and 31%, respectively, of samples. Fentanyl was present in 15 (47%) syringes. Lastly, the most detected drugs in aluminum foil were fentanyl alone (18%) and fentanyl plus fentalogs plus methamphetamine (21%). Of the 3 illicit pills, we found that 1 contained methamphetamine, 1 fentanyl, and 1 a combination of fentanyl and cocaine. The other 12 pills were miscellaneous prescription substances, such as gabapentin, methylphenidate, and licit benzodiazepines.

Drug Use

Table 3 displays the demographic characteristics of the decedents in relation to the drugs detected in 1 or more of their DMP items. Of 106 cases in which the DMP included fentanyl, 82 (77%) were contributed by males, and 24 (23%) were contributed by females. Of methamphetamine- (n_{case} = 58), cocaine- (n_{case} = 68), and fentalog- (n_{case} = 33)

TABLE 1— Demographic Information per Case of the Fatal Fentanyl Overdose Decedent Corresponding to Sample Type: San Francisco, CA, 2022

	Total	Baggie/ Powder, No. (%)	Nonbulbous Glass Pipe, No. (%)	Bulbous Glass Pipe, No. (%)	Aluminum Foil, No. (%)	Syringe, No. (%)	Crystalline Substance, No. (%)	Straw, No. (%)	Pill, No. (%)	Cooper Pad, No. (%)	Cooker, No. (%)	Pushers/ Plungers/ Poker, No. (%)	Miscellaneous., No. (%)
Total	137	81	45	24	29	20	14	16	9	7	8	8	9
Gender													
Male	105 (77)	64 (79)	31 (69)	18 (75)	23 (79)	8 (40)	12 (86)	12 (75)	7 (78)	6 (86)	4 (50)	4 (50)	6 (67)
Female	32 (23)	17 (21)	14 (31)	6 (25)	6 (21)	12 (60)	2 (14)	4 (25)	2 (22)	1 (14)	4 (50)	4 (50)	3 (33)
Age, y													
15–24	3 (2)	2 (2)	...	...	2 (7)	...	...	2 (13)	...	...	...	...	...
25–34	27 (20)	18 (22)	2 (4)	5 (21)	13 (45)	5 (25)	2 (14)	4 (25)	3 (33)	2 (29)	3 (38)	1 (13)	1 (11)
35–44	36 (26)	20 (25)	9 (20)	8 (33)	7 (24)	9 (45)	8 (57)	6 (38)	1 (11)	1 (14)	1 (13)	2 (25)	3 (33)
45–54	32 (23)	18 (22)	12 (27)	6 (25)	7 (24)	2 (10)	2 (14)	2 (13)	3 (33)	...	2 (25)	1 (13)	1 (11)
55–64	29 (21)	16 (20)	15 (33)	5 (21)	...	3 (15)	2 (14)	2 (13)	2 (22)	2 (29)	1 (13)	3 (38)	2 (22)
≥ 65	10 (7)	7 (9)	7 (16)	...	...	1 (5)	...	...	...	2 (29)	1 (13)	1 (13)	2 (22)
Race													
Asian	5 (4)	2 (2)	1 (2)	2 (8)	1 (3)	...	...	...	...	1 (14)	...	...	...
Black	41 (30)	22 (27)	14 (31)	6 (25)	11 (38)	8 (40)	...	5 (31)	2 (22)	3 (43)	3 (38)	4 (50)	5 (56)
Latinx	13 (9)	7 (9)	5 (11)	2 (8)	1 (3)	2 (10)	1 (7)	1 (6)	1 (11)	2 (29)	1 (13)	1 (13)	...
White	72 (53)	46 (57)	23 (51)	13 (54)	14 (48)	9 (45)	12 (86)	8 (50)	6 (67)	1 (14)	4 (50)	3 (38)	4 (44)
Other	6 (4)	4 (5)	2 (4)	1 (4)	2 (7)	1 (5)	1 (7)	2 (13)	...	...	...	...	...
Fixed Address													
Yes	91 (66)	60 (74)	35 (78)	11 (46)	12 (41)	9 (45)	6 (43)	6 (38)	7 (78)	4 (57)	5 (63)	6 (75)	7 (78)
No	46 (34)	21 (26)	10 (22)	13 (54)	17 (59)	11 (55)	8 (57)	10 (63)	2 (22)	3 (43)	3 (38)	2 (25)	2 (22)

Note. The sample size was n = 137. Many cases had more than 1 sample type present, causing the total for all sample types (n = 270) to be greater than the total number of cases (n = 137). Furthermore, we counted multiple items of the same sample type in 1 case as 1, so that the total number of drug material and paraphernalia (n = 409) exceeds the total for all sample types (e.g., 6 syringes and 2 glass pipes from 1 case count as 1 syringe and 1 glass pipe).

TABLE 2— Common Drugs Detected in Drug Material and Paraphernalia, Total, Individually, or in Combination: San Francisco, CA, 2022

	Total, No. (%)	Baggie/ Powder, No. (%)	Nonbulbous Glass Pipe, No. (%)	Aluminum Foil, No. (%)	Bulbous Glass Pipe, No. (%)	Syringe, No. (%)	Straw, No. (%)	Crystalline Substance, No. (%)	Pill, No. (%)	Pusher/ Plunger/ Poker, No. (%)	Cooker, No. (%)	Copper Pad, No. (%)	Miscellaneous,[a] No. (%)
Total	409	121 (30)	86 (21)	38 (9)	37 (9)	32 (8)	20 (5)	20 (5)	15 (4)	13 (3)	9 (2)	7 (2)	11 (3)
Individual drugs													
Fentanyl													
Total	219 (53)	77 (64)	49 (57)	28 (74)	14 (38)	15 (47)	14 (70)	2 (10)	2 (13)	6 (46)	5 (56)	2 (29)	5 (45)
Alone	41 (10)	28 (23)	1 (1)	7 (18)	. . .	2 (6)	2 (10)	. . .	1 (7)	. . .	. . .	. . .	. . .
Methamphetamine													
Total	146 (36)	28 (23)	10 (12)	19 (50)	33 (89)	20 (63)	8 (40)	17 (85)	1 (7)	2 (15)	4 (44)	2 (29)	2 (18)
Alone	55 (13)	9 (7)	1 (1)	1 (3)	19 (51)	10 (31)	. . .	12 (60)	1 (7)	. . .	1 (11)	1 (14)	. . .
Cocaine													
Total	167 (41)	41 (34)	78 (91)	2 (5)	6 (16)	2 (6)	8 (40)	3 (15)	1 (7)	11 (85)	4 (44)	4 (57)	7 (64)
Alone	29 (7)	6 (5)	15 (17)	. . .	. . .	. . .	1 (5)	2 (10)	. . .	3 (23)	. . .	2 (29)	. . .
FAN													
Total	91 (22)	26 (21)	21 (24)	15 (39)	7 (19)	5 (16)	9 (45)	2 (10)	. . .	2 (15)	2 (22)	1 (14)	1 (9)
Alone	5 (1)	2 (2)	. . .	1 (3)	. . .	1 (3)	1 (5)	. . .	. . .	. . .	. . .	. . .	. . .
Drug combinations													
Fentanyl + cocaine	48 (12)	17 (14)	21 (24)	. . .	1 (3)	1 (3)	1 (5)	. . .	1 (7)	3 (23)	. . .	1 (14)	2 (18)
Fentanyl + methamphetamine	23 (6)	6 (5)	1 (1)	6 (16)	4 (11)	5 (16)	1 (5)	. . .	. . .	. . .	. . .	. . .	. . .
Fentanyl + FAN	18 (4)	11 (9)	1 (1)	4 (11)	1 (3)	1 (3)	. . .	. . .	. . .	. . .	. . .	. . .	. . .
Fentanyl + methamphetamine + FAN	20 (5)	3 (2)	. . .	8 (21)	1 (3)	3 (9)	1 (5)	2 (10)	. . .	1 (8)	. . .	1 (14)	. . .
Fentanyl + cocaine + FAN	26 (6)	3 (2)	15 (17)	1 (3)	1 (3)	. . .	3 (15)	. . .	. . .	1 (8)	2 (22)	. . .	. . .
Fentanyl + xylazine[b]	16 (4)	2 (2)	3 (3)	1 (3)	2 (5)	2 (6)	4 (20)	. . .	. . .	1 (8)	. . .	. . .	1 (9)
Miscellaneous[c]	112 (27)	29 (24)	28 (33)	5 (13)	8 (22)	5 (16)	3 (15)	4 (20)	12 (80)	3 (23)	6 (67)	1 (14)	8 (73)
None detected	16 (4)	5 (4)	. . .	4 (11)	. . .	2 (6)	3 (15)	. . .	. . .	1 (8)	. . .	1 (14)	. . .

Note. FAN = fentanyl analog. The sample size was n = 409.

[a]Miscellaneous includes bindle with nonpowder (black tarry substance), a baggie of nonpowder (mushrooms), brown substance (n = 3), green vegetable material (n = 2), a joint (n = 2), a razor blade, and a vape pen.

[b]Fentanyl/xylazine either alone or with other substances (commonly methamphetamine or cocaine).

[c]Miscellaneous drugs and drug combinations are further detailed in Table E (available as a supplement to the online version of this article at http://www.ajph.org).

TABLE 3— Demographic Information of the Fatal Fentanyl Overdose Decedent Corresponding to the Drugs That Were Present in 1 or More of Their Respective Drug Material and Paraphernalia, Total, Alone, or in Combination: San Francisco, CA, 2022

	Total, No. (%)	Gender, No. (%)		Age, Years, No. (%)						Race/Ethnicity, No. (%)					Fixed Address, No. (%)	
		Male	Female	15–24	25–34	35–44	45–54	55–64	≥65	Asian	Black	Latinx	White	Other	Yes	No
Individual drugs																
Fentanyl	137	105 (77)	32 (23)	3 (2)	27 (20)	36 (26)	32 (23)	29 (21)	10 (7)	5 (4)	41 (30)	13 (9)	72 (53)	6 (4)	91 (66)	46 (34)
Total	106 (77)	82 (77)	24 (23)	3 (3)	22 (21)	27 (25)	25 (24)	21 (20)	8 (8)	3 (3)	33 (31)	12 (11)	52 (49)	6 (6)	72 (68)	34 (32)
Alone	35 (26)	25 (71)	10 (29)	1 (3)	7 (20)	10 (29)	8 (23)	8 (23)	1 (3)	1 (3)	11 (31)	3 (9)	17 (49)	3 (9)	24 (69)	11 (31)
Methamphetamine																
Total	58 (42)	41 (71)	17 (29)	1 (2)	13 (22)	16 (28)	14 (24)	10 (17)	4 (7)	3 (5)	18 (31)	2 (3)	33 (57)	2 (3)	30 (52)	28 (48)
Alone	25 (18)	17 (68)	8 (32)	. . .	6 (24)	8 (32)	6 (24)	5 (20)	. . .	1 (4)	5 (20)	2 (8)	16 (64)	1 (4)	9 (36)	16 (64)
Cocaine																
Total	68 (50)	52 (76)	16 (24)	2 (3)	7 (10)	15 (22)	15 (22)	21 (31)	8 (12)	3 (4)	22 (32)	7 (10)	33 (49)	3 (4)	54 (79)	14 (21)
Alone	18 (13)	12 (67)	6 (33)	1 (6)	1 (6)	3 (17)	2 (11)	9 (50)	2 (11)	1 (6)	4 (22)	4 (22)	8 (44)	1 (6)	14 (78)	4 (22)
FAN																
Total	33 (24)	28 (85)	5 (15)	1 (3)	9 (27)	9 (27)	7 (21)	3 (9)	4 (12)	1 (3)	8 (24)	4 (12)	19 (58)	1 (3)	21 (64)	12 (36)
Alone	4 (3)	4 (100)	. . .	1 (25)	1 (25)	1 (25)	. . .	1 (25)	. . .	. . .	. . .	. . .	4 (100)	. . .	2 (50)	2 (50)
Xylazine[a]	14 (10)	9 (64)	5 (36)	. . .	3 (21)	4 (29)	5 (36)	2 (14)	. . .	1 (7)	5 (36)	1 (7)	7 (50)	. . .	8 (57)	6 (43)
Drug combinations																
Fentanyl + cocaine	29 (27)	23 (79)	6 (21)	1 (3)	3 (10)	9 (31)	3 (10)	9 (31)	4 (14)	1 (3)	9 (31)	2 (7)	14 (48)	3 (10)	25 (86)	4 (14)
Fentanyl + methamphetamine	16 (15)	11 (69)	5 (31)	1 (6)	6 (38)	6 (38)	1 (6)	2 (13)	. . .	1 (6)	7 (44)	1 (6)	7 (44)	. . .	5 (31)	11 (69)
Fentanyl + FAN	14 (10)	13 (93)	1 (7)	. . .	4 (29)	4 (29)	4 (29)	1 (7)	1 (7)	. . .	3 (21)	4 (29)	6 (43)	1 (7)	10 (71)	4 (29)
Fentanyl + cocaine + FAN	13 (9)	11 (85)	2 (15)	1 (8)	2 (15)	3 (23)	3 (23)	2 (15)	2 (15)	1 (8)	4 (31)	1 (8)	7 (54)	. . .	8 (62)	5 (38)
Fentanyl + methamphetamine + FAN	9 (7)	7 (78)	2 (22)	. . .	3 (33)	2 (22)	3 (33)	. . .	1 (11)	. . .	2 (22)	. . .	6 (67)	1 (11)	4 (44)	5 (56)
Miscellaneous[b]	26 (19)	21 (81)	5 (19)	1 (4)	6 (23)	7 (27)	5 (19)	3 (12)	4 (15)	. . .	6 (23)	2 (8)	18 (69)	. . .	19 (73)	7 (27)

Note. FAN = fentanyl analog. The sample size was n = 137. Many cases had more than 1 drug present, resulting in the total for all drugs present (n = 305) being greater than the total number of cases (n = 137).

[a]Xylazine detected with other substances (always with fentanyl, also commonly with methamphetamine or cocaine). No cases contained just xylazine (i.e., xylazine alone).

[b]Includes miscellaneous drugs and drug combinations (e.g., heroin, ketamine, mescaline, THC [tetrahydrocannabinol], fentanyl, and cocaine/heroin).

positive cases, males contributed 41 (71%), 52 (76%), and 28 (85%), respectively, whereas females contributed 17 (29%), 16 (24%), and 5 (15%), respectively. The number of times we detected each drug from these 137 fatal fentanyl overdose cases is displayed in Table D (available as a supplement to the online version of this article at http://www.ajph.org).

Fentanyl. We detected fentanyl either alone or in combination with another substance in 77% of cases (n_{case} = 106; n_{sample} = 219) and did not detect it in 23% of cases. Fentanyl was the most common drug detected alone in 26% of cases (n_{case} = 35; n_{sample} = 41). The most instances of fentanyl alone were in baggies and powders (n_{sample} = 28) and aluminum foil (n_{sample} = 7). We detected fentanyl alone in 2 syringes, 2 straws, 1 pill, and 1 nonbulbous glass pipe. We did not detect fentanyl alone in bulbous glass pipes, crystalline substances, cookers, copper pads, or pushers, plungers, or pokers.

Fentanyl analogs. In 24% of cases (n_{case} = 33; n_{sample} = 91), we detected fentalogs, and in 4 of these cases, (n_{sample} = 5) we did not detect fentanyl or any other substances; thus we detected fentalogs alone in only 5% of samples. In cases in which we detected fentalogs alone, we detected *para*-fluoro fentanyl in 4, methoxyacetyl fentanyl in 2, and acryl fentanyl and furanyl ethyl fentanyl in 1. All fentalogs detected are displayed in Table D along with their prevalence, the most common being fluorofentanyl. We detected the most instances of fentalogs in baggies and powders, nonbulbous glass pipes, and aluminum foil.

Methamphetamine. We detected methamphetamine alone in 18% of cases (n_{case} = 25; n_{sample} = 55). Amphetamine was present in 13 cases, always in the presence of methamphetamine. Bulbous glass pipes had a higher instance of methamphetamine (n_{sample} = 19) alone than did nonbulbous pipes (n_{sample} = 1), as these pipes are more commonly used to smoke methamphetamine. In our analysis of syringes, we observed a higher instance of methamphetamine alone (n_{sample} = 10) than any other drug. Additionally, 60% (n_{sample} = 12) of crystalline substances and 9 baggies and powders samples were positive for methamphetamine alone.

Cocaine. We detected cocaine alone in 13% of cases (n_{case} = 18; n_{sample} = 29). We detected anhydroecgonine methyl ester, a product of cocaine pyrolysis and therefore an indication of smoking cocaine, in 138 samples, and benzoylecgonine, which is formed by the hydrolysis of cocaine, in 14 samples. There were no instances of cocaine alone in syringes, suggesting that injecting cocaine is not common. We found that pipes without bulbs are more commonly used to smoke cocaine, as evidenced by the 15 cases in which we identified cocaine in nonbulbous glass pipes and the absence of cocaine in bulbous glass pipes.

Other common drugs. We detected heroin in 2 cases alone (n_{sample} = 4) and in conjunction with cocaine, methamphetamine, or fentanyl in 9 cases (n_{sample} = 19). We often observed morphine, codeine, papaverine, and noscapine, all opium alkaloids, with the heroin samples. We detected THC alone in 6 cases (n_{sample} = 6) and in conjunction with cocaine, methamphetamine, or fentanyl in 17 cases (n_{sample} = 23). We often observed cannabinol, cannabidiol, and cannabichromene, naturally occurring cannabinoids, in these samples. We detected ketamine in 3 cases, psilocin in 1 case, and the veterinary tranquilizer xylazine, which was always in combination with fentanyl, in 14 cases.

Polysubstance occurrence. Apparent co-use of drugs across different drug classes was highly prevalent in the DMP, as we detected 2 or more substances in 235 (57%) DMP samples. We detected fentanyl and cocaine combinations in 12% of samples (n_{sample} = 48; 21% of cases), whereas we detected fentanyl plus methamphetamine combinations in 6% of samples (n_{sample} = 23; 12% of cases). The combination trio of fentanyl, methamphetamine, and cocaine was less common, which we detected in only 1 case. We often detected fentalogs alongside fentanyl (n_{sample} = 18; 10% of cases) or in combination with fentanyl and either methamphetamine (n_{sample} = 20; 7% of cases) or cocaine (n_{sample} = 26; 9% of cases).

We observed more combinations of fentanyl and cocaine than of fentanyl and methamphetamine in every sample type except aluminum foil, syringes, and bulbous glass pipes. We detected fentanyl plus cocaine in 21 nonbulbous glass pipes and 17 baggies and powders, whereas we found fentanyl plus methamphetamine in only 1 nonbulbous glass pipe and 6 baggies and powders. We observed syringes to have a higher instance of fentanyl plus methamphetamine (n_{sample} = 5; 16%) than other combinations: fentanyl plus cocaine (2%); fentanyl, methamphetamine, and cocaine (1%). Bulbous glass pipes had a higher instance of fentanyl plus methamphetamine than did nonbulbous pipes, which had a higher instance of fentanyl plus cocaine.

Overall, methamphetamine plus cocaine combinations were rare, as were fentanyl, methamphetamine, and cocaine combinations.

Cutting agents. Common cutting agents we observed in DMP were lidocaine (77 samples), mannitol (36), ibuprofen (18), levamisole (14), acetaminophen (12), gabapentin (3), phenacetin (2), and diphenhydramine (1). Lidocaine was the most common cutting agent for cocaine (n = 70 samples), and we rarely detected cutting agents with methamphetamine. We found that mannitol was a common cutting agent with fentanyl (n = 36 samples).

DISCUSSION

Monitoring DMP from overdose decedents can provide useful information to public health and safety officials about drug availability and use, including the combinations of substances, how people who use drugs (PWUD) are either concurrently or separately using fentanyl and stimulants and other drug combinations, and how these substances move across regions. This joins several other drug use–monitoring techniques, including emergency department monitoring, wastewater surveillance, controlled substance (e.g., drug material) seizures,[14–16] accidental drug overdose investigation,[17,18] and self-reporting or voluntary paraphernalia submissions to drug-checking services in harm reduction programs.[7,19–22]

Fentanyl was the drug we detected the most, expectedly, as the samples were from fentanyl-involved fatal accidental drug overdoses. However, we did not detect fentanyl in 23% of cases, presumably owing to 1 of the following scenarios: the decedent disposed of the DMP they used containing fentanyl at a location different from where they were found, another individual's DMP was used to consume fentanyl, consumption occurred without DMP, the DMP used to consume fentanyl was not collected, or DMP nearby were incorrectly assumed to be the decedent's and were collected. These scenarios may apply to all drugs, in addition to fentanyl.

We detected several fentalogs or their precursors in this study, the most common being fluorofentanyl and its precursor despropionyl fluorofentanyl. Many of these fentalogs have been reported previously in the literature, specifically fluorofentanyl, acrylfentanyl, and methoxyacetyl fentanyl, although they are found primarily in biological material, seldom DMP. We present the first, to our knowledge, detection in San Francisco of most of these fentalogs, along with an in-depth study on 2022 San Francisco fatal accidental overdoses that reveals and discusses the prevalence of these novel synthetic opioids, specifically fluorofentanyl.[5] Furthermore, we reveal that xylazine in DMP has spread across the United States from the East Coast.

Polysubstance use with fentanyl is commonly reported in the literature,[2,3,19] consistent with our findings, in which 21% of cases were positive for fentanyl plus cocaine and 12% of cases were positive for fentanyl plus methamphetamine. We detected fentanyl combined with cocaine or methamphetamine in patterns consistent with the fourth wave of the opioid crisis, which Ciccarone describes as rising morbidity and mortality from the combined use of opioids and psychostimulants.[2] In Indiana, a comparison of postmortem toxicology results and drug paraphernalia analysis in overdose deaths involving opioids and a stimulant showed that the deaths were largely the result of the course of opioids and stimulants separately, rather than the use of those 2 drug categories combined.[6] Our study was not intended to discern such factors.

However, that we detected fentanyl alone in a small number of glass pipes may indicate that PWUD are smoking fentanyl mixed with a stimulant or that the stimulant drug is residual. Individuals consuming fentanyl may also be using a nonbulbous glass pipe as a straw to inhale the drug and then using the same pipe to consume other drugs, such as cocaine. This scenario may explain why we detected high levels of both drugs in this DMP category. We detected fentanyl alone most frequently in baggies and powder and in aluminum foil, suggesting that smoking fentanyl using aluminum foil or snorting the powder are the most popular routes of administration in San Francisco.

We found that nonbulbous pipes were used more often for fentalogs than were bulbous glass pipes; we detected the combination of fentanyl, fentalog, and cocaine in 15 samples, demonstrating that fentalogs plus cocaine are a more common combination. However, this could be owing to fentanyl being adulterated with fentalogs. As with fentanyl, we detected the highest instances of fentalogs in baggies and powders, aluminum foil, and nonbulbous glass pipes, which suggests that snorting or smoking fentalogs in powder form using foil or nonbulbous glass pipes is similarly the most popular route of administration. However, many decedents and PWUD in general are most likely unknowingly consuming fentalogs, explaining the high incidence of fentanyl plus fentalog in the same DMP type.

Syringe surveillance or needle exchange programs allow drug use monitoring. Research conducted in New York City and Washington, DC, through these programs found that fentanyl is the most common drug detected: 17% of syringes in New York City and 41% in Washington, DC, were found to contain fentanyl alone.[7,20] Of the 32 syringes we analyzed in this study, fentanyl was present in 15 (47%). An increase of 74% in smoking administration and a decrease of 29% in injection among overdose decedents was observed throughout the United States from 2020 to 2022.[12] In King County, Washington, from 2019 to 2022, drug use evidence collected from overdose death scenes showed that fentanyl was the most common drug in powder (n = 158; 17.3%), M30 pills (n = 264; 43.9%), straws (n = 241; 27.5%), pen barrels (n = 46; 24.9%), and foil (n = 172; 22.9%).[8]

Our findings are consistent with previous reports identifying smoking or snorting as the most common routes of fentanyl administration in San Francisco. Kral et al. reported a steady decrease in the number of people who inject drugs in San Francisco, from a median of 92 injections in 2018 to 17 injections in 2020.[11] Kral et al. also observed that the rate of opioid injections was reduced by half, as many PWUD stated that they were switching from injecting tar heroin to smoking fentanyl mainly because of difficulty accessing veins. In interviews with 34 PWUD in San Francisco, 15 individuals reported injecting fentanyl, whereas 28 individuals reported smoking fentanyl.[23] Motivations to transition from injecting to smoking fentanyl in this study included difficulty injecting and fear of overdose.

We found that syringes made up only 10% of the DMP collected at overdose scenes in 2022, supporting the notion that injecting drugs has become less common despite illicit opioids such as heroin and fentanyl historically being administered by injection.[21,24–26] However, this assumption relies on investigators collecting syringe samples, which may be less common than other sample types because of biohazardous concerns. Palamar et al. examined seizure data on fentanyl-containing powders across the United States from 2017 to 2023 and observed an increase in the number of powder seizures containing fentanyl.[27] During these years, the number of powder fentanyl seizures in the United States increased from 1171 to 11 980, with the West having the steepest increase (adjusted annual percentage change = 95%); this is consistent with our detecting fentanyl mostly in powdered form.

A Centers for Disease Control and Prevention report observed that evidence of counterfeit pill use in overdose deaths tripled in 8 Western US states from July to September 2019 through October to December 2021, and 56% of overdose deaths with evidence of counterfeit pill use occurred in Western jurisdictions.[28] The number of pill seizures in the United States increased from 134 in 2017 to 11 537 in 2023 (a higher than 8500% increase), with the Western region experiencing the largest increase.[27] The Drug Enforcement Administration has recognized that proximity to the Mexican border increases the chance of illicit fentanyl pill availability in California, as Mexico is a primary manufacturing site for counterfeit fentanyl-laced pills.[29,30] In Arizona, another border state, seizures of counterfeit pharmaceutical pills that contain fentanyl have increased more than 700%.[22] Of note, we detected only 3 illicit pills in this study, with 2 containing fentanyl.

Limitations

Limitations of this study include our inability to determine whether drugs were mixed intentionally before use, whether the drugs were already mixed in a sample (whether the individual knew or not), whether detected drugs were residual from previous use, and whether the DMP was used by more than 1 individual or belonged to a different individual entirely. Additionally, more DMP may have been present at the scene of death but not collected, as many decedents' residences were cluttered, increasing the chance that DMP was not retrieved. Furthermore, a decedent could have been using another individual's DMP or using drugs at a location other than the place of death.

Another limitation of this study is the variation in drug concentrations across different DMP items, which may affect detection sensitivity. Fentalogs, in particular, may go undetected unless standard drug material amounts are tested. Additionally, this study has limited external validity: the study population (i.e., individuals who died from fentanyl-involved accidental overdoses in San Francisco for whom DMP was collected) may not fully represent the broader population of PWUD in San Francisco.

Public Health Implications

As the complex drug overdose epidemic continues, it is important to identify which substances contribute to fatal overdoses. We observed a high instance of fentanyl alone and in combination with either methamphetamine or cocaine. We detected several fentalogs, along with xylazine, typically in combination with fentanyl, suggesting that fentanyl is being laced with more emerging substances. We observed an increase in smoking fentanyl and a subsequent decrease in the injection of illicit drugs.

We provide objective data demonstrating the prevalence of illicit drug use, including potent synthetic opioids. This information can aid in strengthening harm reduction and public health services to better address the ongoing drug overdose epidemic and identify emerging substances. AJPH

ABOUT THE AUTHORS

All authors are with the Office of the Chief Medical Examiner, San Francisco, CA. Luke N. Rodda is also with the Department of Laboratory Medicine, University of California, San Francisco.

CORRESPONDENCE

Correspondence should be sent to Luke N. Rodda, PhD, Office of the Chief Medical Examiner, 1 Newhall St, San Francisco, CA 94124 (e-mail: luke.rodda@sfgov.org). Reprints can be ordered at https://www.ajph.org by clicking the "Reprints" link.

PUBLICATION INFORMATION

Full Citation: Diekhans K, Yu J, Pearring S, Almeida R, Rodda LN. The fourth wave of the opioid epidemic: increasing combination of fentanyl with stimulants. *Am J Public Health*. 2025;115(4):555–565.

Acceptance Date: November 16, 2024.

DOI: https://doi.org/10.2105/AJPH.2024.307948

ORCID iDs:

Katie Diekhans https://orcid.org/0009-0005-7546-5499

Jihau Yu https://orcid.org/0009-0007-0224-4083

Sue Pearring https://orcid.org/0000-0002-1501-112X

Robert Almeida https://orcid.org/0009-0001-6617-9547

Luke N. Rodda https://orcid.org/0000-0001-8660-6481

CONTRIBUTORS

K. Diekhans collected and analyzed the data and wrote the original draft of the article. L. N. Rodda conceptualized the study, acquired funding, and supervised and administrated the project. All authors designed the methodology and thoroughly reviewed and revised the article and approved this version.

ACKNOWLEDGMENTS

This work was supported by the California Department of Public Health, Substance and Addiction Prevention Branch (Enhance Forensic Toxicology grant 21-10808).

CONFLICTS OF INTEREST

The authors have no conflicts of interest to disclose.

HUMAN PARTICIPANT PROTECTION

No protocol approval was necessary because no human participants were involved in this study.

REFERENCES

1. Centers for Disease Control and Prevention. Provisional drug overdose death counts. January 15, 2025. Available at: https://www.cdc.gov/nchs/nvss/vsrr/drug-overdose-data.htm. Accessed January 22, 2025.
2. Ciccarone D. The rise of illicit fentanyls, stimulants and the fourth wave of the opioid overdose crisis. *Curr Opin Psychiatry*. 2021;34(4):344–350. https://doi.org/10.1097/YCO.0000000000000717
3. West KL, Lindquist K, Rodda LN. Fentanyl epidemic hits the US West Coast: opioid-related deaths in San Francisco from 2009–2019. *Int J Drug Policy*. 2021;95:103402. https://doi.org/10.1016/j.drugpo.2021.103402
4. San Francisco Office of the Chief Medical Examiner. Accidental overdose reports. Available at: https://sf.gov/resource/2020/ocme-accidental-overdose-reports. Accessed January 22, 2025.
5. Yu J, Diekhans K, Tsang A, Rodda LN. Fluorofentanyl and novel synthetic opioids in accidental overdose deaths. *J Anal Toxicol*. 2024;48(8):573–581. https://doi.org/10.1093/jat/bkae062
6. Lockwood TE, Huynh P, Richard A, et al. Community overdose surveillance: comparing substances collected from the death scene investigation to toxicology results. *Drug Alcohol Depend*. 2021;224:108722. https://doi.org/10.1016/j.drugalcdep.2021.108722
7. Evans A, Krause M, Leach S, Levitas M, Nguyen L, Short LC. Analysis of drug residue in needle-exchange syringes in Washington, D.C. *Forensic Sci Int*. 2021;329:111083. https://doi.org/10.1016/j.forsciint.2021.111083
8. Harruff R, Simpson CM, Gifford AL, Yarid N, Barbour WL, Heidere C. Evaluation of "real-time" fatal drug overdose surveillance by King County Medical Examiner's Office, Seattle, Washington. *Am J Forensic Med Pathol*. 2023;44(1):11–16. https://doi.org/10.1097/PAF.0000000000000798
9. Centers for Disease Control and Prevention. Trends and geographic patterns in drug and synthetic opioid overdose deaths—United States, 2013–2019. *MMWR Morb Mortal Wkly Rep*. 2021;70(6):202–207. https://doi.org/10.15585/mmwr.mm7006a4
10. Bradley H, Hall EW, Asher A, et al. Estimated number of people who inject drugs in the United States. *Clin Infect Dis*. 2023;76(1):96–102. https://doi.org/10.1093/cid/ciac543
11. Kral AH, Lambdin BH, Browne EN, et al. Transition from injecting opioids to smoking fentanyl in San Francisco, California. *Drug Alcohol Depend*. 2021;227:109003. https://doi.org/10.1016/j.drugalcdep.2021.109003
12. Centers for Disease Control and Prevention. Routes of drug use among drug overdose deaths—United States, 2020–2022. *MMWR Morb Mortal Wkly Rep*. 2024;73(6):124–130. https://doi.org/10.15585/mmwr.mm7306a2
13. Diekhans K, Yu J, Farley M, Rodda LN. Analysis of over 250 novel synthetic opioids and xylazine by LC-MS-MS in blood and urine. *J Anal Toxicol*. 2024;48(3):150–164. https://doi.org/10.1093/jat/bkae009
14. Palamar JJ, Ciccarone D, Rutherford C, Keyes KM, Carr TH, Cottler LB. Trends in seizures of powders and pills containing illicit fentanyl in the United States, 2018 through 2021. *Drug Alcohol Depend*. 2022;234:109398. https://doi.org/10.1016/j.drugalcdep.2022.109398
15. Park JN, Rashidi E, Foti K, Zoorob M, Sherman S, Alexander GC. Fentanyl and fentanyl analogs in the illicit stimulant supply: results from US drug seizure data, 2011–2016. *Drug Alcohol Depend*. 2021;218:108416. https://doi.org/10.1016/j.drugalcdep.2020.108416
16. Rosenblum D, Unick J, Ciccarone D. The rapidly changing US Illicit drug market and the potential for an improved early warning system: evidence from Ohio drug crime labs. *Drug Alcohol Depend*. 2020;208:107779. https://doi.org/10.1016/j.drugalcdep.2019.107779
17. Centers for Disease Control and Prevention. SUDORS dashboard: fatal drug overdose data. December 12, 2024. Available at: https://www.cdc.gov/overdose-prevention/data-research/facts-stats/sudors-dashboard-fatal-overdose-data.html. Accessed January 22, 2025.
18. Centers for Disease Control and Prevention. National Vital Statistics System. 2022. Available at: https://www.cdc.gov/nchs/nvss/index.htm. Accessed January 22, 2025.
19. Shearer RD, Howell BA, Bart G, Winkelman TNA. Substance use patterns and health profiles among US adults who use opioids, methamphetamine, or both, 2015–2018. *Drug Alcohol Depend*. 2020;214:108162. https://doi.org/10.1016/j.drugalcdep.2020.108162
20. Blachman-Forshay J, Nolan ML, McAteer JM, Paone D. Estimating the risk of exposure to fentanyl in New York City: testing drug residue in used syringes. *Am J Public Health*. 2018;108(12):1666–1668. https://doi.org/10.2105/AJPH.2018.304694
21. Buresh M, Genberg BL, Astemborski J, Kirk GD, Mehta SH. Recent fentanyl use among people who inject drugs: results from a rapid assessment in Baltimore, Maryland. *Int J Drug Policy*. 2019;74:41–46. https://doi.org/10.1016/j.drugpo.2019.08.006
22. Daniulaityte R, Sweeny K, Ki S, Doebbeling BN, Mendoza N. "They say it's fentanyl, but they honestly look like Perc 30s": initiation and use of counterfeit fentanyl pills. *Harm Reduct J*. 2022;19(1):52. https://doi.org/10.1186/s12954-022-00634-4
23. Ciccarone D, Holm N, Ondocsin J, et al. Innovation and adaptation: the rise of a fentanyl smoking culture in San Francisco. *PLoS One*. 2024;19(5):e0303403. https://doi.org/10.1371/journal.pone.0303403
24. Strang J, Griffiths P, Powis B, Abbey J, Gossop M. How constant is an individual's route of heroin administration? Data from treatment and non-treatment samples. *Drug Alcohol Depend*. 1997;46(1–2):115–118. https://doi.org/10.1016/S0376-8716(97)00035-5
25. Jarlais DC, Arasteh K, Feelemyer J, et al. From long-term injecting to long-term non-injecting heroin and cocaine use: the persistence of

changed drug habits. *J Subst Abuse Treat*. 2016;71:48–53. https://doi.org/10.1016/j.jsat.2016.08.015

26. Lankenau SE, Teti M, Silva K, Jackson Bloom J, Harocopos A, Treese M. Initiation into prescription opioid misuse amongst young injection drug users. *Int J Drug Policy*. 2012;23(1):37–44. https://doi.org/10.1016/j.drugpo.2011.05.014
27. Palamar JJ, Fitzgerald N, Carr TH, Cottler LB, Ciccarone D. National and regional trends in fentanyl seizures in the United States, 2017–2023. *Int J Drug Policy*. 2024;104417:104417. https://doi.org/10.1016/j.drugpo.2024.104417
28. Centers for Disease Control and Prevention. Drug overdose deaths with evidence of counterfeit pill use—United States, July 2019–December 2021. *MMWR Morb Mortal Wkly Rep*. 2023;72(35):949–956. https://doi.org/10.15585/mmwr.mm7235a3
29. Lassi N. Strengthening pill press control to combat fentanyl: legislative and law enforcement imperatives. *Explor Res Clin Soc Pharm*. 2023;11:100321. https://doi.org/10.1016/j.rcsop.2023.100321
30. US Department of Justice. Drug Enforcement Administration, National Drug Threat Assessment 2024. Available at: https://www.dea.gov/sites/default/files/2024-05/NDTA_2024.pdf. Accessed January 22, 2025.

State Child Abuse and Mandated Reporting Policies for Prenatal Substance Use and Congenital Syphilis Case Rates: United States, 2018–2022

Anna E. Austin, PhD, MPH, Kevin O'Callaghan, MB BCh BAO, Julie Rushmore, PhD, DVM, Ryan Cramer, JD, MPH, Robert McDonald, MD, MPH, and Emily R. Learner, PhD, MPH

Objectives. To estimate the association of state policies that define prenatal substance use as child abuse and mandate that health care professionals report prenatal substance use to child protective services with congenital syphilis case rates.

Methods. We used 2018 to 2022 US data on congenital syphilis case notifications to the National Notifiable Diseases Surveillance System. We conducted linear regression with a generalized estimating equation approach to compare congenital syphilis case rates in states with a child abuse policy only, a mandated reporting policy only, and both polices to rates in states with neither policy.

Results. After adjustment for confounders, the rate of congenital syphilis cases was, on average, 23.5 (95% confidence interval = 2.2, 44.8) cases per 100 000 live births higher in states with both a child abuse policy and a mandated reporting policy for prenatal substance use than in states with neither policy. Rates were similar in states with a child abuse policy only and a mandated reporting policy only compared to states with neither policy.

Conclusions. The combination of state child abuse policies and mandated reporting policies for prenatal substance use potentially contributes to higher congenital syphilis case rates. (*Am J Public Health*. 2025;115(4):566–574. https://doi.org/10.2105/AJPH.2024.307951)

AJPH April 2025, Vol. 115, No. 4

Cases of congenital syphilis have rapidly escalated over the past decade in the United States. From 2013 to 2022, the number of cases increased more than 10 times, from 362 in 2013 to 3755 in 2022, representing an increase from 9.2 to 102.5 cases per 100 000 live births.[1] Increases in congenital syphilis cases mirror increases in syphilis infections among pregnant women,[2] which, if untreated, can be transmitted to the fetus during pregnancy or at birth. Congenital syphilis can cause miscarriage, stillbirth, and neonatal death and result in adverse health and developmental outcomes among surviving infants.[3,4]

Substance use is associated with syphilis and congenital syphilis infection. Increases in substance use, particularly methamphetamine, heroin, and injection drug use, are correlated with recent increases in syphilis infections among women and heterosexual men.[5,6] This may be attributable to associations of substance use with sexual behaviors (e.g., inconsistent condom use, transactional sex) that increase the risk for syphilis transmission.[6] Among pregnant women with syphilis, substance use is nearly twice as high among those with a congenital syphilis pregnancy outcome (48%) than those without this outcome (25%),[7] underscoring an important association between prenatal substance use and congenital syphilis.

Congenital syphilis is preventable. Timely testing to identify syphilis infections during pregnancy and adequate treatment of identified syphilis infections can prevent perinatal transmission.[8] Leading medical and public health organizations recommend testing for syphilis infection in all pregnancies as early as possible or at the first prenatal visit.[8,9]

State prenatal substance use policies, including policies that define substance use during pregnancy as child abuse (i.e., child abuse policies) and policies that require health care professionals to report substance use during pregnancy to child protective services (CPS) agencies (i.e., mandated reporting policies), can create barriers to health care services[10–12] and may preclude receipt of timely syphilis testing and treatment during pregnancy.

In states with child abuse and mandated reporting policies, pregnant women engaging in substance use initiate prenatal care later and are less likely to have adequate prenatal care than those in states without these policies.[10] Receipt of substance use disorder treatment is also lower among pregnant women in states with these policies than among those in states without these policies.[11] Pregnant women using substances report delaying or avoiding prenatal care and other health care services because of the potential consequences of prenatal substance use, including CPS involvement and loss of infant custody.[12–16] Thus, state child abuse and mandated reporting policies for prenatal substance use may create barriers to health care engagement and, by extension, inhibit receipt of timely syphilis testing and treatment. This may be of particular concern for pregnant women engaging in substance use, a population at increased risk for syphilis during pregnancy and congenital syphilis as a pregnancy outcome.[7]

The primary aim of this study was to estimate the association of state child abuse policies and mandated reporting policies for prenatal substance use with rates of congenital syphilis cases. Because previous research shows delays and reductions in prenatal care and other health care services during pregnancy in states with these policies and these interactions are critical to ensuring timely syphilis testing and treatment, we hypothesized that states with child abuse policies and mandated reporting policies for prenatal substance use would have higher rates of congenital syphilis cases than states without these policies. The secondary aim was to describe missed congenital syphilis prevention opportunities by state policy context to provide actionable information for public health and clinical prevention efforts.

METHODS

We examined congenital syphilis case rates and state child abuse policies and mandated reporting policies for prenatal substance use during 2018 to 2022. We selected these years because they represent a period of rapid escalation in congenital syphilis case rates.[17]

Data Sources and Measures

We identified the years from 2018 to 2022 in which states had a child abuse policy and a mandated reporting policy for prenatal substance use using information from the Child Welfare Information Gateway, official state policy text from the Guttmacher Institute and available online from state agencies, and published studies that have reconciled differences across sources, including through direct contact with CPS agencies.[18–20] We categorized each state and year as having a child abuse policy only, a mandated reporting policy only, both policies, or neither policy (Appendix Table A, available as a supplement to the online version of this article at http://www.ajph.org).

For our primary analyses, we considered states to have a child abuse policy if prenatal substance use was criminalized or defined as child abuse or neglect under civil child welfare statutes, considered to be grounds for termination of parental rights, used as evidence to substantiate reports of child abuse or neglect, or resulted in placement on a CPS registry.[19] We considered states to have a mandated reporting policy if health care providers were required to report suspected or confirmed prenatal substance use to CPS agencies.[10]

Congenital syphilis is a reportable condition in all 50 states and the District of Columbia and is a nationally notifiable disease. All US jurisdictions voluntarily provide case notifications to the Centers for Disease Control and Prevention (CDC) through the National Notifiable Diseases Surveillance System using the Council of State and Territorial Epidemiologists case definition. We used 2018 to 2022 National Notifiable Diseases Surveillance System data on the annual number of congenital syphilis cases for all 50 states and the District of Columbia.

We created a conceptual diagram of factors likely operative in associations between these state policies and congenital syphilis case rates using existing empirical evidence and our subject matter expertise (Appendix Figure A, available as a supplement to the online version of this article at http://www.ajph.org). On the basis of our conceptual diagram, we adjusted analyses for time-varying indicators of the state health policy context (state Medicaid expansion, income thresholds for Medicaid eligibility for pregnant and postpartum women, percentage of adult women 19 to 64 years of age without health insurance, number of obstetricians/gynecologists per 100 000 live births, and policies specifying priority access to substance use disorder treatment for pregnant women) and state demographics (percentage of the population unemployed, percentage of the population in poverty, and race and ethnicity).

Statistical Analysis

We examined congenital syphilis case rates per 100 000 live births by year and state policy category. We calculated rates using live birth data from the National Center for Health Statistics. We also examined the distribution (mean, median, 25th percentile, and 75th percentile) of indicators of the state health policy context and state demographics over the entire study period by state policy category.

To compare congenital syphilis case rates in states with a child abuse policy only, a mandated reporting policy only, and both policies to rates in states with neither policy, we conducted linear regression with a generalized estimating equation approach and an exchangeable correlation matrix to account for repeated measures within states over time. Generalized estimating equations are a set of equations applied to regression models to estimate model coefficients and their standard errors when the outcomes are not independent, for example when there is clustering of data (e.g., repeated measures within states over time).[21] They are used to obtain population average estimates while accounting for the fact that outcomes within clusters (e.g., within states) are likely to be more similar than those between clusters (e.g., between states).[21] We adjusted regression models for the confounders noted previously and a linear time trend to account for secular trends over time.

We did not use a quasi-experimental study design, such as a difference-in-differences approach, as there was no prepolicy time for most states. Forty-eight of the states and the District of Columbia first implemented child abuse or mandated reporting policies before 2018 (Appendix Table A). Prepolicy time is necessary for conducting a difference-in-differences analysis as this approach leverages policy changes both over time and between states to generate estimates.[22]

The CDC uses National Notifiable Diseases Surveillance System case notification data and a stepwise analytic framework[23] to classify congenital syphilis cases by type of missed prevention opportunity. This framework classifies missed prevention opportunities as follows: (1) among all congenital syphilis cases, the number that had a nondocumented or nontimely test or late identification of seroconversion in pregnancy; (2) among cases with a timely test, the number with inadequate treatment or no or nondocumented treatment; and (3) among cases in which there was adequate treatment, the number with clinical evidence of congenital syphilis despite adequate treatment or with an unclear indication for inclusion as a reportable congenital syphilis case. We used information on missed prevention opportunities to create Sankey diagrams visualizing the number of missed prevention opportunities by state policy category and to calculate the unadjusted percentage of cases by type of missed prevention opportunity.

Sensitivity Analyses

We conducted multiple sensitivity analyses. First, given that some state child abuse policies have less severe consequences (e.g., placement on a CPS registry), we conducted analyses in which we classified only states with policies that criminalized prenatal substance use, defined it as child abuse or neglect, or considered it grounds for termination of parental rights as having a child abuse policy (Appendix Table A). Second, given that some state mandated reporting policies are less stringent and require reporting of prenatal substance use to CPS only if there is also suspicion of child abuse or neglect, we conducted analyses in which we classified states as having a mandated reporting policy if prenatal substance use alone was sufficient to require reporting (Appendix Table A).

Third, given the onset of the COVID-19 pandemic and acute disruptions to health care access in 2020, we conducted analyses excluding 2020. Fourth, we adjusted for the rate of primary and secondary syphilis infections among women 15 to 44 years of age per 100 000 population as a proxy for the incidence of syphilis in each state (Appendix Figure A).

Fifth, we adjusted for whether states required syphilis testing during the third trimester of pregnancy, overall or only for populations at increased risk, as of 2018.[24] Although this requirement is unlikely to affect whether states have a child abuse policy or mandated reporting policy for prenatal substance use, it is likely to affect receipt of syphilis testing and treatment during pregnancy. Finally, to assess whether our results were disproportionately influenced by states with high congenital syphilis case rates, we conducted analyses excluding California, a state with a child abuse policy only, and Florida and Texas, states with a mandated reporting policy only.

RESULTS

From 2018 to 2022, 10 states had a child abuse policy only, 8 had a mandated reporting policy only, 14 had both policies, and 16 had neither policy (Figure 1 and Appendix Table B, available as a supplement to the online version of this article at http://www.ajph.org). Three states initially had only one policy but switched to both policies in later years.

There were 12 009 congenital syphilis cases between 2018 and 2022. Rates of congenital syphilis cases per 100 000 live births increased steadily each year in all state policy categories (Figure 2 and Appendix Table A). In comparison to states with neither policy, rates of congenital syphilis cases were consistently higher in states with a child abuse policy only, states with a mandated reporting policy only, and states with both policies (52.8 vs 137.2, 102.1, and 109.8 cases per 100 000 live births in 2022, respectively).

Relative to other state policy categories, a higher average percentage of the population was American Indian/Alaska Native in states with a child abuse policy only, a mandated reporting policy only, or both policies; a higher average percentage of the population was Black in states with both policies; and a higher average percentage of the population was of Hispanic ethnicity in states with a child abuse policy only (Appendix Table C, available as a supplement to the online version of this article at http://www.ajph.org). There was higher average percentage of adult women without health insurance and a lower average number of obstetricians/gynecologists per 100 000 live births in states with a child abuse policy only than in other state policy categories. There were higher average percentages of years with state Medicaid expansion in states with a mandated reporting policy only and lower average percentages of years with an income threshold for Medicaid eligibility for pregnant and postpartum women that was above the US median in states with neither policy than in other state policy categories.

Adjusted models showed that the rate of congenital syphilis cases was, on average, 23.5 (95% confidence interval [CI] = 2.2, 44.8) cases per 100 000 live births higher in states with both a child

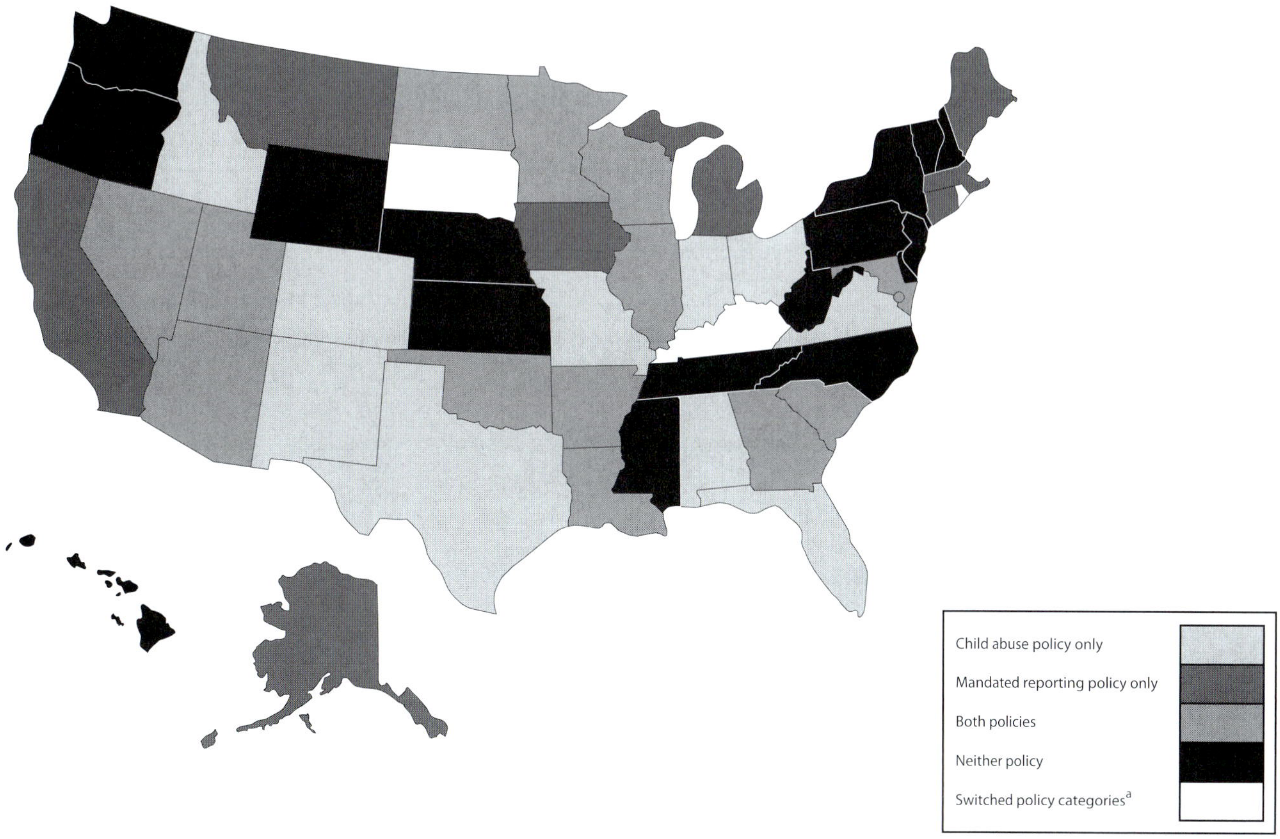

FIGURE 1— State Child Abuse and Mandated Reporting Policies for Prenatal Substance Use: United States, 2018–2022

[a]Three states initially had only one policy but then switched to both policies in later years.

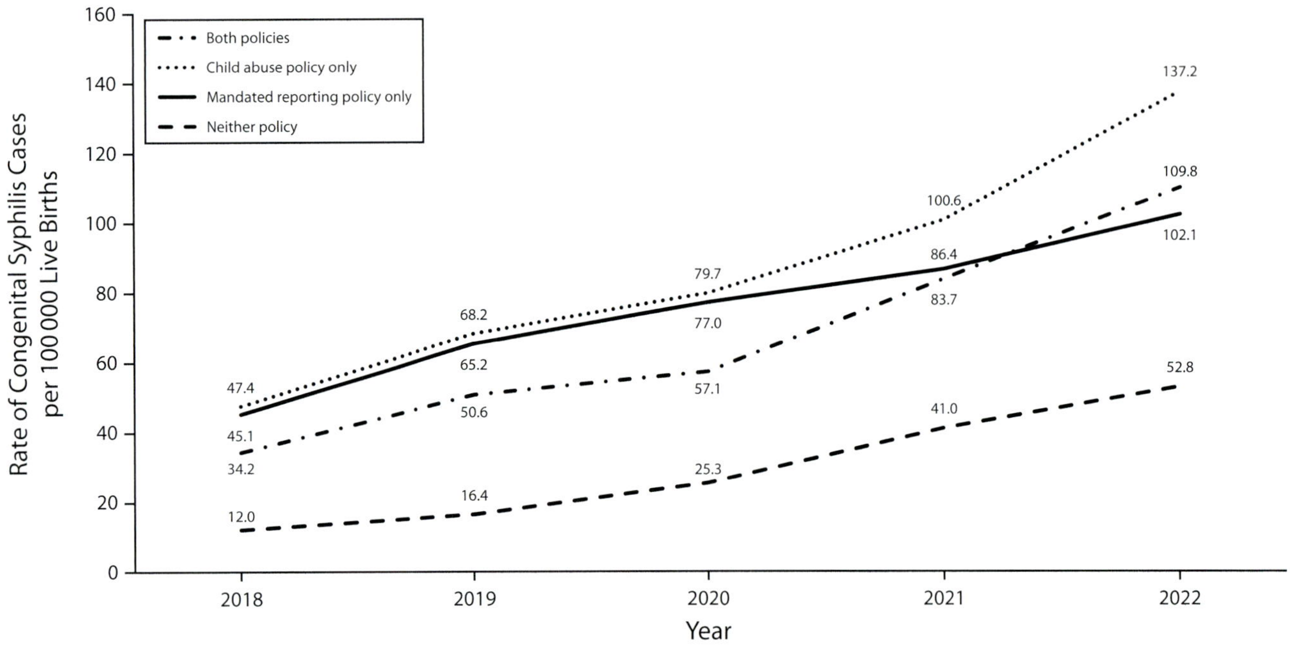

FIGURE 2— Rates of Congenital Syphilis Cases per 100 000 Live Births by State Prenatal Substance Use Policy Category: United States, 2018–2022

Note. Rates were calculated by summing numerators (number of congenital syphilis cases) and denominators (number of live births) across states in each category.

abuse policy and a mandated reporting policy for prenatal substance use than in states with neither policy (Table 1 and Figure 3). The rate of congenital syphilis cases was similar in states with a child abuse policy only (B = −0.4; 95% CI = −15.2, 14.5) and states with a mandated reporting policy only (B = 2.0; 95% CI = −11.0, 15.0) compared to states with neither policy.

The results were similar in sensitivity analyses in which

1. narrower definitions of state child abuse policies were used (Appendix Table D, available as a supplement to the online version of this article at http://www.ajph.org),
2. narrower definitions of state mandated reporting policies were used (Appendix Table E, available as a supplement to the online version of this article at http://www.ajph.org),
3. the year 2020 was excluded (Appendix Table F, available as a supplement to the online version of this article at http://www.ajph.org),
4. there was adjustment for the rate of syphilis infections among women 15 to 44 years of age (Appendix Table G, available as a supplement to the online version of this article at http://www.ajph.org),
5. there was adjustment for whether states required third-trimester syphilis testing (Appendix Table H, available as a supplement to the online version of this article at http://www.ajph.org),

TABLE 1— Mean Difference in Rates of Congenital Syphilis Cases per 100 000 Live Births by State Prenatal Substance Use Policy Category: United States, 2018–2022

State Policy Category	Unadjusted B (95% CI)	Adjusted B[a] (95% CI)
Neither policy (Ref)	0	0
Mandated reporting policy only	3.2 (−21.6, 28.1)	2.0 (−11.0, 15.0)
Child abuse policy only	18.6 (−16.6, 53.7)	−0.4 (−15.2, 14.5)
Both policies	41.7 (12.9, 70.5)	23.5 (2.2, 44.8)

Note. CI = confidence interval.
[a]Adjusted for a linear time trend and state Medicaid expansion, threshold for Medicaid eligibility for pregnant and postpartum people, percentage of women aged 19 to 64 years who were uninsured, number of obstetricians/gynecologists per 100 000 live births, policies specifying priority access to substance use disorder treatment for pregnant women, percentage of the population that was unemployed, percentage of the population in poverty, and percentage of the population by race and ethnicity.

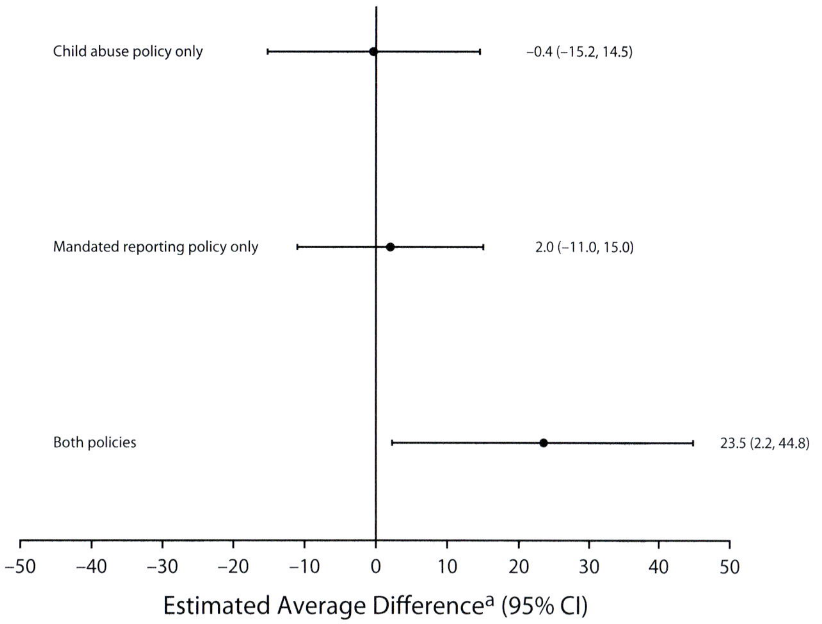

FIGURE 3— Average Difference in Rates of Congenital Syphilis Cases per 100 000 Live Births by State Prenatal Substance Use Policy Category: United States, 2018–2022

Note. CI = confidence interval.
[a]Adjusted for a linear time trend and state Medicaid expansion, threshold for Medicaid eligibility for pregnant and postpartum women percentage of women 19 to 64 years of age who are uninsured, number of obstetricians/gynecologists per 100 000 live births, policies specifying priority access to substance use disorder treatment for pregnant women percentage of the population that is unemployed, percentage of the population in poverty, and percentage of the population by race and ethnicity.

6. California was excluded (Appendix Table I, available as a supplement to the online version of this article at http://www.ajph.org), and
7. Florida and Texas were excluded (Appendix Table J, available as a supplement to the online version of this article at http://www.ajph.org).

Lack of timely testing and lack of adequate treatment were the most common missed congenital syphilis prevention opportunities in all state policy categories (Appendix Figures B–E and Appendix Table K, available as supplements to the online version of this article at http://www.ajph.org). Lack of timely testing among all congenital syphilis cases was highest in states with a mandated reporting policy only (59.0%), followed by states with neither policy (43.5%), states with both policies (38.0%), and states with a child abuse policy only (23.9%). Lack of treatment or inadequate treatment among cases with timely testing was high in all state policy categories. The percentage of cases with no or inadequate treatment was highest in states with a mandated reporting policy only (92.6%) and a child abuse policy only (91.8%), followed by states with neither policy (79.3%) and states with both policies (77.8%).

DISCUSSION

From 2018 to 2022, congenital syphilis case rates increased annually and were consistently higher in states with prenatal substance use policies (including states with a child abuse policy only, a mandated reporting policy only, and both policies) than in states with neither policies. In adjusted analyses, congenital syphilis case rates were higher in states with both a child abuse policy and a mandated reporting policy for prenatal substance use than in states with neither policy. On average, there were 23.5 more cases of congenital syphilis per 100 000 live births in states with both policies than in states with neither policy. In all state policy categories, lack of timely syphilis testing and lack of adequate treatment were key missed opportunities to prevent congenital syphilis cases.

Although states with both a child abuse policy and a mandated reporting policy for prenatal substance use had higher average congenital syphilis case rates than states with neither policy, adjusted analyses showed that case rates were similar in states with a child abuse policy only and a mandated reporting policy, compared to states

AJPH April 2025, Vol. 115, No. 4

with neither policy. Substance use during pregnancy is associated with syphilis and congenital syphilis infections.[5,7] Pregnant women engaging in substance use report that they avoid interacting with health care professionals who may detect their substance use, fearing that detection will result in CPS involvement and loss of infant custody.[12–16] In states with both a child abuse policy and a mandated reporting policy for prenatal substance use, there may be a clearer path to these feared outcomes than in states with only one of these policies. Specifically, in most states with both policies, not only are health care professionals required to report confirmed or suspected prenatal substance use to CPS, but prenatal substance use in and of itself can be used as grounds to substantiate abuse or neglect or to terminate parental rights.

In states with a mandated reporting policy only, health care professionals must report prenatal substance use to CPS, but this may not result in substantiated abuse or neglect or in termination of parental rights. In states with a child abuse policy only, prenatal substance use can be grounds for substantiating abuse or neglect or terminating parental rights, but it may not necessarily be reported to CPS. The synergistic combination of the 2 policies may be more likely to result in consequences that are perceived as punitive, amplifying fears among pregnant women and discouraging health care engagement.

A Massachusetts health center recently implemented new guidelines for health care responses to prenatal substance use that include a focus on providing trauma-informed care and substance use disorder treatment and require CPS reporting only if infant safety concerns are identified.[25] Recent research shows that implementation of these guidelines resulted in reductions in the number of prenatal substance use cases reported to CPS without corresponding increases in adverse short-term outcomes.[25] These results highlight the promise of trauma- and treatment-focused policies for prenatal substance use.

Of note, our analyses included all reported congenital syphilis cases and were not restricted to cases among pregnant women engaging in substance use, the population most likely to be affected by these state policies. Our results may underestimate associations between these policies and congenital syphilis case rates among pregnant women engaging in substance use. Previous research shows stronger associations of state child abuse policies with measures of prenatal care among pregnant women reporting substance use[10] than among the entire population of all live births.[19] It is possible that states with a child abuse policy only or a mandated reporting policy only have higher rates of congenital syphilis cases among pregnant women engaging in substance use than states with neither policy. Data on congenital syphilis case rates among pregnant women engaging in substance use are not currently available.

Across state policy categories, one fourth to more than one half of congenital syphilis cases did not have timely syphilis testing during pregnancy. Among cases that did receive timely testing, most did not receive adequate syphilis treatment. Lack of timely testing and lack of adequate treatment are key missed opportunities to prevent congenital syphilis. Promoting access to and engagement in prenatal care is a critical component of efforts to ensure timely syphilis testing and treatment.[26] Ensuring that syphilis testing is accessible in other community and clinical care settings, such as syringe service programs and emergency departments, and through point of care testing is also critical.[27] Reductions and delays in prenatal care and other health care services in states with child abuse policies and mandated reporting policies for prenatal substance use[10,19] may limit opportunities for syphilis testing and treatment.

Importantly, our results show that a higher percentage of the population was Black or American Indian/Alaska Native in states with both a child abuse policy and a mandated reporting policy for prenatal substance use than in states with neither policy. Disproportionate exposure to these policies among Black and American Indian/Alaska Native pregnant women has the potential to exacerbate existing disparities in prenatal care,[28] syphilis and congenital syphilis infections,[29] and CPS involvement.[30]

Limitations

This study has limitations. First, this was an ecological study conducted at the state level. The results do not allow for casual inferences regarding the potential impact of living in a state with a child abuse policy or a mandated reporting policy for prenatal substance use on congenital syphilis as a pregnancy outcome at the individual level. Second, although we adjusted for a comprehensive set of potential confounders, there may be unmeasured confounding. Specifically, because we were not able to use a quasi-experimental study design such as a difference-in-differences approach, there is the potential for unmeasured confounding resulting from differences in state contexts.

Third, there is some variation across states in the specifics of their child abuse policies and mandated reporting policies. However, our results were robust to sensitivity analyses incorporating narrower definitions of these policies. Fourth, how states implement child abuse policies and mandated reporting policies likely varies. Future research can further our understanding of differences in policy implementation across states and the potential implications of these differences for behaviors and receipt of health care services among pregnant women.

Finally, pregnant women may not necessarily be aware of specific state policies. However, pregnant women using substances report that they avoid health care interactions because they are afraid of detection and punishment, including CPS involvement and loss of infant custody.[12–16] They often note that these fears are based on their own experiences during previous pregnancies and knowledge of their family's and friends' experiences,[12–16] suggesting an overall awareness of the context and consequences created by child abuse policies and mandated reporting policies for prenatal substance use. Existing evidence aligns with these fears, showing higher rates of CPS reports[18] and foster care entries[31] among infants in states with these policies than in states without them.

Public Health Implications

Congenital syphilis is a serious condition that is preventable though timely syphilis testing and adequate treatment of infection during pregnancy. Rapidly increasing congenital syphilis case rates indicate an urgent need to reduce barriers to prenatal care, a critical opportunity for testing and treatment. Leading medical and public health organizations have issued statements recommending against child abuse policies and mandated reporting policies for prenatal substance use, noting that these policies can create barriers to care and subsequent harms to maternal and infant health.[32–34] Our results align with these statements, demonstrating elevated congenital syphilis case rates in states with both a child abuse policy and a mandated reporting policy for prenatal substance use. AJPH

ABOUT THE AUTHORS

At the time of the study, Anna E. Austin was with the University of North Carolina at Chapel Hill and the National Center for Injury Prevention and Control, Centers for Disease Control and Prevention, Atlanta, GA. Kevin O'Callaghan, Julie Rushmore, Ryan Cramer, Robert McDonald, and Emily R. Learner were with the Division of STD Prevention, Centers for Disease Control and Prevention. The findings and conclusions of this study are those of the authors and do not represent the official position of the Centers for Disease Control and Prevention.

CORRESPONDENCE

Correspondence should be sent to Anna Austin, PhD, MPH, National Center for Injury Prevention and Control,4770 Buford Hwy, Atlanta, GA 30341 (e-mail: une1@cdc.gov). Reprints can be ordered at https://www.ajph.org by clicking the "Reprints" link.

PUBLICATION INFORMATION

Full Citation: Austin AE, O'Callaghan K, Rushmore J, Cramer R, McDonald R, Learner ER. State child abuse and mandated reporting policies for prenatal substance use and congenital syphilis case rates: United States, 2018–2022. *Am J Public Health*. 2025;115(4):566–574.

Acceptance Date: November 18, 2024.

DOI: https://doi.org/10.2105/AJPH.2024.307951

ORCID iDs:

Anna E. Austin https://orcid.org/0000-0001-6605-363X

Kevin O'Callaghan https://orcid.org/0000-0002-0432-9730

Emily R. Learner https://orcid.org/0000-0003-3778-8631

CONTRIBUTORS

A. E. Austin conceptualized and designed the study, conducted the data analyses, interpreted results, and drafted the initial article. K. O'Callaghan conceptualized and designed the study, acquired the data, interpreted results, and revised the article for important intellectual content. J. Rushmore, R. Cramer, R. McDonald, and E. R. Learner conceptualized and designed the study, interpreted results, and revised the article for important intellectual content.

CONFLICTS OF INTEREST

The authors have no conflicts of interest to report.

HUMAN PARTICIPANT PROTECTION

Because all data were deidentified and aggregated at the state level, this study was not considered human participant research and thus did not require institutional review board approval.

REFERENCES

1. Centers for Disease Control and Prevention. Sexually transmitted infection surveillance, 2022. Available at: https://www.cdc.gov/std/statistics/2022/default.htm. Accessed May 29, 2024.
2. Gregory ECW, Ely DM. Trends and characteristics in maternal syphilis rates during pregnancy: United States, 2016–2022. Available at: https://www.cdc.gov/nchs/products/databriefs/db496.htm#:~:text=natality%20data%20file.-,Summary,and%20nearly%20all% 20reporting%20areas. Accessed May 29, 2024.
3. Centers for Disease Control and Prevention. About congenital syphilis. Available at: https://www.cdc.gov/syphilis/about/about-congenital-syphilis.html. Accessed May 29, 2024.
4. David M, Hcini N, Mandelbrot L, Sibiude J, Picone O. Fetal and neonatal abnormalities due to congenital syphilis: a literature review. *Prenat Diagn.* 2022; 42(5):643–655. https://doi.org/10.1002/pd.6135
5. Kidd SE. Increased methamphetamine, injection drug, and heroin use among women and heterosexual men with primary and secondary syphilis—United States, 2013–2017. *MMWR Morb Mortal Wkly Rep.* 2019;68(6):144–148. https://doi.org/10.15585/mmwr.mm6806a4
6. Copen CE, Brookmeyer KA, Haderxhanaj LT, Hogben M, Torrone EA. Sexual risk behaviors among persons diagnosed with primary and secondary syphilis who reported high-risk substance use: data from the National Notifiable Diseases Surveillance System, 2018. *Sex Transm Dis.* 2022; 49(2):99–104. https://doi.org/10.1097/OLQ.0000000000001546
7. Carlson JM. Substance use among persons with syphilis during pregnancy—Arizona and Georgia, 2018–2021. *MMWR Morb Mortal Wkly Rep.* 2023; 72(3):63–67. https://doi.org/10.15585/mmwr.mm7203a3
8. Curry SJ, Krist AH, Owens DK, et al. Screening for syphilis infection in pregnant women: US Preventive Services Task Force reaffirmation recommendation statement. *JAMA.* 2018;320(9):911–917. https://doi.org/10.1001/jama.2018.11785
9. Workowski KA. Centers for Disease Control and Prevention sexually transmitted diseases treatment guidelines. *Clin Infect Dis.* 2015;61(suppl 8): S759–S762. https://doi.org/10.1093/cid/civ771

10. Austin AE, Naumann RB, Simmons E. Association of state child abuse policies and mandated reporting policies with prenatal and postpartum care among women who engaged in substance use during pregnancy. *JAMA Pediatr*. 2022;176(11):1123–1130. https://doi.org/10.1001/jamapediatrics.2022.3396
11. Atkins DN, Durrance CP. State policies that treat prenatal substance use as child abuse or neglect fail to achieve their intended goals: study examines the effect of state policies that treat prenatal substance use as child abuse or neglect on the incidence of neonatal abstinence syndrome and other factors. *Health Aff (Millwood)*. 2020;39(5):756–763. https://doi.org/10.1377/hlthaff.2019.00785
12. Stone R. Pregnant women and substance use: fear, stigma, and barriers to care. *Health Justice*. 2015;3(1):2. https://doi.org/10.1186/s40352-015-0015-5
13. Syvertsen JL, Toneff H, Howard H, Spadola C, Madden D, Clapp J. Conceptualizing stigma in contexts of pregnancy and opioid misuse: a qualitative study with women and healthcare providers in Ohio. *Drug Alcohol Depend*. 2021;222:108677. https://doi.org/10.1016/j.drugalcdep.2021.108677
14. Park E, Yip J, Harville E, et al. Gaps in the congenital syphilis prevention cascade: qualitative findings from Kern County, California. *BMC Infect Dis*. 2022;22(1):129. https://doi.org/10.1186/s12879-022-07100-3
15. Leiner C, Cody T, Mullins N, Ramage M, Ostrach BMM. "The elephant in the room;" a qualitative study of perinatal fears in opioid use disorder treatment in Southern Appalachia. *BMC Pregnancy Childbirth*. 2021;21(1):143. https://doi.org/10.1186/s12884-021-03596-w
16. Roberts S, Pies C. Complex calculations: how drug use during pregnancy becomes a barrier to prenatal care. *Matern Child Health J*. 2011;15(3):333–341. https://doi.org/10.1007/s10995-010-0594-7
17. McDonald R. Vital signs: missed opportunities for preventing congenital syphilis—United States, 2022. *MMWR Morb Mortal Wkly Rep*. 2023;72(46):1269–1274. https://doi.org/10.15585/mmwr.mm7246e1
18. Maclean JC, Witman A, Durrance CP, Atkins DN, Meinhofer A. prenatal substance use policies and infant maltreatment reports: study examines prenatal substance use policies and infant maltreatment reports. *Health Aff (Millwood)*. 2022;41(5):703–712. https://doi.org/10.1377/hlthaff.2021.01755
19. Meinhofer A, Witman A, Maclean JC, Bao Y. Prenatal substance use policies and newborn health. *Health Econ*. 2022;31(7):1452–1467. https://doi.org/10.1002/hec.4518
20. Tabatabaeepour N, Morgan JR, Jalali A, Kapadia SN, Meinhofer A. Impact of prenatal substance use policies on commercially insured pregnant females with opioid use disorder. *J Subst Abuse Treat*. 2022;140:108800. https://doi.org/10.1016/j.jsat.2022.108800
21. Gardiner JC, Luo Z, Roman LA. Fixed effects, random effects and GEE: what are the differences? *Stat Med*. 2009;28(2):221–239. https://doi.org/10.1002/sim.3478
22. French B, Stuart EA. Study designs and statistical methods for studies of child and adolescent health policies. *JAMA Pediatr*. 2020;174(10):925–927. https://doi.org/10.1001/jamapediatrics.2020.3408
23. O'Callaghan KP, Jones MLJ, McDonald R, et al. The congenital syphilis prevention cascade: reimagining a missed prevention opportunities framework for effective intervention. *Sex Transm Dis*. 2024;51(1):8–10.
24. Centers for Disease Control and Prevention. State statutory and regulatory language regarding prenatal syphilis screenings in the United States, 2018. Available at: https://www.cdc.gov/syphilis/media/pdfs/2024/07/Prenatal-Syphilis-Screening-Laws-Web-Document-25-July-2024-final.pdf. Accessed November 5, 2024.
25. Khazanchi R, Wachman EM, Schiff DM, Modest A, Saia KA, Hsu HE. Mandatory child protective services reporting for substance-exposed newborns and peripartum outcomes: a difference-in-differences analysis. *JAMA Pediatr*. 2024;178(7):719–722. https://doi.org/10.1001/jamapediatrics.2024.0903
26. Plotzker RE, Murphy RD, Stoltey JE. Congenital syphilis prevention: strategies, evidence, and future directions. *Sex Transm Dis*. 2018;45(suppl 9):S29–S37. https://doi.org/10.1097/OLQ.0000000000000846
27. National Syphilis and Congenital Syphilis Syndemic Federal Task Force. Considerations for the implementation of point of care tests for syphilis. Available at: https://www.hhs.gov/sites/default/files/nscss-considerations-for-the-implementation-of-syphilis-poc-tests.pdf. Accessed November 5, 2024.
28. Gadson A, Akpovi E, Mehta PK. Exploring the social determinants of racial/ethnic disparities in prenatal care utilization and maternal outcome. *Semin Perinatol*. 2017;41(5):308–317. https://doi.org/10.1053/j.semperi.2017.04.008
29. Martin EG, Ansari B, Rosenberg ES, et al. Variation in patterns of racial and ethnic disparities in primary and secondary syphilis diagnosis rates among heterosexually active women by region and age group in the United States. *Sex Transm Dis*. 2022;49(5):330–337. https://doi.org/10.1097/OLQ.0000000000001607
30. Kim H, Wildeman C, Jonson-Reid M, Drake B. Lifetime prevalence of investigating child maltreatment among US children. *Am J Public Health*. 2017;107(2):274–280. https://doi.org/10.2105/AJPH.2016.303545
31. Atkins DN, Durrance CP. The impact of state-level prenatal substance use policies on infant foster care entry in the United States. *Child Youth Serv Rev*. 2021;130:106194. https://doi.org/10.1016/j.childyouth.2021.106194
32. Patrick SW, Schiff DM. A public health response to opioid use in pregnancy. *Pediatrics*. 2017;139(3):e20164070. https://doi.org/10.1542/peds.2016-4070
33. American College of Obstetricians and Gynecologists Committee on Health Care for Underserved Women. Substance abuse reporting and pregnancy: the role of the obstetrician-gynecologist. Available at: https://www.acog.org/clinical/clinical-guidance/committee-opinion/articles/2011/01/substance-abuse-reporting-and-pregnancy-the-role-of-the-obstetrician-gynecologist. Accessed May 29, 2024.
34. Faherty LJ, Stein BD, Terplan M. Consensus guidelines and state policies: the gap between principle and practice at the intersection of substance use and pregnancy. *Am J Obstet Gynecol MFM*. 2020;2(3):100137. https://doi.org/10.1016/j.ajogmf.2020.100137

Syndromic Surveillance and Case Identification for Varicella Among Recent Immigrants: New York City, 2023

Melanie S. Askari, PhD, MPH, Robert J. Arciuolo, MPH, Olivia Matalka, MPH, Krishika A. Graham, MD, MPH, Beth M. Isaac, MPH, Ramona Lall, PhD, MS, Antonine Jean, MPH, and Jennifer B. Rosen, MD

Objectives. To determine utility of syndromic surveillance in improving varicella case detection during an outbreak among recent immigrants to New York City (NYC).

Methods. During March through August 2023, the NYC Health Department received varicella reports from routine sources and syndromic surveillance from emergency department visits with varicella as a chief complaint or discharge diagnosis. Reports were reviewed to determine if individuals met criteria for confirmed or probable varicella cases and if cases were outbreak-associated. We calculated positive predictive value (PPV) and timeliness of syndromic surveillance reports and compared them with routine surveillance reports.

Results. The health department received 639 unique varicella reports. Of 513 varicella cases, 247 (48.1%) were from syndromic surveillance alone, 194 (37.8%) from routine sources alone, and 72 (14.0%) from both sources. PPV was higher for syndromic surveillance (89.1%) versus routine surveillance (74.7%). Among 310 outbreak-associated cases, 139 were identified through syndromic surveillance (44.8%); syndromic surveillance was the only reporting source for 75 (24.2%). Syndromic surveillance was more timely than routine reporting (median = 3 days; range = 1–27 vs 5 days; range = 0–52).

Conclusions. NYC syndromic surveillance improved varicella case detection during this outbreak. (*Am J Public Health*. 2025;115(4):575–578. https://doi.org/10.2105/AJPH.2024.307961)

AJPH April 2025, Vol. 115, No. 4

Varicella (chickenpox) is a vaccine-preventable disease, but outbreaks still occur because of incomplete vaccination coverage globally.[1] Varicella is a contagious viral infection characterized by a generalized rash that can include complications such as pneumonia.[2] Before availability of a vaccine in the United States beginning in 1995, the majority of persons acquired varicella during childhood and developed lifelong immunity.[2] Since a vaccine has been available, varicella incidence in the United States has declined by more than 97%.[3] In New York State, 2 doses of varicella vaccine are required to attend school.[4] Until December 20, 2023, providers were required to report varicella outbreaks, but individual cases of varicella were not reportable to public health departments in New York.[5]

During October 2022, the New York City (NYC) Health Department identified a varicella outbreak among persons residing in temporary housing who recently immigrated to NYC, primarily from Central and South American countries that do not have routine or have disrupted varicella immunization programs. Approximately 900 varicella cases were identified as of March 2024.[6] Outbreak control measures included contact tracing, recommendations for isolation and quarantine, vaccine administration, and provision of guidance to exposure settings.

We evaluated utility of emergency department (ED) syndromic surveillance data as a supplemental tool for identifying any new cases and outbreak-associated cases.

METHODS

The NYC Health Department routinely received reports of varicella during this outbreak from NYC shelters and residential facilities, schools, field investigations, health care facilities, and laboratories (defined as "routine sources"). After receiving a varicella report, NYC Health Department staff conducted patient interviews and reviewed medical, laboratory, and immunization records to determine if the person's illness met the Council of State and Territorial Epidemiologists' definition of a confirmed or probable case (referred to as "case").[7] Cases were investigated to determine whether they were associated with this outbreak among recently arrived immigrants, defined as occurring in a person who arrived to the United States and NYC since June 2022 or with an epidemiological link to an outbreak-associated case.

During this outbreak, NYC syndromic surveillance from ED visit data[8] was added as a supplemental surveillance tool on March 1, 2023. This was done to identify additional cases that might not have been proactively reported to the NYC Health Department through routine reporting sources. Syndromic surveillance data included ED visits with a varicella discharge diagnosis code (i.e., B01) or mentions of varicella or pox in the chief complaint.

Reports of varicella identified by syndromic surveillance and by routine reporting sources during March 1 through August 31, 2023, were included in the evaluation. Number and proportion of all cases and of outbreak-associated cases identified by report source (i.e., syndromic surveillance only, routine surveillance only, or both reporting sources) were calculated. We calculated the positive predictive value (PPV), defined as proportion of varicella reports classified as cases, separately for syndromic surveillance and routine surveillance reports. Non–outbreak-associated cases were included in PPV calculation to enhance generalizability beyond this outbreak. We calculated the percentage increase in case ascertainment resulting from cases identified only through syndromic surveillance separately for all varicella cases and for outbreak-associated cases. We calculated timeliness (median time from rash onset to Health Department receipt of first report) for outbreak-associated cases and compared them by reporting source (i.e., syndromic surveillance first vs routine surveillance first).

RESULTS

The NYC Health Department received 639 unique varicella reports during March 1 through August 31, 2023, from syndromic surveillance and routine reporting sources (Figure 1). Of the 639 reports from all sources, 513 were classified as varicella cases, including 247 (48.1%) reported from syndromic surveillance alone (increasing case ascertainment by 93%), 194 (37.8%) from routine reporting sources alone, and 72 (14.0%) from both sources.

For reports from syndromic surveillance, 319 of 358 were classified as cases (PPV = 89.1%), compared with 266 of 356 reports from routine surveillance that were classified as cases (PPV = 74.7%). Among 310 outbreak-associated cases, 139 (44.8%) were reported by syndromic surveillance (75 reported only by syndromic surveillance, increasing ascertainment of outbreak cases by 32%, and 64 reported by both routine sources and syndromic surveillance; Figure 1). Time from varicella rash onset to Health Department receipt of first report for outbreak-associated cases was shorter for syndromic surveillance (median = 3 days; range = 1–27 days), compared with those reported by routine reporting sources first (median = 5 days; range = 0–52 days).

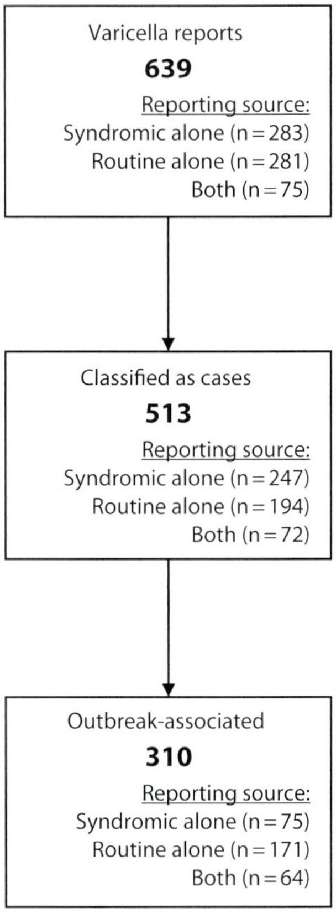

FIGURE 1— Varicella Reports Received by the New York City Health Department by Case Classification, Outbreak Association, and Reporting Source: New York City, March 1–August 31, 2023

Note. Routine reporting sources included residential facilities, schools, field investigations, health care facilities, and laboratory reports. Cases included confirmed or probable cases classified based on the Council for State and Territorial Epidemiologists case definitions. Outbreak-associated cases were defined as those occurring in persons who arrived in the United States and New York City since June 2022 or with an epidemiological link to an outbreak-associated case.

DISCUSSION

NYC syndromic surveillance demonstrated its utility in varicella surveillance during an outbreak. It improved completeness of overall case ascertainment by more than 90%, identifying 247 cases that were not reported through routine surveillance and increased detection of outbreak-associated cases by approximately 30%. Additional effort to determine outbreak association was not resource intensive. Approximately 90% of reports from syndromic surveillance were classified as cases, which makes resources spent on investigation of syndromic reports worthwhile. As of 2020, there were 39 states with case-based varicella reporting.[9] Because case-based varicella reporting by providers was not required in New York State until after the evaluation period,[5] the possibility exists that syndromic surveillance was the sole source of reports for a greater proportion of cases compared with states with case-based varicella reporting. However, provider reporting for communicable diseases is often incomplete, despite case-based reporting requirements.[10] In addition, syndromic surveillance increased the timeliness of case identification.

A limitation of ED-based syndromic surveillance is that it would only identify patients who sought ED-level care (e.g., cases involving more severe symptoms or patients without health insurance). Because most persons with varicella do not require ED-level care, we would not expect syndromic surveillance to identify all outbreak-associated cases. The proportion of outbreak-associated cases identified by syndromic surveillance during the evaluation period (45%) might be higher in this recently arrived immigrant population compared with other populations. This is because many persons in this outbreak do not have existing connections to primary care on arrival to NYC or might be more likely to be uninsured, so they might be more likely to seek health care in an ED setting. Future evaluations should assess demographic and social characteristics of cases captured by syndromic surveillance versus routine sources to characterize differences between types of patients captured. A limitation of this analysis is that routine surveillance report documentation might have been incomplete, particularly when the report was already identified by syndromic surveillance. Syndromic surveillance was timelier, and populated into our database automatically, whereas other sources (e.g., provider phone call) required manual entry. Thus, the percentage of outbreak-associated cases identified only by syndromic surveillance might be overestimated.

PUBLIC HEALTH IMPLICATIONS

Syndromic surveillance allowed for earlier and more complete identification of cases associated with the varicella outbreak. Identification of outbreak-associated cases facilitated implementation of control measures, including contact tracing, recommendations for isolation and quarantine, vaccine administration, and provision of guidance to exposure settings. Timely varicella reporting is important because postexposure prophylaxis includes varicella vaccination within 5 days of exposure. Although investigating reports of varicella is resource-intensive, reports received through syndromic surveillance were predominantly classified as cases, and additional effort to determine outbreak association was minimal. Syndromic surveillance might be valuable for jurisdictions regardless of whether they have case-based varicella surveillance, as NYC has demonstrated in this report, given improved timeliness and underreporting of varicella even in jurisdictions with case-based surveillance. This might also serve as a model for using syndromic surveillance for other vaccine-preventable diseases in NYC and other jurisdictions. AJPH

ABOUT THE AUTHORS

Melanie S. Askari is with the Epidemic Intelligence Service at the Centers for Disease Control and Prevention (CDC) and the New York City Health Department, Long Island City, NY. Robert J. Arciuolo, Olivia Matalka, Krishika A. Graham, Beth M. Isaac, Ramona Lall, Antonine Jean, and Jennifer B. Rosen are with the New York City Health Department, Bureau of Immunization, Long Island City.

Note. The findings and conclusions in this report are those of the authors and do not necessarily represent the official position of the CDC.

PUBLICATION INFORMATION

Full Citation: Askari MS, Arciuolo RJ, Matalka O, et al. Syndromic surveillance and case identification for varicella among recent immigrants: New York City, 2023. *Am J Public Health*. 2025; 115(4):575–578.

Acceptance Date: November 25, 2024.

DOI: https://doi.org/10.2105/AJPH.2024.307961

ORCID iDs:

Melanie S. Askari https://orcid.org/0000-0002-7700-0872

Robert J. Arciuolo https://orcid.org/0000-0002-5140-6209

Olivia Matalka https://orcid.org/0009-0000-9067-7100

Krishika A. Graham https://orcid.org/0009-0006-7117-2530

Ramona Lall https://orcid.org/0000-0003-4079-4610

Antonine Jean https://orcid.org/0009-0009-3581-8316

CORRESPONDENCE

Correspondence should be sent to Melanie S. Askari, 42-09 28th St, Long Island City, NY 11101 (e-mail: maskari@health.nyc.gov). Reprints can be ordered at https://www.ajph.org by clicking the "Reprints" link.

CONTRIBUTORS

M. S. Askari conducted the analyses; contributed to the conceptualization, design, and interpretation of data; and drafted and revised the article. R. J. Arciuolo curated the data set for the evaluation, advised on the analyses, and contributed to the conceptualization and design or analysis and interpretation of data, the drafting or revision of the article, and the approval of the final version. J. B. Rosen provided supervision of the analyses and writing, and contributed to the conceptualization and design or analysis and interpretation of data, the drafting or revision of the article, and the approval of the final version. O. Matalka, K. A. Graham, B. M. Isaac, R. Lall, and A. Jean contributed to the conceptualization and design or analysis and interpretation of data, the drafting or revision of the article, and the approval of the final version.

CONFLICTS OF INTEREST

The authors report no conflicts of interest.

HUMAN PARTICIPANT PROTECTION

This activity was reviewed by the CDC, deemed not research, and was conducted consistent with applicable federal law and CDC policy. (See, e.g., 45 CFR part 46.102(l)(2); 21 CFR part 56; 42 USC §241(d); 5 USC §552a; 44 USC §3501 et seq.) The NYC Health Department also reviewed this activity and determined it to be nonresearch public health surveillance (institutional review board 23-075).

REFERENCES

1. Varela FH, Pinto LA, Scotta MC. Global impact of varicella vaccination programs. *Hum Vaccin Immunother.* 2019;15(3):645–657. https://doi.org/10.1080/21645515.2018.1546525
2. Lopez A, Harrington T, Marin M. Varicella. In: Hall E, Wodi AP, Hamborsky J, Morelli V, Schillie S. *The Pinkbook.* Available at: https://www.cdc.gov/vaccines/pubs/pinkbook/varicella.html. Accessed November 16, 2023.
3. Marin M, Leung J, Anderson TC, Lopez AS. Monitoring varicella vaccine impact on varicella incidence in the United States: surveillance challenges and changing epidemiology, 1995–2019. *J Infect Dis.* 2022;226(suppl 4):S392–S399. https://doi.org/10.1093/infdis/jiac221
4. New York State Department of Health. New York State School Vaccine Requirements. Available at: https://www.health.ny.gov/prevention/immunization/schools/school_vaccines. Accessed October 29, 2024.
5. New York Department of State. Section 2.1 of Title 10 (Health) of the Official Compilation of Codes, Rules, and Regulations of the State of New York. December 20, 2023;XLV(51). Available at: https://dos.ny.gov/system/files/documents/2023/12/122023.pdf. Accessed October 29, 2024.
6. Graham KA, Arciuolo RJ, Matalka O, et al. Varicella outbreak among recent arrivals to New York City, 2022–2024. *MMWR Morb Mortal Wkly Rep.* 2024;73(21):478–483. https://doi.org/10.15585/mmwr.mm7321a1
7. Centers for Disease Control and Prevention. Varicella/chickenpox 2010 case definition. Available at: https://ndc.services.cdc.gov/case-definitions/varicella-2010. Accessed October 29, 2024.
8. Heffernan R, Mostashari F, Das D, et al. Syndromic surveillance in public health practice, New York City. *Emerg Infect Dis.* 2004;10(5):858–864. https://doi.org/10.3201/eid1005.030646
9. Centers for Disease Control and Prevention. Varicella reporting and surveillance. Available at: https://www.cdc.gov/chickenpox/php/conducting-surveillance/?CDC_AAref_Val=https://www.cdc.gov/chickenpox/health-departments/conducting-surveillance.html. Accessed October 29, 2024.
10. Revere D, Hills RH, Dixon BE, Gibson PJ, Grannis SJ. Notifiable condition reporting practices: implications for public health agency participation in a health information exchange. *BMC Public Health.* 2017;17(1):247. https://doi.org/10.1186/s12889-017-4156-4

Population-Level Risks for HIV Mortality During the COVID-19 Pandemic in the United States by Demographic Characteristics and Medicaid Access, 2020–2021

Donrie Purcell, PhD, MPH, Wayne A. Duffus, MD, PhD, Maisha Standifer, PhD, MPH, Robert Mayberry, PhD, MS, MPH, and Sonja S. Hutchins, MD, DrPH, MPH

Objectives. To evaluate the impact of the COVID-19 pandemic on HIV mortality rates with a focus on demographic predictors and Medicaid access.

Methods. Using Wide-Ranging Online Data for Epidemiologic Research, we conducted a descriptive study comparing HIV mortality in the United States 2 years before the COVID-19 pandemic (2018–2019) and the initial 2 years of the pandemic (2020–2021), and identifying HIV mortality factors during the pandemic.

Results. During the first 2 years of the pandemic, crude HIV death rates increased and then decreased marginally. COVID-19 and HIV together contributed to 11% of the HIV death rate. While African Americans had a higher HIV mortality rate, there was a slight decrease during the pandemic. Nonelderly adults in Medicaid expansion states had lower HIV mortality than those in nonexpansion states.

Conclusions. Contrary to initial concerns, we found no substantial increase in HIV mortality. A slight decrease was observed with persisting racial disparities in mortality and lower mortality in states that expanded Medicaid.

Public Health Implications. The study findings can inform the development of policies to address demographic disparities in HIV mortality through targeted system-level interventions for vulnerable populations, such as Medicaid expansion and Ryan White Program services. (*Am J Public Health.* 2025;115(4):579–587. https://doi.org/10.2105/AJPH.2024.307916)

AJPH April 2025, Vol. 115, No. 4

The emergence of the COVID-19 pandemic, attributed to severe acute respiratory syndrome coronavirus 2 (SARS-CoV-2), has profoundly impacted global health care systems.[1] By the close of 2021, the cumulative number of confirmed COVID-19 cases surpassed an alarming 278 million, accompanied by more than 5.4 million recorded fatalities worldwide.[2] Notably, the United States witnessed a staggering toll, with more than 55 million documented cases and 824 000 associated deaths by December 31, 2021.[3]

While individuals across all demographics are susceptible to COVID-19, extensive research indicates that those with comorbidities face a significantly heightened risk of adverse outcomes.[4–6] Furthermore, the immunocompromised population emerged as a particularly vulnerable cohort for COVID-19.[1]

Surprisingly, in the United States, persons with HIV have not exhibited substantially elevated incidence rates of respiratory viral infections like influenza or COVID-19 when compared with the US general population. However, Spinelli et al. posit that although people with HIV infection (PWH) do not demonstrate heightened susceptibility to SARS-CoV-2, they do face an elevated risk of experiencing severe COVID-19 outcomes upon exposure.[7] Conversely, a significant study by Turtle et al. underscores those immunocompromised patients, including PWH, remain at a persistently elevated risk of mortality associated with COVID-19.[8]

Furthermore, the World Health Organization confirms that PWH are at increased risk for severe COVID-19 and mortality, particularly those with comorbidities.[9]

Given concerns about increased risk of severe COVID-19 outcomes among those who are immunocompromised and particularly among PWH, we examined predictors of HIV mortality such as age, race, ethnicity, geographic region, and access to Medicaid to critically understand the nuanced dynamics of US HIV mortality during the COVID-19 pandemic.

METHODS

In 2023, we used Wide-Ranging Online Data for Epidemiologic Research (WONDER), an online data analysis system from the Centers for Disease Control and Prevention (CDC),[10] to conduct a descriptive study. Data were from 2018 to 2021, including the first 2 years of the COVID-19 pandemic from 2020 to 2021. To provide context of previous HIV mortality, we initially present HIV mortality trends from 1999 to 2021. Detailed methods for WONDER are described elsewhere.[11] Briefly, WONDER provided the number of deaths from the National Vital Statistics System and the midyear US population from the Census Bureau, and computed crude and age-adjusted death rates. The WONDER data set used was the "Multiple causes of deaths."

HIV deaths were defined as the underlying causes of death based on the *International Classification of Diseases, 10th Revision* (*ICD-10*; Geneva, Switzerland: World Health Organization; 1992) codes B20–B24. The HIV deaths linked to COVID-19 deaths were defined as COVID-19 deaths as the underlying cause of death using *ICD-10* code U07.1 and HIV as the contributing cause on the death certificate. Crude death rates were obtained from WONDER instead of age-adjusted rates to assess the actual impact of the COVID-19 mortality across the age span and not to duplicate provisional age-adjusted analysis by the CDC. Crude HIV-related death rates during the COVID-19 pandemic from 2020 to 2021 were defined as the combined HIV death rate with HIV as the underlying cause of death plus the crude death rate with COVID-19 as the underlying cause of death and HIV as the contributing cause of death. Definitions of race and ethnicity were those from the Office of Management and Budget and included non-Hispanic African Americans, non-Hispanic Whites, non-Hispanic American Indian/Alaska Natives, non-Hispanic Asians, non-Hispanic Native Hawaiian and other Pacific Islanders, non-Hispanic persons with multiple races (multiracial persons), and Hispanics.[10]

We further described HIV mortality or death rates by age, sex, region, and race/ethnicity. Next, we assessed racial and ethnic differences in HIV mortality before and during the pandemic and then by region and residence in Medicaid expansion versus nonexpansion states among the nonelderly population. We defined the period before the pandemic as 2 years from 2018 to 2019, and we defined the period during the pandemic as 2020 to 2021. Census regions in the United States were examined: Northeast, Midwest, South, and West. HIV mortality by residence of population in Medicaid expansion and nonexpansion states was limited to nonelderly adults aged 19 to 64 years residing in those states by January 1, 2014, a date by which health plans were required to include essential preventive and treatment services because of the Patient Protection and Affordable Care Act.[12] Nonelderly adults were examined only because adults aged 65 years or older were likely to receive Medicare and gain access to medical care through that health insurance, whereas a substantial number of low-income nonelderly adults who did not have employer-based health insurance were unlikely to gain access to medical care unless they lived in a Medicaid expansion state.

Status of Medicaid expansion was obtained from the Kaiser Family Foundation.[13] Medicaid expansion states were California, Colorado, Connecticut, Delaware, Hawaii, Illinois, Maryland, Massachusetts, Minnesota, Nevada, New Jersey, New Mexico, New York, North Dakota, Ohio, Oregon, Rhode Island, Vermont, Washington, and West Virginia, as well as the District of Columbia. Nonexpansion states were Alabama, Florida, Georgia, Kansas, Mississippi, North Carolina, South Carolina, South Dakota, Tennessee, Texas, Wisconsin, and Wyoming. Death rates among nonelderly adults were examined for all 20 states and the District of Columbia classified as Medicaid expansion states and compared with death rates among nonelderly adults from the 12 states defined as nonexpansion states. Eighteen states were excluded from this analysis, because those states were in various stages of implementing Medicaid expansion; these states either began Medicaid expansion after January 1, 2014, or were implementing Medicaid expansion through waivers (Appendices A and B, available as supplements to the online version of this article at https://ajph.org).

The distribution of available demographic characteristics of all nonelderly adults residing in Medicaid expansion states were similar to those adults residing in nonexpansion states by age and most racial/ethnic populations (Appendix B). There were some differences in that a slightly greater proportion of non-Hispanic Asians resided in Medicaid expansion than nonexpansion states. More of the nonelderly adults also resided in the Northeast and Midwest census regions of the United States compared with those adults residing in nonexpansion states. Nearly all of these adults in nonexpansion states resided in the South.

Statistical Analysis

Crude mortality was computed in WONDER, because this measure provides the actual risk of dying, and age-adjusted estimates were essentially similar. Because crude mortality or death rate was computed from the total number of deaths divided by the total midyear US population and not considered a sample, "statistics" accounting for uncertainty in sample estimates such as confidence intervals and *P* values were not required, even though the estimated intercensal midyear populations by year were from populations in the census years of 2000, 2010, or 2020. Observed mortality was the actual measure and not an estimate.[14] Temporal trends in HIV mortality did not include age-adjusted mortality as mentioned previously.

RESULTS

Crude HIV mortality rates in the United States decreased from 5.3 deaths per 100 000 population in 1999 to 2.7 per 100 000 by 2010, and by 2019, before the COVID-19 pandemic, the mortality rate further decreased to 1.5 per 100 000 (Figure 1). Compared with the 2-year period before the COVID-19 pandemic (2018–2019), temporal trends in crude HIV mortality rate showed an increase during 2020 and a decrease during 2021 to below the prepandemic level of 2018 (Figure 1). In fact, during the pandemic, the HIV mortality rate changed slightly, ranging from 1.8 per 100 000 in 2020 to 1.7 per 100 000 in 2021 (Figure 1). Deaths directly attributed to both COVID-19 and HIV in an individual represented 11% of the HIV death rate (0.2 deaths per 100 000 in 2020 and 2021; Figure 1). Populations with the greatest HIV mortality were African American, male, aged 65 years and older followed by aged 19 to 64 years, and living in the South (Table 1).

During the pandemic, there was a slight increased HIV mortality for all racial and ethnic populations combined compared with the period before the pandemic (Table 2). For example, among African Americans, a 5.8% increase was found during the pandemic compared with the period before the pandemic (Table 2).

AJPH April 2025, Vol. 115, No. 4

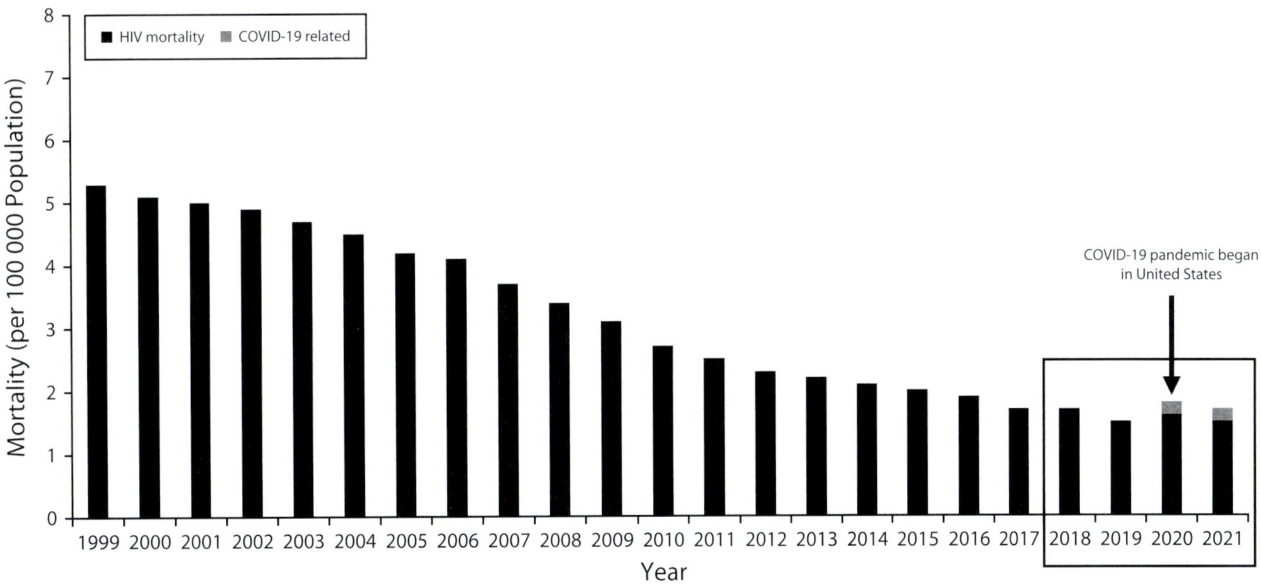

FIGURE 1— Crude HIV Mortality (Per 100 000 Population) by Year: United States, 1999–2021

Note. COVID-19 mortality related to HIV is defined as underlying cause of death as COVID-19 and HIV as a contributing cause. HIV mortality (per 100 000 population) is defined as HIV as underlying cause of death. The box serves to highlight the study period of 2 years before the COVID-19 pandemic (2018–2019) and the initial 2 years of the pandemic (2020–2021).

TABLE 1— Crude HIV Mortality (Per 100 000 Population) by Year, Race/Ethnicity, Sex, Age and Region: United States, 2018–2021

Characteristics	Average Total Population	Mortality per 100 000 Population[a]			
		2018	2019	2020	2021
Race/ethnicity[b,c]					
African American	41 333 897	6.7	6.2	7.2	6.6
White	197 115 763	0.9	0.8	0.9	0.9
AI/AN	2 434 133	1.6	1.3	1.4	1.5
Asian	19 171 913	0.3	0.3	0.3	0.4
NHOPI	605 502	[d]	[d]	[d]	[d]
Multiple races	7 434 022	0.4	0.3	0.4	0.4
Hispanic	61 100 977	1.2	1.2	1.5	1.4
Sex					
Female	166 839 470	0.8	0.8	0.9	0.8
Male	162 356 737	2.5	2.3	2.7	2.6
Age, y					
< 19	77 463 806	[d]	[d]	[d]	[d]
19–64	197 233 707	2.3	2.0	2.2	2.2
≥ 65	54 499 194	1.9	1.9	2.5	2.3
Region					
Northeast	27 493 448	2.2	2.2	2.6	2.3
Midwest	33 852 893	1.5	1.2	1.7	1.4
South	61 839 607	3.4	3.2	3.6	3.6
West	39 170 789	2.1	1.9	2.3	2.3

Note. AI/AN = American Indian/Alaska Native; NHOPI = Native Hawaiian and other Pacific Islander.
[a]Crude HIV mortality is defined as the number of HIV deaths divided by midyear population (per 100 000 population); HIV deaths during 2018–2019 are defined as underlying cause of death as HIV (*International Classification of Diseases, 10th Revision* [Geneva, Switzerland: World Health Organization; 1992], codes B20–B24) and during 2020–2021 is defined as combined COVID-19 deaths as underlying cause and HIV as a contributing cause plus HIV deaths as underlying cause of death.
[b]All "races" are non-Hispanic.
[c]May include more than the total of non-Hispanic and Hispanic because missing race/ethnicity (< 1% of total: 33 849–36 381 annually).
[d]Defined as number of deaths < 10 (suppressed by Wide-Ranging Online Data for Epidemiologic Research [WONDER]) or number of deaths < 20 (defined as unreliable by WONDER).

HIV mortality rate increased from 6.5 deaths per 100 000 population from 2018 to 2019 to 6.9 deaths per 100 000 population from 2020 to 2021 (Table 1). HIV mortality also increased slightly in the White population, but the absolute increase was much less compared with most other populations except for Asian and multiracial populations. Among all racial and ethnic populations examined, the percentage increase in HIV mortality of 5.8% among African Americans was the smallest percentage.

Compared with the period before the pandemic, temporal trends in the increased HIV mortality rates during the individual years of the pandemic varied by race and ethnicity (Table 1). Among African Americans, the rate increased in 2020 followed by a decreased rate in 2021 to the prepandemic rate in 2018. Among Whites and those with multiple races, the rate slightly increased during both years of the pandemic from 2020 to 2021 to the prepandemic rate in 2018. Among American Indian/Alaska Natives, the rate increased from 2019 during both pandemic years but remained less than the rate in 2018 (Table 1). Among Asians, the rate remained constant until a slight increase was observed in 2021. In addition, among Hispanics, the rate increased during both years of the pandemic from 2020 to 2021 and remained greater than the rates during prepandemic years. Although the 6- to 7-fold greater death rate among African Americans compared with other racial and ethnic

TABLE 2— Change in Crude HIV Mortality (Per 100 000 Population) During COVID-19 Pandemic Compared With Period Before by Race/Ethnicity: United States, 2018–2021

Race[a]/Ethnicity	Total Population, Mortality per 100 000 Population[b]		Mortality[b] Change,[c] Difference (% Difference)
	Before Pandemic (2018–2019)	During Pandemic (2020–2021)	
African American	82 049 711 (6.5)	83 285 877 (6.9)	+0.4 (+5.8)
White	394 856 229 (0.9)	393 606 821 (1.1)	+0.2 (+18.2)
AI/AN	4 852 279 (1.4)	4 884 254 (1.5)	+0.1 (+6.7)
Asian	37 634 554 (0.3)	39 053 098 (0.3)	0.0 (0.0)
NHOPI	1 182 254 ([d])	1 239 753 ([d])	[d] ([d])
Multiple races	14 387 947 (0.3)	15 348 142 (0.4)	+0.1 (+25.0)
Hispanic	120 443 983 (1.2)	123 959 923 (1.4)	+0.2 (+14.3)
Total[e]	655 406 957 (1.6)	661 377 868 (1.7)	+0.1 (+5.9)

Note. AI/AN = American Indian/Alaska Native; NHOPI = Native Hawaiian and other Pacific Islander.
[a]All "races" are non-Hispanic.
[b]Crude HIV mortality is defined as the number of HIV deaths divided by midyear population (per 100 000 population); HIV deaths during 2018–2019 are defined as underlying cause of death as HIV (*International Classification of Diseases, 10th Revision* [Geneva, Switzerland: World Health Organization; 1992], codes B20–B24) and during 2020–2021 are defined as COVID-19 deaths as underlying cause and HIV as a contributing cause.
[c]Mortality change is defined as mortality during the pandemic (2020–2021) minus mortality before the pandemic (2018–2019); percentage change is defined as the change divided by mortality during the pandemic multiplied by 100.
[d]Defined as number of deaths fewer than 10 (suppressed by Wide-Ranging Online Data for Epidemiologic Research [WONDER]) or number of deaths < 20 (defined as unreliable by WONDER).
[e]May include more than the total of non-Hispanic and Hispanic because missing race/ethnicity (< 1% of total: 33 849–36 381 annually).

TABLE 3— Difference in Crude HIV Mortality (per 100 000 Population) Among Adults Aged 19–64 Years During the COVID-19 Pandemic by Residence in Medicaid Expansion Versus Nonexpansion States: United States, 2020–2021

Race[a]/Ethnicity	Total Population, Mortality per 100 000 Population[b]		Mortality[b] Difference,[c] Difference (% Difference)
	Medicaid Expansion States	Nonexpansion States	
African American	17 935 254 (8.3)	22 461 219 (10.1)	+1.8 (+19.8)
White	95 966 930 (1.0)	66 527 039 (1.5)	+0.5 (+33.3)
AI/AN	1 015 272 ([d])	[d] ([d])	[d] ([d])
Asian	17 077 944 (0.4)	4 737 456 ([d])	[d] ([d])
NHOPI	[d] ([d])	[d] ([d])	[d] ([d])
Multiple races	3 823 986 (0.9)	1 685 073 ([d])	[d] ([d])
Hispanic	39 028 380 (2.1)	25 919 104 (1.9)	−0.2 (−10.5)
Total[e]	175 381 704 (2.0)	122 078 594 (3.1)	+1.1 (+35.5)

Note. AI/AN = American Indian/Alaska Native; NHOPI = Native Hawaiian and other Pacific Islander.
[a]All "races" are non-Hispanic.
[b]Crude HIV mortality is defined as the number of HIV deaths divided by midyear population (per 100 000 population).
[c]Difference is defined as mortality in Medicaid nonexpansion states minus mortality in Medicaid expansion states; percentage difference is defined as the difference divided by mortality in nonexpansion states multiplied by 100.
[d]Defined as number of deaths < 10 (suppressed by Wide-Ranging Online Data for Epidemiologic Research [WONDER]) or number of deaths < 20 (defined as unreliable by WONDER).
[e]May include more than the total of non-Hispanic and Hispanic because missing race/ethnicity (< 1% of total: 33 849–36 381 annually).

populations decreased slightly in 2021, the large mortality difference remained compared with other racial and ethnic populations (Table 1).

During the pandemic, the available HIV mortality rate among nonelderly racial and ethnic adults aged 19 to 64 years residing in nonexpansion states compared with those adults residing in Medicaid expansion states was in general greater except for the rate in the Hispanic population (Table 3). Overall, among nonelderly adults, the HIV mortality rate was 1.1 deaths per 100 000 population greater in nonexpansion states than among nonelderly adults who resided in Medicaid expansion states (a 35.5% increase). Of the available mortality, the greatest absolute difference was among nonelderly African Americans. The HIV mortality rate among nonelderly African American adults who resided in nonexpansion states was 10.1 deaths per 100 000 population compared with 8.3 deaths per 100 000 population among nonelderly adults who resided in Medicaid expansion states. Among nonelderly Hispanics, the slight absolute difference was much lower (–0.2 deaths per 100 000 population).

DISCUSSION

In this study, we used the WONDER online data analysis system to assess the impact of the COVID-19 pandemic on HIV mortality rates among PWH in the United States, examining demographic factors such as age, race, ethnicity, region, and Medicaid access.

From 1999 to 2019, crude HIV death rates substantially decreased because of various factors, including treatment advancements and preventive measures.[15–17] Surprisingly, from our analysis, the COVID-19 pandemic did not substantially increase HIV mortality with an actual decrease in mortality in 2021 among African Americans. Possible reasons include health care system adaptability, innovative care approaches (telemedicine, home-based services) ensuring that individuals with HIV continued to receive necessary medical attention and antiretroviral therapy,[18] and COVID-19 control measures such as vaccination early when available as PWH are considered a high-risk population for severe disease and have been prioritized for vaccination.

In addition, some of the risk factors for severe outcomes in both COVID-19 and HIV, such as age and underlying health conditions, might have led to a more cautious approach among individuals with HIV. For instance, individuals aware of their HIV status may have taken extra precautions to protect themselves from COVID-19. Scientific and public health communities likely intensified their efforts to understand the intersection of COVID-19 and HIV, leading to targeted interventions and guidance to minimize the impact of both diseases.[19] It is essential to note that the relationship between the COVID-19 pandemic and HIV is complex and multifaceted. Other investigations have demonstrated an association with worse outcomes when comorbidities are present during COVID-19 and HIV dual infections.[20–24] The impact may vary across populations and regions, and ongoing research is necessary to comprehensively understand the consequences of the COVID-19 pandemic on various health outcomes, including HIV mortality.

Individuals infected with both COVID-19 and HIV contributed to 11% of the HIV death rate, and this should raise alarm for public health officials because it represents a threat to the progress made in HIV care and treatment.[9] Our data did not contain vireo-immunologic parameters or antiretroviral status, and we cannot comment if these were potentiating factors influencing mortality outcomes. However, managing both health challenges simultaneously increases strain on health care systems, affecting staff, intensive care unit beds, medications, surveillance, outbreak response, public health messaging, and recommendations.

Integrated health care services addressing both diseases are crucial, emphasizing the need for coordinated testing, treatment, and follow-up care. Allocating resources effectively requires balancing COVID-19 response with ongoing HIV services. Public health strategies should include targeted campaigns promoting preventive measures such as vaccination for COVID-19, adherence to HIV treatment, and regular check-ups. The Ryan White Program likely played an outsized role in mitigating the consequences of dual infection through streamlining services to improve access to prevention and treatment.[25,26] Efforts must address social determinants (e.g., age, race/ethnicity, geography, and insurance status), ensuring equitable care for vulnerable populations. Ongoing research, surveillance systems, and international collaboration are vital to understand the dual impact and optimize public health responses. Mental health support services should be integrated to address the well-being of individuals with both conditions. In summary, a comprehensive and integrated approach is essential to address the dual impact of COVID-19 and HIV deaths effectively.[19,27,28]

Our data also demonstrate that the demographic groups that experienced the highest HIV mortality rates during the COVID-19 pandemic were male, certain age groups (19–64 years and 65 years and older), and individuals residing in the South. The potential reasons behind these disparities are manyfold: historically, male individuals, particularly men who have sex with men, have been disproportionately affected by HIV/AIDS. This disparity may be attributed to factors such as higher rates of certain risk behaviors, stigma affecting testing and treatment-seeking behaviors, and challenges in accessing health care services. During the COVID-19 pandemic, if these patterns persisted, male persons, especially men who have sex with men, might have continued to experience higher HIV mortality rates.

The impact of HIV/AIDS on different age groups can vary. Younger individuals (aged 19–64 years) may face challenges related to risk behaviors, awareness, and access to prevention and treatment services. Older individuals (aged 65 years and older) may face unique challenges, including potential comorbidities and age-related health issues. Disparities in mortality rates could be influenced by differences in health care–seeking behavior, comorbidity management, and social support networks. The southern United States has historically seen higher HIV incidence and mortality rates compared with other regions.[29,30] Factors contributing to this disparity include socioeconomic challenges, limited access to health care, higher rates of certain risk behaviors, and stigma associated with HIV. During the COVID-19 pandemic, existing health disparities may have been exacerbated, potentially leading to higher HIV mortality rates in the southern states.[28,29]

Racial disparities persisted, with African Americans facing a 6- to 7-fold greater HIV death rate, albeit with a 5.8% increase overall from 2020 to 2021 and a slight decrease in 2021. Contributing factors include socioeconomic challenges, limited health care access, stigma, and historical higher HIV incidence.[30] The percentage decrease in 2021 during the pandemic may be influenced by improved health care access, awareness, and HIV treatment advancements. Efforts to enhance health care infrastructure and address social determinants of health during the pandemic likely positively impacted HIV outcomes. The intersectionality of HIV and COVID-19 interventions may have inadvertently improved HIV outcomes among African Americans. To address persistent disparities, careful examination and ongoing research, surveillance, and comprehensive public health strategies are vital.[31]

Our data revealed higher HIV mortality among nonelderly adults in Medicaid nonexpansion states, suggesting a link to limited health care access. Medicaid expansion, a key Patient Protection and Affordable Care Act provision, targets increased health care access for low-income individuals,[32,33] potentially benefiting HIV testing, treatment, and prevention. Other authors have presented data supporting evidence that insurance and health care access prevented mortality for some individuals because of Medicaid expansion.[34,35] Regional HIV mortality disparities stem from variations in health care access, policy decisions, and demographics. States not expanding Medicaid may delay HIV testing, diagnosis, and treatment because of limited health care access. Advocating Medicaid expansion in nonexpansion states is crucial for addressing this issue. Health care policy complexity underscores that Medicaid expansion likely impacts HIV outcomes but is only 1 facet. Comprehensive strategies addressing social determinants, reducing disparities, and enhancing overall access to care are pivotal for nationwide HIV improvement.

Limitations

This study had a few limitations. First, differences in state responses (such as stay-at-home orders),[36] as well as adaptations in service delivery by HIV clinics made early in the pandemic, may have influenced which regions and populations were impacted. Second, we did not utilize electronic health records, which may capture COVID-19 genomic surveillance data. The individuals in our cohort may have been infected with different variants over time, which likely impacted disease severity and outcomes in different populations. Third, the data set does not report individual-level data (e.g., HIV treatment history and type of antiretroviral therapy, duration of HIV infection, viral load, or CD4 cell count) and so we cannot determine the factors that likely impacted outcome[37] such as the proportions of people with advanced HIV, those not receiving care, or, in contrast, those who were virologically suppressed. Fourth, our analysis used crude death rates instead of adjusted death rates. It is possible that the relationship between HIV infection and COVID-19 mortality may differ after certain effect modifiers and confounding factors (e.g., race, ethnicity, age) are adjusted for by multivariate models.[24] Fifth, the observed difference in rates between the prepandemic and pandemic periods cannot be solely attributed to the impact of the pandemic, as the analysis does not account for time trends. As such, no causality relationship is implied. Last, the first COVID-19 vaccines received emergency use authorization in December 2020, and uptake likely impacted outcomes during our study year 2021. However, we have no data differentiating uptake by geographic region or by populations within those areas.

Public Health Implications

The study findings can inform the development of policies to address demographic disparities in HIV mortality—for example, through targeted system-level interventions for vulnerable populations, such as Medicaid expansion. In addition, modifications to the Ryan White Program policies (e.g., waiving laboratory test requirements for recertification, expanded telehealth, mail order medications) helped maintain access to care during an extraordinary health crisis, and stakeholders should seriously consider making permanent many of these modifications to further improve access to prevention and treatment services.[18,25,26] Medicaid expansion may play a crucial role in mitigating HIV mortality by advocating broader health care access to reduce disparities, especially in nonexpansion states. Most of the nonexpansion states are in the southern United States, where HIV infection rates and AIDS cases are higher than in any of the other 3 regions. The decision not to expand Medicaid in the South could negatively affect the states' economy and population health well-being in the long term because undiagnosed HIV cases could lead to unrecognized transmission and more serious AIDS symptoms. Further research is needed to understand the complex interplay between COVID-19 and HIV outcomes and to inform public health policies tailored to diverse demographic populations. AJPH

ABOUT THE AUTHORS

Donrie Purcell is with the Satcher Health Leadership Institute, Morehouse School of Medicine (MSM), Atlanta, GA. Wayne A. Duffus is with the Department of Medicine, Division of Infectious Diseases, University of South Carolina School of Medicine, Columbia. Maisha Standifer is with the Satcher Health Leadership Institute and Department of Community Health and Preventive Medicine, MSM. Robert Mayberry is with the Department of Community Health and Preventive Medicine and the MSM Research Design and Biostatistics Core, MSM. Sonja S. Hutchins is with the Department of Community Health and Preventive Medicine, MSM.

CORRESPONDENCE

Correspondence should be sent to Wayne A. Duffus, MD, PhD, Department of Medicine, Division of Infectious Diseases, University of South Carolina School of Medicine, One Medical Park, Suite 420, Columbia, SC 29203 (e-mail: wayne.duffus@prismahealth.org). Reprints can be ordered at https://www.ajph.org by clicking the "Reprints" link.

PUBLICATION INFORMATION

Full Citation: Purcell D, Duffus WA, Standifer M, Mayberry R, Hutchins SS. Population-level risks for HIV mortality during the COVID-19 pandemic in the United States by demographic characteristics and Medicaid access, 2020–2021. *Am J Public Health*. 2025;115(4):579–587.

Acceptance Date: November 4, 2024.

DOI: https://doi.org/10.2105/AJPH.2024.307916

ORCID iDs:

Donrie Purcell https://orcid.org/0000-0002-4710-9412

Wayne A. Duffus https://orcid.org/0000-0002-0014-2856

CONTRIBUTORS

All authors contributed to the concept and design. D. Purcell, W. A. Duffus, and R. Mayberry contributed the interpretation of data, writing, and editing. M. Standifer contributed the interpretation of data. S. S. Hutchins contributed to data analyses and interpretation, writing, and editing.

ACKNOWLEDGMENTS

Funding for this article was supported in part by the Dr Daniel S. Blumenthal Endowed Fund of the Morehouse School of Medicine.

CONFLICTS OF INTEREST

The authors declare no conflicts of interest.

HUMAN PARTICIPANT PROTECTION

No human participants were enrolled for this study, and the de-identified data provided for this secondary analysis is publicly available and originally collected for public health activities and purposes. All methods were carried out in accordance with relevant guidelines and regulations, including the Declaration of Helsinki. Reasonable data access requests can be made by applying to the Centers for Disease Control and Prevention.

REFERENCES

1. Baek MS, Lee MT, Kim WY, et al. COVID-19-related outcomes in immunocompromised patients: a nationwide study in Korea. *PLoS One*. 2021;16(10):e0257641. https://doi.org/10.1371/journal.pone.0257641
2. World Health Organization. COVID-19 Dashboard. Available at: https://data.who.int/dashboards/covid19/cases?n=o. Accessed February 5, 2025.
3. Johns Hopkins University. Coronavirus Resource Center: data timeline 2023. Available at: https://coronavirus.jhu.edu/region/united-states. Accessed February 5, 2025.
4. Cho SI, Yoon S, Lee HJ. Impact of comorbidity burden on mortality in patients with COVID-19 using the Korean health insurance database. *Sci Rep*. 2021;11(1):6375. https://doi.org/10.1038/s41598-021-85813-2
5. Osibogun A, Balogun M, Abayomi A, et al. Outcomes of COVID-19 patients with comorbidities in southwest Nigeria. *PLoS One*. 2021;16(3):e0248281. https://doi.org/10.1371/journal.pone.0248281
6. Sanyaolu A, Okorie C, Marinkovic A, et al. Comorbidity and its impact on patients with COVID-19. *SN Compr Clin Med*. 2020;2(8):1069–1076. https://doi.org/10.1007/s42399-020-00363-4
7. Spinelli MA, Jones BLH, Gandhi M. COVID-19 outcomes and risk factors among people living with HIV. *Curr HIV/AIDS Rep*. 2022;19(5):425–432. https://doi.org/10.1007/s11904-022-00618-w
8. Turtle L, Thorpe M, Drake TM, et al. Outcome of COVID-19 in hospitalized immunocompromised patients: an analysis of the WHO ISARIC CCP-UK prospective cohort study. *PLoS Med*. 2023;20(1):e1004086. https://doi.org/10.1371/journal.pmed.1004086
9. World Health Organization. WHO warns that HIV infection increases risk of severe and critical COVID-19. July 15, 2021. Available at: https://www.who.int/news/item/15-07-2021-who-warns-that-hiv-infection-increases-risk-of-severe-and-critical-covid-19. Accessed September 24 2024.
10. Centers for Disease Control and Prevention, National Center for Health Statistics. About underlying cause of death, 2018–2023, single race. Available at: http://wonder.cdc.gov/ucd-icd10-expanded.html. Accessed November 1, 2023.
11. Centers for Disease Control and Prevention. CDC WONDER: Multiple Cause of Death by Single Race 2018–2023. Available at: https://wonder.cdc.gov/wonder/help/mcd-expanded.html. Accessed February 5, 2025.
12. Implementing the ACA's Medicaid-Related Health Reform provisions after the Supreme Court's decision. KFF. August 1, 2012. Available at: https://www.kff.org/health-reform/issue-brief/implementing-the-acas-medicaid-related-health-reform. Accessed April 19, 2023.
13. Kaiser Family Foundation. Status of state Medicaid expansion decisions: interactive map. The Henry J. Kaiser Family Foundation. March 13, 2020. Available at: https://www.kff.org/medicaid/

issue-brief/status-of-state-medicaid-expansion-decisions-interactive-map. Accessed April 19, 2023.

14. Glen S. Census in statistics: simple definition. Statistics How To. February 3, 2023. Available at: https://www.statisticshowto.com/what-is-a-census. Accessed April 20, 2023.
15. Dasgupta S, Tie Y, Beer L, Weiser J. Unmet needs for ancillary care services are associated with HIV clinical outcomes among adults with diagnosed HIV. *AIDS Care.* 2022;34(5):606–614. https://doi.org/10.1080/09540121.2021.1946001
16. Cohen MS, Chen YQ, McCauley M, et al. Prevention of HIV-1 infection with early antiretroviral therapy. *N Engl J Med.* 2011;365(6):493–505. https://doi.org/10.1056/NEJMoa1105243
17. The White House. National HIV/AIDS Strategy for the United States 2022–2025. Available at: https://www.hiv.gov/federal-response/national-hiv-aids-strategy/national-hiv-aids-strategy-2022-2025. Accessed February 5, 2025.
18. Armstrong WS, Agwu AL, Barrette EP, et al. Innovations in human immunodeficiency virus (HIV) care delivery during the coronavirus disease 2019 (COVID-19) pandemic: policies to strengthen the Ending the Epidemic Initiative—a policy paper of the Infectious Diseases Society of America and the HIV Medicine Association. *Clin Infect Dis.* 2021;72(1):9–14. https://doi.org/10.1093/cid/ciaa1532
19. Meyer D, Slone SE, Ogungbe O, Duroseau B, Farley JE. Impact of the COVID-19 pandemic on HIV healthcare service engagement, treatment adherence, and viral suppression in the United States: a systematic literature review. *AIDS Behav.* 2023;27(1):344–357. https://doi.org/10.1007/s10461-022-03771-w
20. Liang X, Shi L, Wang Y, et al. The association of hypertension with the severity and mortality of COVID-19 patients: evidence based on adjusted effect estimates. *J Infect.* 2020;81(3):e44–e47. https://doi.org/10.1016/j.jinf.2020.06.060
21. Deiana G, Azara A, Dettori M, et al. Deaths in SARS-CoV-2 positive patients in Italy: the influence of underlying health conditions on lethality. *Int J Environ Res Public Health.* 2020;17(12):4450. https://doi.org/10.3390/ijerph17124450
22. Emami A, Javanmardi F, Akbari A, et al. Survival rate in hypertensive patients with COVID-19. *Clin Exp Hypertens.* 2021;43(1):77–80. https://doi.org/10.1080/10641963.2020.1812624
23. Filardo TD, Khan MR, Krawczyk N, et al. Comorbidity and clinical factors associated with COVID-19 critical illness and mortality at a large public hospital in New York City in the early phase of the pandemic (March–April 2020). *PLoS One.* 2020;15(11):e0242760. https://doi.org/10.1371/journal.pone.0242760
24. Han X, Hou H, Xu J, et al. Significant association between HIV infection and increased risk of COVID-19 mortality: a meta-analysis based on adjusted effect estimates. *Clin Exp Med.* 2023;23(3):689–700. https://doi.org/10.1007/s10238-022-00840-1
25. Trepka MJ, Ward MK, Ladner RA, et al. HIV care access during the COVID-19 pandemic as perceived by racial/ethnic minority groups served by the Ryan White Program, Miami-Dade County, Florida. *J Int Assoc Provid AIDS Care.* 2022;21:23259582221084536. https://doi.org/10.1177/23259582221084536
26. Patel P, Kerzner M, Reed JB, Sullivan PS, El-Sadr WM. Public health implications of adapting HIV pre-exposure prophylaxis programs for virtual service delivery in the context of the COVID-19 pandemic: systematic review. *JMIR Public Health Surveill.* 2022;8(6):e37479. https://doi.org/10.2196/37479
27. Hanson HA, Kim E, Badowski ME. A systematic review: impact of SARS-CoV-2 infection on morbidity, mortality, and viral suppression in patients living with HIV. *SN Compr Clin Med.* 2023;5(1):144. https://doi.org/10.1007/s42399-023-01480-6
28. Spence AB, Desale S, Lee J, et al. COVID-19 outcomes in a US cohort of persons living with HIV (PLWH). *Reports (MDPI).* 2022;5(4):41. https://doi.org/10.3390/reports5040041
29. Adimora AA, Ramirez C, Schoenbach VJ, Cohen MS. Policies and politics that promote HIV infection in the Southern United States. *AIDS.* 2014;28(10):1393–1397. https://doi.org/10.1097/QAD.0000000000000225
30. Poteat T, Millett GA, Nelson LE, Beyrer C. Understanding COVID-19 risks and vulnerabilities among Black communities in America: the lethal force of syndemics. *Ann Epidemiol.* 2020;47:1–3. https://doi.org/10.1016/j.annepidem.2020.05.004
31. Montano M. Pressing questions and challenges in the HIV-1 and SARS-CoV-2 syndemic. *AIDS Res Hum Retroviruses.* 2021;37(8):589–600. https://doi.org/10.1089/aid.2021.0005
32. Griffith K, Evans L, Bor J. The Affordable Care Act reduced socioeconomic disparities in health care access. *Health Aff (Millwood).* 2017;36(8):1503–1510. https://doi.org/10.1377/hlthaff.2017.0083
33. Buchmueller TC, Levy HG. The ACA's impact on racial and ethnic disparities in health insurance coverage and access to care: an examination of how the insurance coverage expansions of the Affordable Care Act have affected disparities related to race and ethnicity. *Health Aff (Millwood).* 2020;39(3):395–402. https://doi.org/10.1377/hlthaff.2019.01394
34. Auty SG, Aswani MS, Wahbi RN, Griffith KN. Changes in health care access by race, income, and Medicaid expansion during the COVID-19 pandemic. *Med Care.* 2023;61(1):45–49. https://doi.org/10.1097/MLR.0000000000001788
35. Rakus A, Soni A. Association between state Medicaid expansion status and health outcomes during the COVID-19 pandemic. *Health Serv Res.* 2022;57(6):1332–1341. https://doi.org/10.1111/1475-6773.14044
36. Feyman Y, Bor J, Raifman J, et al. Effectiveness of COVID-19 shelter in-place orders varied by state. *PLoS One.* 2020;15(12):e0245008. https://doi.org/10.1371/journal.pone.0245008
37. Tesoriero JM, Swain CE, Pierce JL, et al. COVID-19 outcomes among persons living with or without diagnosed HIV infection in New York State. *JAMA Netw Open.* 2021;4(2):e2037069. https://doi.org/10.1001/jamanetworkopen.2020.37069

OSHA Injury Data: An Opportunity for Improving Work Injury Prevention

David Michaels, PhD, MPH, and Gregory R. Wagner, MD

Millions of US workers are seriously injured on the job annually. These injuries have a significant and deleterious impact on injured workers, their families, and their communities. The limitations of the historical work injury surveillance systems have constrained research into the distribution and determinants of work injuries and efforts to improve allocation of limited injury prevention resources. Most work injury data sets suffer from significant limitations and fail to include a sizable proportion of work injuries.

In recent years, the Occupational Safety and Health Administration has begun to collect and make available to the public more detailed data on work injuries at thousands of high hazard establishments. These data sets provide the opportunity to greatly improve our work injury surveillance system. Researchers are now using these data to investigate and compare injury risk in industries and high-hazard firms where workers are at increased risk of musculoskeletal disorders. However, these rich data sets are underused.

Maintaining and facilitating access to accurate, current data can contribute to improved prevention of work-related injuries and deaths. (*Am J Public Health*. 2025;115(4):588–595. https://doi.org/10.2105/AJPH.2024.307934)

AJPH April 2025, Vol. 115, No. 4

Workers in the United States face unacceptably high risks of work-related injury. Although most employers have the legal responsibility to provide workplaces free of recognized, serious hazards, millions of workers are injured on the job each year. Despite efforts by government agencies such as the Occupational Safety and Health Administration (OSHA), employers, labor, and public health professionals over the past decade, the rate of fatal injuries has not decreased.[1] This appears to also be true for the rate of nonfatal injuries, but these injuries are so significantly undercounted that the true number and rate of work injuries are unknown.[2]

The fact that we do not have even close to accurate estimates of the number and distribution of workplace injuries is a significant barrier to understanding and addressing the causes and distribution of injuries and deaths from work.[3] With the exception of events such as mine collapses or explosions that kill several workers at once, workplace fatalities receive little public attention. If a workplace death receives any public notice at all, at most there will be a small media report of the event, often concluding with a statement that the police determined that the incident was an "accident" (meaning that it was unintentional) and that no criminal investigation would take place. The initial statements by employer representatives often attribute the incident to mistakes made by the worker: "human error."

Although work injuries are rarely in the public's consciousness, they often have a profound impact on injured workers, their families, and their communities. Beyond the human costs of injuries, the financial costs are subsidized by injured workers, their families, and other taxpayer-supported components of the social safety net.[4–6] For many injured workers and their families, a workplace injury creates a trap in which they are less able to save for the future or to make investments in skills and education that provide the opportunity for advancement, contributing to income inequality and poverty. Many injured workers, even those awarded workers' compensation, end up disabled and receiving often meager Social Security Disability Insurance benefits, resulting in taxpayer subsidization of high-hazard employers.[7,8]

A recent consensus study report issued by the National Academy of Sciences, Engineering, and Medicine recommended prioritizing and strengthening work injury and illness surveillance. The conclusion of the report was that the nation clearly needs a smarter occupational safety and health surveillance system for the 21st century.[2]

CURRENT INJURY SURVEILLANCE SYSTEMS

The Bureau of Labor Statistics (BLS) operates the 2 leading annual national work injury surveillance systems, the Census of Fatal Occupational Injuries (CFOI) and the Survey of Occupational Injuries and Illnesses (SOII). The BLS compiles the CFOI from many data sources and requires 3 pieces of confirmatory data for inclusion of a single case. The CFOI includes fatal injuries that employers under OSHA's jurisdiction are required to report, as well as fatalities that occur among employees of firms covered by other agencies such as the Mine Safety and Health Administration and workers who are self-employed or whose employer has no regulatory coverage such as some state and local government agencies.[9] During 2023, the most recent year for which statistics are available, the BLS reported that about 5300 workers were fatally injured on the job.[1]

The SOII is, by definition, a survey and not a census. Thus, the SOII can provide an estimate of the annual number and rate of injuries and illnesses derived from data recorded on forms that OSHA requires employers to maintain to track workplace injuries and illnesses. To create the SOII, the BLS first identifies a stratified sample from across all industries that considers industry, ownership, and establishment size. The agency then instructs these employers to maintain and submit the relevant data after the end of the calendar year. Because OSHA does not require small establishments (10 or fewer employees), firms covered by the Mine Safety and Health Administration and other regulatory agencies, some public sector agencies and establishments, and establishments in certain low-hazard industries to maintain OSHA logs, the BLS requests a sample of establishments in these categories to maintain the logs and send the content to the agency.

In addition, the BLS codes and checks the accuracy of injury data, reporting injury numbers and rates by industry, occupation, state, establishment size, and nature and severity of the injury. Using these employer reports, the BLS estimated that, among workers employed by private sector employers in 2023, there were 2.4 million serious injuries (a rate of 2.2 cases per 100 full-time-equivalent workers) that required treatment beyond first aid; as discussed subsequently, however, this is likely a significant underestimate given that many work injuries are not recorded by employers.[10] The nonmandatory injury reports of public sector and small establishments also result in significant underestimates.[11]

To protect the confidentiality of employers that submit data, the BLS restricts researchers' access to the CFOI and SOII data sets. Researchers must work through and closely with the BLS to access the data, and analyses can be performed only at the BLS or other tightly controlled facilities. In their publications, researchers may not reveal the identity of the employer or establishment. As a result, BLS data are useful in understanding injury incidence rates within or across industries over time but are of more limited value in conducting research on injury causation or providing information that enables microtargeting of prevention resources.

Workers' compensation cases are another source of data on injuries, although these data are often difficult to compare because they are not collected and reported consistently across the more than 50 US workers' compensation systems. To date, attempts to standardize and provide comprehensive comparative workers' compensation reporting statistics on the types and causes of injuries across the United States have not been successful. Although these data are often used to estimate the number and rate of worker injuries, statistics based on injury cases that are filed or compensated also provide an incomplete picture because a sizable proportion of injured workers do not apply for compensation and their injuries are never registered in that system.[12–14]

Finally, although OSHA's requirement is for recording both injuries and illnesses and workers' compensation insurance programs are meant to provide benefits for employees with work-related illnesses, it is widely recognized that both the recording and compensation of work illnesses are particularly incomplete.[2,15,16] Chronic disease may occur long after exposure ends, and claims are often denied by employers even if the disease manifests while the worker is employed. Musculoskeletal disorders are recorded infrequently, as are cases of hearing loss and chronic work-related asthma. Historically, employers have rarely noted the occurrence of illnesses other than the immediate effects of exposures to the skin or acute toxic inhalational injuries.

This changed somewhat during the COVID-19 pandemic. OSHA requires employers to record COVID-19 cases if the employee who had the disease while on the job had frequent, close contact with the general public in a locality with ongoing community transmission and there was no alternative explanation for the disease.[17] It is clear that recording was inconsistent and that many work-related COVID-19 cases were not recorded. For these reasons, we focus here only on work injuries.

USING DATA TO PREVENT FUTURE WORK INJURIES

In contrast to the human, social, and financial impact of this large number of work injuries, the resources devoted to researching the causation and prevention of work injuries are modest. Primary responsibility for conducting and supporting workplace injury prevention research resides with the National Institute for Occupational Safety and Health (NIOSH), organizationally located within the Centers for Disease Control and Prevention (CDC). Only approximately 4% of the CDC budget is directed to NIOSH, whose overall budget in 2023 of $362.8 million was about $2.16 per worker in the nation's civilian workforce. Within that budget, NIOSH funds intramural field and laboratory research as well as workplace injury surveillance, including supporting 23 states to conduct state-based targeted work injury and illness surveillance.[18]

Data collection varies widely from state to state, access to relevant statistical information in many states is challenging for outside researchers, and the completeness and accuracy of the data are rarely evaluated. Insurance companies that provide liability and compensation policies for employers often collect and analyze data relevant to workplace injuries. Access to these data, for example those compiled by the National Council on Compensation Insurance, is generally restricted to member organizations and is not easily available to independent researchers.

The Council of State and Territorial Epidemiologists has established and disseminated "occupational health indicators" to assist and guide state public health agencies that choose to track workplace injury and health information.[19] Tracking and reporting of these indicators vary widely among states.

INJURY DATA AS AN UNDERUSED RESOURCE

Since its beginning in 1971, OSHA has required employers to report fatal injuries to the agency. Recently, OSHA has begun to collect and make public additional data that may be useful in conducting studies that can contribute to injury prevention. Although OSHA's data are primarily self-reported by employers and have some of the limitations described earlier, they are much more extensive and easier to access than data from the BLS or state workers' compensation systems.

In the sections to follow, we discuss 3 types of injury data available from OSHA covering fatal injuries, severe injuries (amputations and hospitalizations), and injuries recorded on OSHA logs and provide examples of how they have been used. All of these data are amenable to analysis by researchers using Excel or other spreadsheet programs.

OSHA Fatality Data

Employers covered by OSHA are required to report workplace fatalities to the agency within 8 hours of the event. The agency opens a case file for each report and in many instances conducts an inspection as well. Most work fatalities reported to OSHA are caused by traumatic injuries; the data set also includes fatalities related to extreme heat, chemical releases, and other nontraumatic causes of death. Employers are not required to report a fatality if it was caused by a motor vehicle crash unless it occurred in a construction work zone. However, employers are required to record fatal injuries on their injury log if they are among the employers required to maintain such a log. On its Web site, OSHA lists more than 7500 fatalities reported to the agency since 2017, linking each to the record of the inspection if one was conducted.[20] Additional information for many fatal and severe injuries can be obtained from OSHA inspections of the establishments where the worker was hurt. Reports of fatalities that occurred between 2009 and 2017 are archived elsewhere on the OSHA Web site.[21]

Researchers have used these data, often in combination with case data from other sources, to examine risk factors for high-hazard industries such as oil and gas extraction,[22] tree felling, and arboricultural operations[23,24] or the impact of exposure to specific hazards such as extreme heat.[25] These data, although very useful, do not include deaths of workers whose employers are under the safety and health authority of other agencies or who are not covered by OSHA such as workers employed by certain state and local government agencies, by independent contractors, or through platforms such as Uber or TaskRabbit. Injuries among temporary workers employed by staffing agencies but supervised by the host employer are required by OSHA to be combined with injuries among those who are "direct hires" by the host employer; thus, injury rates among these workers may be obscured.

OSHA's Severe Injury Reporting Program

Since 2015, employers have been required to report amputations and inpatient hospitalizations to OSHA within 24 hours of occurrence. Previously, employers were required to report nonfatal events only when 3 or more workers were hospitalized. Under its Severe Injury Reporting program, the agency received about 75 000 reports between 2015 and 2021 from employers in states under the authority of federal OSHA, covering about half of the nation's workforce. Less than half of the reports resulted in an OSHA inspection. In most of the other cases, OSHA instructed the employer to conduct its own investigation into the incident and share its findings with the agency. The employer is required to provide an abatement certification signed by an official of the company that details the abatement measures that have been implemented to correct the conditions that caused the injury.[26] Complete data from these reports, including descriptions of the incident and the name and address of the establishment where it occurred, are available for downloading and analysis.[27]

Many eligible hospitalizations and amputations are not reported to OSHA. One study of reports of worker hospitalizations in Michigan showed an overall compliance rate of 45.1%, with significant variability. For example, employers in manufacturing reported 64.7% of cases, while construction employers reported 38.2% and employers in agriculture, forestry, fishing, and hunting reported 8.2%.[28]

These data have been useful to OSHA in identifying industries that had not previously been prioritized. For example, the SOII reports that supermarkets generally have low injury rates, but after OSHA received numerous reports of amputations among deli slicers and meat counter workers, the agency increased its attention to preventing those events.[29]

Severe Injury Reporting program data have been analyzed for time trends and seasonality and to examine injury causation in specific industries and firms[30] and compare amputation and hospitalization rates among different employers and industries. For example, using the data, investigative journalists with NBC News Digital identified the United Parcel Service (UPS) as employing numerous workers who were hospitalized after exposure to extreme heat. These articles were important in encouraging the Teamsters union to make heat an issue in bargaining with UPS, resulting in UPS committing to purchasing air-conditioned trucks.[31]

Academic scientists have also used Severe Injury Reporting program data in studies on the epidemiology of specific hazards or occupations; for example, data have been collected on laborers,[32] oil and gas extraction workers,[33] and operators of skid steers.[34] Recently, OSHA has developed a dashboard to facilitate downloading and analyzing data from the program.[35]

Injury Data From OSHA's Injury Tracking Application

OSHA requires most establishments with more than 10 employees to keep a record (often called the OSHA log) of serious work-related injuries and illnesses. Certain lower risk industries are exempted, and large categories of workers, including independent contractors, many state and county employees, and those employed in the gig economy, are not within OSHA's jurisdiction. Workers employed in mines are covered by the Mine Safety and Health Administration, which requires all covered employers to report injuries, fatalities, and illnesses to the agency. Operator injury reporting data and workplace safety violations are publicly available in searchable databases maintained by that agency.

The OSHA reporting requirement is establishment or workplace based rather than employer based. Although many larger employers track injuries centrally, they must maintain a record of injuries for each establishment. These data serve as the primary basis for BLS SOII estimates.

One of the objectives of this recording requirement is to help OSHA, employers, workers, and unions prevent future injuries in each establishment. OSHA inspectors examine the logs at the start of an inspection because they identify the locations of some of the most serious hazards, ones that have already injured workers.

OSHA issued a regulation in 2016 requiring certain employers with 20 or more employees in higher risk industries to electronically report the establishment-specific summary data to the agency, along with the number of hours worked at the establishment, enabling injury rate (number of injuries per 100 full-time-equivalent employees) calculation. The agency also developed the Injury Tracking Application to facilitate employers reporting data and making the data available to the public in electronic format.[36]

OSHA's primary objective in making these data publicly available derived from studies done in the behavioral sciences revealing that public disclosure of some types of data can cause behavior change in the party making the disclosure.[37,38] For example, under the Environmental Protection Agency's Toxic Release Inventory, some establishments are required to report the amounts of toxic chemicals released each year. Public disclosure of these data has contributed to significant reductions in releases.[39] Similarly, posting of restaurant letter grades given by public health inspectors has contributed to improved sanitary practices and reductions in food-borne illnesses.[40]

There are several mechanisms through which public reporting on injury rates could lead to increased injury prevention without OSHA conducting additional inspections:

- Lower injury rates provide a comparative advantage for employers trying to hire high-skill employees in competitive markets.
- Employers and workers could compare establishments' safety record with other establishments in their industry, potentially stimulating modification of safety practices and policies.
- Researchers may be able to identify previously unrecognized patterns of injuries across establishments where workers are exposed to similar hazards and evaluate the effectiveness of workplace safety activities in reducing the number or severity of work injuries or illnesses.
- Workplace safety professionals could identify establishments with high injury rates, which could benefit from their services.
- Low injury rates might improve employers' reputation among investors and consumers.

OSHA developed the Injury Tracking Application to facilitate electronic collection of these data and to enable employers to upload data files. Establishment-specific summary injury data are available for years subsequent to 2016, although they do not represent the complete set of data OSHA should have received and the agency does not check the data for accuracy or completeness before posting them.[36] The Government Accountability Office reported that 42% and 46% of establishments sent the required data to OSHA in 2017 and 2018, respectively.[41]

Although these data are useful in benchmarking overall safety performance and helping to identify facilities with particularly effective or ineffective injury prevention programs, there is compelling evidence that statistics derived from employer self-reports significantly underestimate the actual burden of injuries occurring among the nation's workers.[13–15] The BLS commissioned a series of studies by academic researchers to estimate the percentage of work-related injuries reported by employers. All of these studies showed that a significant proportion of work injuries (30% to more than 60%) were not included in employer reports, with underreporting varying by employer and type of injury.[13]

To date, summary injury data have been used by researchers, journalists, and public health activists to better understand the relative risk of injuries in several high-hazard industries. Studies incorporating these data have shown, for example, that workers at Amazon fulfillment centers are at greater risk of injury than workers at comparable facilities operated by other firms[42,43] and that injury risk increases significantly during high-volume events such as Prime Day and Cyber Monday.[44] Researchers have also used information collected in the CFOI, SOII, and Injury Tracking Application data sets to examine injury trends among parcel delivery drivers.[45] Elevated worker injury rates gleaned from Injury Tracking Application data, as well as the firm's failure to report injuries in some years, were central in a recent report by Reuters on safety hazards at SpaceX[46] and a *Wall Street Journal* investigation into injuries suffered by aviation industry ground workers who refuel planes, handle baggage, and help move aircraft around the tarmac.[47]

Because many employers who are required to send their data to OSHA fail to do so, examining the employers that report their data to the agency and the ones that do not can also provide useful insights. Researchers have looked at the impact of unionization on establishments reporting injury data to OSHA, finding that unionization increases injury reporting.[48]

The availability of establishment-specific injury rates and granular information on large numbers of establishments provides researchers with the ability to conduct more in-depth analyses of a wide range of topics. It might be productive, for example, to link the Injury Tracking Application data set with other establishment- or corporation-specific data sets that focus on union status, management structure and characteristics, amount of overtime work, corporate financial health, ownership (public vs private), workers' compensation insurance carrier, chemical emissions, Environmental

Protection Agency violations, or other variables.

To further increase the value of these data in injury prevention, it would be worthwhile for OSHA to prioritize issuing citations and fines to employers that do not report and publicizing their names. Although the monetary penalties for not reporting are relatively low, this may encourage some firms to report to avoid reputational damage.

AVAILABILITY OF INJURY CASE DATA

OSHA now requires establishments in higher hazard industries with 100 or more workers to electronically submit case data on each injury.[49] Data from almost 900 000 injuries and illnesses recorded and reported by more than 350 000 establishments in 2023 have been posted by OSHA. These data include the date and time of the incident (if known) and text fields that provide additional information about the injury or illness, the parts of the body affected, and the objects or substances that directly injured or made the person ill. OSHA has redacted certain information from the text fields to protect the confidentiality of injured workers.[36]

For research purposes, the data in the deidentified text fields will become much more useful when they are coded into the variables commonly used in injury categories. The BLS has developed an automated coding system for converting text descriptions of injuries into coding text in the standard categories used in reporting injury data (e.g., nature of injury, part of body injured).[50] OSHA has plans to provide tools to make the data easier to search and download and is working with the BLS to develop a system to code the Injury Tracking Application data. NIOSH has developed an automated system to code records for industries and occupations.[51,52]

Establishment-specific data also have significant limitations. Injury rates are lagging indicators and provide limited information about the presence of hazards that could contribute to future injuries. In addition, most injuries reported by employers are caused by ergonomic hazards or are types of personal injuries sometimes called "slips, trips, and falls." Injuries associated with process safety hazards (those that occur when there is an explosion, fire, or chemical release) are far less frequent events. Low injury rates are sometimes misinterpreted to suggest that process safety hazards are well controlled. Famously, BP executives gave an award for low injury rates to the team operating the Deepwater Horizon drilling rig the day before the rig exploded, killing 11 workers, injuring 17, and releasing the millions of barrels of oil that devastated the ecosystem of much of the Gulf of Mexico.[53]

Even with these caveats, the existence and accessibility of the new OSHA data sets provide an important opportunity to improve our understanding and prevention of work injuries. Establishment-specific data could be cross-linked with information from other data sets to compare the characteristics of establishments that that do similar work but have dissimilar rates of different types of injuries. Employers can now benchmark their injury rates with other firms in their industry. Establishment-specific data can also be used to improve the targeting of prevention efforts. These efforts would be strengthened if OSHA is able to increase compliance with its regulations on recording and reporting work injuries and to make efforts to improve the accuracy and completeness of data.

In summary, when identifying areas in which additional research could have a significant public health impact, work injuries are low-hanging fruit. We believe that increased research into the distribution and determinants of work injuries, especially using data sets that OSHA now makes publicly available and linking them with other databases, can make an important contribution to increased prevention of work-related injuries and fatalities. Maintaining and promoting access to these data are critical. AJPH

ABOUT THE AUTHORS

David Michaels is with the George Washington University Milken Institute School of Public Health, Washington, DC. Gregory R. Wagner is with the Harvard T. H. Chan School of Public Health, Boston, MA.

CORRESPONDENCE

Correspondence should be sent to David Michaels, PhD, MPH, Environmental & Occupational Health Department, George Washington University Milken Institute School of Public Health, 950 New Hampshire Ave NW, Washington, DC 20052 (e-mail: drdavidmichaels@gmail.com). Reprints can be ordered at https://www.ajph.org by clicking the "Reprints" link.

PUBLICATION INFORMATION

Full Citation: Michaels D, Wagner GR. OSHA injury data: an opportunity for improving work injury prevention. *Am J Public Health*. 2025;115(4):588–595.

Acceptance Date: November 11, 2024.

DOI: https://doi.org/10.2105/AJPH.2024.307934

ORCID iDs:

David Michaels https://orcid.org/0000-0001-8558-7733

Gregory R. Wagner https://orcid.org/0000-0003-4165-7079

CONTRIBUTORS

D. Michaels and G. R. Wagner were co-first authors and contributed equally to all aspects of the article.

ACKNOWLEDGMENTS

We acknowledge financial support from the McElhattan Foundation. David Michaels also receives financial support from the Health Action Alliance.

We thank Kenneth Rosenman for his advice on work injury and illness data and Vana Brookins for assistance with the article. We are also grateful to the leadership and staff of the Occupational Safety and Health Administration and the Bureau of Labor Statistics for their continued commitment to the safety and health of the nation's workers.

CONFLICTS OF INTEREST

The authors report no conflicts of interest.

HUMAN PARTICIPANT PROTECTION

No human participants were involved in this research.

REFERENCES

1. US Bureau of Labor Statistics. Census of fatal occupational injuries summary, 2023. Available at: https://www.bls.gov/news.release/cfoi.nr0.htm. Accessed January 21, 2025.
2. National Academies of Sciences, Engineering, and Medicine. *A Smarter National Surveillance System for Occupational Safety and Health in the 21st Century*. Washington, DC: National Academies Press; 2024.
3. Spieler EA, Wagner GR. Counting matters: implications of undercounting in the BLS survey of occupational injuries and illnesses. *Am J Ind Med*. 2014;57(10):1077–1084. https://doi.org/10.1002/ajim.22382
4. Leigh JP, Marcin J. Workers' compensation benefits and shifting costs for occupational injury and illness. *J Occup Environ Med*. 2012;54(4):445–450. https://doi.org/10.1097/JOM.0b013e3182451e54
5. Leigh JP. Economic burden of occupational injury and illness in the United States. *Milbank Q*. 2011;89(4):728–772. https://doi.org/10.1111/j.1468-0009.2011.00648.x
6. Groenewold MR, Baron SL. The proportion of work-related emergency department visits not expected to be paid by workers' compensation: implications for occupational health surveillance, research, policy, and health equity. *Health Serv Res*. 2013;48(6):1939–1959. https://doi.org/10.1111/1475-6773.12066
7. Michaels D. Adding inequality to injury: the costs of failing to protect workers on the job. Available at: https://www.regulations.gov/document/OSHA-2015-0002-0059. Accessed January 21, 2025.
8. Reville RT, Schoeni RF. The fraction of disability caused at work. *Soc Secur Bull*. 2004;65:31–37.
9. US Bureau of Labor Statistics. Technical notes. Available at: https://www.bls.gov/news.release/cfoi.tn.htm. Accessed October 15, 2024.
10. US Bureau of Labor Statistics. Employer-reported workplace injuries and illnesses, 2023. Available at: https://www.bls.gov/news.release/osh.nr0.htm. Accessed January 21, 2025.
11. Huband EM, Bobbitt PA. Nonresponse bias in the Survey of Occupational Injuries and Illnesses. https://www.bls.gov/osmr/research-papers/2013/pdf/st130170.pdf. Accessed January 21, 2025.
12. Spieler EA. (Re)assessing the grand bargain: compensation for work injuries in the US, 1900–2017. *Rutgers University Law Rev*. 2017;69:891–1014.
13. US Bureau of Labor Statistics. Injuries, illnesses, and fatalities: Survey of Occupation Injuries and Illness Data Quality Research. Available at: https://www.bls.gov/iif/data-quality-research/data-quality.htm. Accessed January 21, 2025.
14. Boden LI, Ozonoff A. Capture-recapture estimates of nonfatal workplace injuries and illnesses. *Ann Epidemiol*. 2008;18(6):500–506. https://doi.org/10.1016/j.annepidem.2007.11.003
15. Azaroff LS, Levenstein C, Wegman DH. Occupational injury and illness surveillance: conceptual filters explain underreporting. *Am J Public Health*. 2002;92(9):1421–1429. https://doi.org/10.2105/AJPH.92.9.1421
16. US Department of Labor, Office of the Assistant Secretary for Policy, Evaluation, and Research. An interim report to Congress on occupational diseases. Available at: https://www.google.com/books/edition/An_Interim_Report_to_Congress_on_Occupat/u3Ype2_9oeAC?hl=en. Accessed January 21, 2025.
17. Kapust PJ. Updated interim enforcement response plan for coronavirus disease 2019 (COVID-19). Available at: https://www.osha.gov/laws-regs/standardinterpretations/2021-07-07. Accessed January 21, 2025.
18. National Institute for Occupational Safety and Health. NIOSH State Occupational Safety and Health Surveillance Program. Available at: https://www.cdc.gov/niosh/extramural-programs/php/about/state-surveillance.html. Accessed January 21, 2025.
19. Council of State and Territorial Epidemiologists. Occupational health indicators. Available at: https://www.cste.org/page/OHIndicators. Accessed January 21, 2025.
20. US Occupational Safety and Health Administration. Fatality inspection data: work-related fatalities for cases inspected by federal or state OSHA. Available at: https://www.osha.gov/fatalities#&sort%5B. Accessed October 15, 2024.
21. US Occupational Safety and Health Administration. Reports of fatalities and catastrophes. Available at: https://www.osha.gov/fatalities/reports/archive. Accessed October 15, 2024.
22. Wingate KC, Ramirez-Cardenas A, Hill R, Ridl S, Hagan-Haynes K. Fatalities in Oil and Gas Extraction Database, an industry-specific worker fatality surveillance system—United States, 2014–2019. *MMWR Surveill Summ*. 2023;72(8, SS-8):1–15. https://doi.org/10.15585/mmwr.ss7208a1
23. Michael J, Gorucu S. Occupational tree felling fatalities: 2010–2020. *Am J Ind Med*. 2021;64(11):969–977. https://doi.org/10.1002/ajim.23286
24. Ball J, Vosberg SJ, Walsh T. A Review of United States arboricultural operation fatal and nonfatal incidents (2001–2017): implications for safety training. Available at: https://tinyurl.com/mu5ubas4. Accessed October 15, 2024.
25. Tustin AW, Cannon DL, Arbury SB, Thomas RJ, Hodgson MJ. Risk factors for heat-related illness in US workers: An OSHA case series. *J Occup Environ Med*. 2018;60(8):e383–e389. https://doi.org/10.1097/JOM.0000000000001365
26. US Occupational Safety and Health Administration. Severe injury report: a seven year lookback. Available at: https://www.osha.gov/sites/default/files/severe-injury-report-2015to2021.pdf. Accessed January 21, 2025.
27. US Occupational Safety and Health Administration. Severe Injury Reports Database. Available at: https://www.osha.gov/sites/default/files/severe_injury.zip. Accessed January 21, 2025.
28. Reilly MJ, Wang L, Rosenman KD. Evaluation of the characteristics of workers injured on the job requiring hospitalization, and employer compliance with OSHA's reporting requirement for these work-related hospitalizations. *Am J Ind Med*. 2023;66(2):109–121. https://doi.org/10.1002/ajim.23447
29. US Occupational Safety and Health Administration. OSHA Fact sheet: preventing cuts and amputations from food slicers and meat grinders. Available at: https://www.osha.gov/sites/default/files/publications/OSHA3794.pdf. Accessed January 21, 2025.
30. Gomes H, Parasram V, Collins J, Socias-Morales C. Time series, seasonality and trend evaluation of 7 years (2015–2021) of OSHA severe injury data. *J Safety Res*. 2023;86:30–38. doi: 10.1016/j.jsr.2023.06.005.PMID: 37718058.
31. McCorvey JJ, Kaplan A, Probert A. UPS drivers on track to get air-conditioned trucks for the first time. Available at: https://www.nbcnews.com/business/business-news/ups-drivers-track-get-air-conditioned-trucks-first-time-ever-rcna88460. Accessed January 21, 2025.
32. Morrissey MC, Kerr ZY, Brewer GJ, Tishukaj F, Casa DJ, Stearns RL. Analysis of exertion-related injuries and fatalities in laborers in the United States. *Int J Environ Res Public Health*. 2023;20(3):2683. https://doi.org/10.3390/ijerph20032683
33. Parasram V, Socias-Morales C, Reichard A. Severe work-related injuries in the oil and gas extraction industry—32 federal Occupational Safety and Health Administration jurisdictions, United States, January 2015–July 2022. *MMWR Morb Mortal Wkly Rep*. 2024;73(5):104–109. https://doi.org/10.15585/mmwr.mm7305a3
34. Gorucu S, Weichelt B, Burk R. Injuries and illnesses related to skid steers: 2015–2020. *Safety (Basel)*. 2022;8(3):56. https://doi.org/10.3390/safety8030056
35. US Occupational Safety and Health Administration. Severe injury reports. Available at: https://www.osha.gov/severe-injury-reports. Accessed January 21, 2025.
36. US Occupational Safety and Health Administration. Injury Tracking Application (ITA) data: establishment and case detail work-related injury and illness data. Available at: https://www.osha.gov/Establishment-Specific-Injury-and-Illness-Data. Accessed January 21, 2025.
37. Fung A, Graham M, Weil D. *Full Disclosure: The Perils and Promise of Transparency*. Cambridge, England: Cambridge University Press; 2007.
38. Johnson MS. Regulation by shaming: deterrence effects of publicizing violations of workplace safety and health laws. *Am Econ Rev*. 2020;110(6):1866–1904. https://doi.org/10.1257/aer.20180501
39. Hamilton JT. *Regulation through Revelation: The Origin, Politics, and Impacts of the Toxics Release Inventory Program*. Cambridge, England: Cambridge University Press; 2005.
40. Kim TN, Edmundson AR, Hedberg CW. Foodborne illness complaint systems detect, and restaurant inspection programs prevent restaurant-associated foodborne illness outbreaks. *Foodborne Pathog Dis*. 2024;21(2):92–98. https://doi.org/10.1089/fpd.2023.0086
41. US Government Accountability Office. Workplace safety and health: actions needed to improve reporting of summary injury and illness data. Available at: https://www.gao.gov/products/gao-21-122. Accessed January 21, 2025.

42. Greene J, Alcantara C. Amazon warehouse workers suffer serious injuries at higher rates than other firms. Available at: https://www.washingtonpost.com/technology/2021/06/01/amazon-osha-injury-rate. Accessed January 21, 2025.
43. Tung I, Tufano A. Amazon workers are injured almost twice as often as other warehouse workers in Massachusetts. Available at: https://www.nelp.org/insights-research/amazon-workers-are-injured-almost-twice-as-often-as-other-warehouse-workers-in-massachusetts. Accessed January 21, 2025.
44. Strategic Organizing Center. Same day injury: Amazon fails to deliver safe jobs. Available at: https://thesoc.org/what-we-do/same-day-injury-amazon-fails-to-deliver-safe-jobs. Accessed January 21, 2025.
45. Iacobucci E, McDonald NC, Naumann RB, Kucera KL. Examining injury trends in parcel delivery drivers in the United States: challenges and opportunities. *Am J Ind Med*. 2023;66(6):441–453. https://doi.org/10.1002/ajim.23473
46. Taylor M. At SpaceX, worker injuries soar in Elon Musk's rush to Mars: a Reuters investigation. Available at: https://www.reuters.com/investigates/special-report/spacex-musk-safety. Accessed January 21, 2025.
47. Katz B. More workers are getting hurt on the tarmac: "it was really frightening." Available at: https://www.wsj.com/business/airlines/airport-ground-workers-safety-airlines-c98e3216. Accessed October 15, 2024.
48. Dean A, McCallum J, Venkataramani AS, Michaels D. The effect of labor unions on nursing home compliance with OSHA's workplace injury and illness reporting requirement. *Health Aff (Millwood)*. 2023;42(9):1260–1265. https://doi.org/10.1377/hlthaff.2023.00255
49. US Department of Labor, US Occupational Safety and Health Administration. Improve tracking of workplace injuries and illnesses. Available at: https://www.federalregister.gov/documents/2023/07/21/2023-15091/improve-tracking-of-workplace-injuries-and-illnesses. Accessed January 21, 2025.
50. US Bureau of Labor Statistics. Injuries, illnesses, and fatalities: automated coding of injury and illness data. Available at: https://www.bls.gov/iif/automated-coding.html. Accessed January 21, 2025.
51. US Centers for Disease Control and Prevention. Modernizing the coding of occupational health data. Available at: https://www.cdc.gov/nndss/in-action/health-data.html. Accessed January 21, 2025.
52. US Centers for Disease Control and Prevention. NIOSH Industry and Occupation Computerized Coding System. Available at: https://csams.cdc.gov/nioccs. Accessed January 21, 2025.
53. Jacobs D. *BP Blowout: Inside the Gulf Oil Disaster*. Washington, DC: Brookings Institution Press; 2016.

Navigating Dual-Harm: Integrating Self- and Other-Harm Into Public Health Inquiry

Diego A. Díaz-Faes, PhD, Sonali Rajan, EdD, and Charles C. Branas, PhD

Dual-harm, the co-occurrence of self- and other-harm, recognizes the overlap between these outcomes of aggressive behavior and their potential shared causes. Little progress has been made in preventing and responding to dual-harm in the broader population, and it remains understudied in public health research.

We posit that the scientific investigation of dual-harm would greatly benefit from the application of public health principles and methods. In this essay, we operationalize dual-harm as a public health problem and identify gaps in knowledge, addressing its conceptual and definitional issues, prevalence estimates, methodological considerations, theoretical foundations, risk factors, and prevention strategies. We also offer a series of recommendations to advance dual-harm study and challenge the notion of conflating nonfatal dual-harm with homicide-suicide as part of a continuum, arguing that they are distinct phenomena. We identify the need for epidemiological studies to characterize those engaging in dual-harm and better understand their mechanisms and outcomes, focusing on adolescence as a critical developmental period.

Future studies should develop, implement, and evaluate targeted intervention and preventive efforts for individuals involved in or at risk for dual-harm. (*Am J Public Health*. 2025;115(4):596–604. https://doi.org/10.2105/AJPH.2024.307940)

AJPH April 2025, Vol. 115, No. 4

Self- and other-harm, outcomes of inward-outward aggression, are typically studied in isolation from one another, treated as separate phenomena, or even seen as opposite. Consequently, individuals who engage in either self- or other-harm are often considered to be 2 discrete populations. However, it is documented that some individuals engage in both.[1,2] This means that self- and other-harm may co-occur or be intertwined. Those involved in dual-harm may share a significant number of etiological pathways and risk factors but also present an exacerbation of such risks.[3] Individuals engaging in dual-harm may share an underlying vulnerability to emotional and behavioral dysregulation that drives aggression while facing long-term life difficulties.[4] Framing self- and other-harm as nonlinked fails to examine the directionality and possible feedback loops between them and overlooks the associated risks. For example, a population-based case–control cohort study found that individuals engaging in dual-harm had a higher risk of death from external causes and a greater prevalence of multiple drug misuse than those with either no history of harm or single-harm involvement.[5]

A significant number of dual-harm studies have been conducted in clinical and forensic settings (e.g., with prisoners and forensic inpatients), focusing on high-risk populations.[1,2] Nonfatal dual-harm incidents that take place in nonclinical settings are equally challenging, and it is important to better understand them; to date, however, there has been limited data or research informing this phenomenon. Only a small proportion of those who harm themselves attend or receive clinical services; that is, most self-harm episodes occur at the community level (i.e., non-high-risk samples, such as adolescents from the general population).[6] Official records provide little insight into aggression among those without contact with the criminal justice system. Additionally, there is very limited research that has framed nonfatal dual-harm via a population-based approach. Incidence and prevalence rates in the general population, as well as their distribution among subgroups, remain unexplored, and longitudinal harm trajectories (i.e., no-harm vs single-harm vs dual-harm) have been barely explored.[7]

For these reasons, we advocate for incorporating the study of dual-harm into the public health research agenda. Decker et al.'s integrated public health approach to interpersonal violence and suicide prevention provides a strong foundation for nonfatal dual-harm prevention, grounded in an intersectional and socioecological framework.[8] Recent research has begun to explore the prevalence, trajectories, and risk factors associated with dual-harm, primarily at the individual level. However, there remains a gap in addressing risk patterns of inward-outward aggression through a multilayered perspective that considers age, gender, sexual orientation, and race/ethnicity. Also lacking is a population-level approach that incorporates social determinants of health, including structural factors (e.g., urban policies like redlining) and community factors (e.g., hazardous conditions, neighborhood collective efficacy) and their impact on dual-harm prevention.[9] Such an approach would help shape an epidemiological characterization of the population that engages in dual-harm, leading to a better understanding of its correlates, pathways, and outcomes, as well as the role of oppression, inequality, and power dynamics. Ultimately, this would allow for the prevention of dual-harm by distinguishing the variables and patterns linked to dual-harm from those associated with single- or no-harm and facilitate the early detection of those involved in dual-harm. This is crucial because self-harm emerges during late childhood and early adolescence,[10] a period when various changes in the patterns and levels of antisocial and criminal behavior also occur and intensify.[11]

In this essay, we review the theoretical and empirical foundations of dual-harm research, and highlight key research in this area to date, gaps in the existing knowledge base, methods of prevention, and suggestions to move new studies forward. We also offer a series of reflections to increase awareness and help further expand public health research and inquiry.

DUAL-HARM: CONCEPTUAL AND DEFINITIONAL ISSUES

The variability in the study on both self- and other-harm is also reflected in the study of dual-harm, referred to as the co-occurrence of self- and other-harm. There is currently no agreed-upon operational definition of dual-harm, which is particularly challenging because of the convergence and exacerbation of issues present in both self- and other-harm literature. We therefore discuss 5 main elements of contention in dual-harm research:

1. the definition of self-harm,
2. other-harm—the specific aggressive behaviors relevant to the dual-harm construct,
3. the role of homicide followed by suicide with dual-harm research,
4. the behavioral time span, and
5. the identification of the harm groups.

Self-Harm

Self-harm refers to nonfatal acts of self-poisoning or self-injury.[12] Yet, there remains an ongoing debate on the definition, boundaries, and taxonomy of self-harm behaviors. Some describe self-harm as occurring regardless of suicidal intent, whereas others define it in the absence of such intent, irrespective of the motivation or degree of suicidal intent.[6,13] This has led to a loose definition of self-harm since, depending on the frame, it can encompass nonsuicidal self-injury (NSSI), indirect self-injury, or a suicide attempt. Presently, 3 leading organizations have addressed the definitional issues. The American Psychiatric Association differentiates between NSSI (self-inflicted damage to the body surface or internal injury) and self-harm with intent to die (i.e., suicide attempt). The Centers for Disease Control and Prevention (CDC) distinguishes suicidal self-directed violence from nonsuicidal self-directed violence; in both cases, behaviors deliberately cause injury, but in nonsuicidal self-directed violence, there is no explicit or implicit suicidal intent (i.e., no fully revealed or expressed intention either implied or inherent in the nature of something, as defined by the CDC).[14] The International Society for the Study of Self-Injury defines NSSI as an intentional or expected self-inflicted injury resulting in immediate physical injury not intended to cause death or based on social or cultural practices,[15] thus delineating NSSI from thoughts or behaviors with suicidal intention. Lack of specificity or uncertainty exists across definitions regarding the required body damage or the level of immediacy of the resulting injury. Consequently, some studies differentiate between NSSI and suicide attempts when considering self-harm, whereas others do not.

From a practical standpoint, to address suicidal-related behaviors,

AJPH April 2025, Vol. 115, No. 4

public health scholars can rely on the conceptualization provided by the International Study of Definitions of English-Language Terms for Suicidal Behaviors (ISDELTSB).[16] It offers a minimum starting consensus covering the views of high-income and low- to middle-income countries. As the ISDELTSB suggested, self-harm involves nonfatal self-inflicted harm where the intent to die is either absent or not observable. If the person reports intent to die, the suicide attempt is the preferred construct. Therefore, a suicide attempt involves self-inflicted harm with intent to die in which the person survives.

Other-Harm

The most accepted definition of human aggression is a goal-directed behavior aimed at causing harm to another person who wants to avoid the harm.[17] Aggression encompasses various modalities, subtypes, motivations, and behavioral patterns, whereas the severity of acts varies widely across its forms. Dual-harm research has utilized either a broad or narrow range of aggressive behaviors toward others, depending on the specific focus of the study. Some have considered multiple forms of aggression, and others focus solely on physical aggression, excluding verbal aggression or property damage. However, the question of which behaviors are pertinent—and why—remains open to interpretation.

Reaching a certain degree of consensus on the aggressive behaviors relevant to dual-harm will be a lengthy process. Although some variability according to context is expected, it would be helpful to outline the core of the phenomena and delve into why self- and other-harm are associated with one another. To advance this early-stage field, we suggest that researchers prioritize interpersonal aggression, adopting a relatively narrow approach to establish a solid foundation. We suggest focusing on direct aggression (behaviors openly aimed at causing physical or psychological harm to others or coercing them[18]) and relational aggression (a nonphysical form of aggression aimed at damaging or threatening to damage relationships[18]). In particular, we emphasize moderate and severe forms of direct physical aggression, which include sexual aggression.

We also consider relational aggression in intimate relationships to be a significant component of dual-harm, although its consistent measurement remains challenging because of several methodological issues associated with relational aggression measures.[19] We recommend including it only if it is assessed adequately.

In contrast, alongside noninterpersonal aggression, we suggest excluding the relational aggression modality of bullying from the core set of behaviors, for several reasons. Although a meta-analytic review has found a relationship between bullying perpetration and dating violence perpetration,[20] the link is weak, largely based on cross-sectional research, and does not account for the relative contributions of bullying subtypes. Bullying is particularly rooted in peer dynamics and group processes, which can encourage bystander involvement, especially in its mild to moderate forms.[21]

An exploratory, data-driven examination of additional behaviors that may expand the dual-harm construct can complement the proposed core set of behaviors. Shafti et al. made an initial attempt to analyze the relationship between self-harm and various types of aggressive behaviors, finding a weak correlation.[22] They concluded that relational aggression, in the forms of bullying and dating violence, should not be included in their definition of dual-harm. Notably, the study assessed bullying and dating violence differently, categorizing both as relational aggression but capturing only physical instances of dating violence, which conflicts with the definition of relational aggression applied in aggression research. We urge researchers to properly capture and describe aggressive behaviors. Additionally, certain types of violence, such as bias-based violence, are uniquely shaped by sex/gender, race/ethnicity, disability, and other intersecting identities, highlighting the need to consider how some forms of violence manifest.[23,24]

Lessons From Homicide-Suicide Literature

Akin to the dimensional model of suicide, it has been suggested that dual-harm can be understood as a continuum based on the level of harm, with homicide-suicide representing its most serious form.[2] Most research on homicide-suicide and nonfatal dual-harm has been conducted independently. Theories addressing dual-harm have arisen from the suicide and extreme aggression framework, whereas less severe forms have received less theoretical attention.[1,2,25] Homicide-suicide presents several conceptual challenges, including the lack of a formal or legal definition, questions about whether it should be limited to intentional homicides, and variability in the time frame of occurrence (typically within 24 hours, but sometimes extending to days, weeks, or without a specific limit).[25,26] Homicide-suicide is an extremely rare event that primarily occurs within the family context.[27] Internationally, the incidences vary around the world, ranging from 0.05 to 0.89 per 100 000 inhabitants.[25] We argue that homicide-suicide may be better understood as a distinct phenomenon from nonfatal dual-harm and that it may constitute distinguishable subpopulations. Even when one considers self- and other-harm in high-risk populations framed within the broader conceptualization of dual-harm, homicide-suicide is regarded somewhat separately.[28] Research in homicide-suicide is framed in death studies, mass murder, femicide, familicide, terrorism, lethal firearm use, or copycat crimes.[26,29] Including homicide-suicide as part of the dual-harm continuum—the hypothesis of escalation—may potentially blur the discussion by considering an outlier with different sociodemographic characteristics, contextual factors, and situational inducement.

Time Span

Another key definitional element with no consensus is the time span in which self- and other-harm must occur to qualify as a dual-harm incident. The emergence of dual-harm among youths is likely to follow a developmental sequence.[30] Individuals typically begin with 1 behavior and transition later to another, as they may serve different functions.[31,32] Dual-harm has been measured either concurrently or sequentially. The 2 systematic reviews covering any form of dual-harm have employed a broad approach to time frames (i.e., lifetime).[1,2] Longitudinal data can help to identify dual-harm progression and to what extent it is sensitive to a specific developmental period, such as adolescence. We suggest that if the assessment is longitudinal, the 12-month window is a usual measure in many cohort studies, allowing one to gather information accurately while reducing recall bias.

Harm Groups

Once the behaviors are identified, cross-tabulation allows for the identification of individuals who engage in harmful behaviors and classify them into the following groups: self-harm, other-harm, and dual-harm. The dual-harm group can be further disaggregated into 2 groups to assess directionality (self-harm to other-harm and other-harm to self-harm) if the study design allows for adequate assessment of the temporal order of events. Similarly, the single-harm group can also be disaggregated between those who engaged in self-harm or other-harm.

PREVALENCE ESTIMATES

Dual-harm prevalence varies according to the narrowness of the definition used, the population studied, and the measures employed: 0.9% of people incarcerated (89.1% no-harm),[33] 11% in a prospective sample of psychiatric inpatients,[34] 13% in a cohort of psychiatric outpatients,[35] 2.8% of adults (aged ≥ 18 years),[36] 0.4% in a population-based cohort of adolescents (14.8% within the self-harm group),[4] 3.7% of youths in a intergenerational cohort study,[37] 4.7% in a cohort of youth twin pairs,[38] 7.2% in a stratified random cohort of adolescents,[39] and 17.1% in another prospective population-based cohort.[40] As observed, there is a wide range of prevalence across studies. Interestingly, the prevalence is surprisingly low in the largest study so far involving incarcerated persons,[33] which defies current dual-harm knowledge[28] and the well-known elevated risk of mortality, morbidity, and behavioral problems among this population.[41] These findings warrant further research.

METHODOLOGICAL CONSIDERATIONS

Most dual-harm investigations heavily rely on cross-sectional designs and relatively small sample sizes.[1,2] Only a handful of cohort studies have started to address the longitudinal course of self-, other-, and dual-harm together.[5,7,33,38,39] Because of definitional and methodological heterogeneity and the implications of the types of measures used (e.g., self-reports or psychophysiological measures), making direct comparisons across studies is challenging. A common approach to nonfatal dual-harm studies is the use of nonvalidated self-report measures to assess harmful behaviors.[2] We suggest using validated measures of aggression and cross-informants' perspectives to capture children's and adolescents' behaviors while being aware of the limitations of identifying causal effects.[42,43]

Level of Analysis

Traditional clinical and epidemiological research is nomothetic (population-based, focused on interindividual variation). Nomothetic knowledge is fundamental, but understanding aggressive behaviors also requires an idiographic (individual-based, focused on intraindividual variation) approach. At the societal level, researchers can address societal factors by examining policies and policing practices, such as health care accessibility, (de)criminalization, income security, crisis support resources, and school-based mental health programs. To assess the influence of cultural norms and beliefs, researchers can use large social or public opinion surveys. This can be combined with individual-level data to examine how broader societal or environmental factors interact with individual characteristics influencing aggressive behaviors and associated outcomes, although it requires data harmonization.[44] At the group level, nomothetic analysis identifies population patterns by examining differences between groups, the primary approach for advancing dual-harm research at this early stage. It helps uncover what differentiates those engaged in dual-harm from those involved in single- or no-harm. Here, researchers can follow our suggestion to find a balance between conceptualization and measurement and how to leverage the existing public health data. At the individual level, idiographic approaches using clinical data can provide insights for more personalized treatment by helping to understand the dynamics underlying mental health issues, identifying the optimal timing for intervention, and uncovering unique symptoms or individual differences that contribute to the outcome.[45] Time series analysis or real-time evaluation, such as ecological momentary assessment, can be a fruitful methodology to capture processes influencing behaviors.

Data Sources

To study human aggression, public health researchers often use a variety of data sources intended for different purposes, such as hospital records, nationally representative surveys via existing surveillance systems, and crime and criminal justice data. These different types of data sources pose different shortcomings. For instance, public health survey data collecting self-harm and suicide exhibit greater variability across data collection levels, procedures, and case classification while relying on self-reports and not capturing fatal instances. Similarly, health care data also underrepresent instances of self-harm, in particular nonfatal attempts. They focus on injuries and immediate medical outcomes but, unlike crime data, often lack a broader psychosocial context. Medical records can also contain stigmatizing language that drives implicit bias.[46] Because of its design, *International Classification of Diseases* (*ICD*) coding has limitations as a tool for determining intentionality and perpetrator relationships. On the other hand, crime and criminal justice data are based on legal definitions that often differ across jurisdictions and from the scientific consensus.[47] Some crimes are not necessarily intended, as incidents can escalate, or the result can be somewhat accidental. The wording can be narrow but inaccurate, overinclusive, or encompassing a broad range of behaviors that vary in severity (e.g., domestic violence).

We suggest that public health researchers employ multiple sources of data not limited to observational accounts and capitalize on nationally representative data sets to epidemiologically characterize the population of those involved in dual-harm and provide more reliable estimates of its incidence and prevalence in the community. Useful references for this endeavor include a review of national data sources on adolescent suicidal ideation and suicide attempts, including related factors such as aggressive behaviors,[48] as well as a systematic review of *ICD-10* codes for all forms of injury.[49] For example, the National Violent Death Reporting System can be used to study homicide-suicide, but also premature or accidental death related to nonfatal dual-harm.

Public health researchers must carefully examine both self- and other-harm and be transparent about the pros and cons of the selected approach to provide evidence to build the scaffolding for a reliable conceptualization of the behaviors and outcomes that are relevant to the dual-harm construct. That said, there are no gold standard measures for all scenarios to capture self- and other-harm and the related risk factors and outcomes. The use of objective and subjective measures has advantages and disadvantages that need to be considered.[50,51] Otherwise, researchers may overlook potential measurement bias. For instance, common method variance can occur in cross-sectional studies when the same method and source are used to capture the variables of interest, such as the relationship between a psychological construct and behavior, leading to potentially detrimental effects (e.g., inflated correlations).

THEORETICAL CONSIDERATIONS

Because of the conceptual problems and limited research, it is still not possible to ascertain whether dual-harm is a separate behavioral construct from self- and other-harm with distinct, unique underlying factors. Current evidence suggests that dual-harm may represent an overlap between self- and other-harm, along with their associated factors, with the exacerbated effect potentially leading to dual-harm.[2] Reflecting a similar foundational idea, the Two-Stage Model of Countervailing Forces[52] posits that there is an innate aggressive impulse that underlies both self- and other-harm, with its expression dependent on the interaction of psychosocial variables that either amplify or attenuate the impulse (Stage I), whereas a second set of variables determines whether the aggression is directed inward toward the self or outward toward others (Stage II). It should be noted that Stage II does not conclusively distinguish chronic trait vulnerabilities for co-occurring self- and other-harm from acute state factors determining the aggression direction (i.e., inward-outward).[1] To offer a model specifically designed for dual-harm, the Cognitive-Emotional Model of Dual-Harm builds upon previous work rooted in the General Aggression Model, emotion regulation, and diathesis-stress models.[53] The model underscores the prospective distal, proximal, and feedback mechanisms involved in dual-harm, as well as the influence of personality style and the potential emotional regulation and interpersonal purposes. As the authors acknowledge,[2] the model represents the first, albeit not an exhaustive, attempt to provide scaffolding for further theoretical developments and empirical tests. For instance, the model does not elaborate on emotional regulation intricacies nor address other functions of self-harm apart from those related to self-regulation purposes.[50] It does not explain what distinguishes dual-harm from other behavioral outcomes or include distal biological factors.[53]

RISK FACTORS

Developmentally, numerous risk factors contribute to self- and other-harm. Nevertheless, the factors' relative contributions vary among individuals. This heterogeneity can be interpreted by means of equifinality (the same variables can lead to different outcomes) and multifinality (different variables can lead to the same outcome).[54] Individuals engaging in dual-harm differ by their cumulative increased risk compared with those involved in no- or single-harm.[2] The reciprocal dynamics in the development of self- and other-harm can be addressed using the developmental cascade framework.[55] This metaphor posits that difficulties in 1 area can trigger a chain reaction, spreading problems across interconnected domains over time through transactional processes. These effects increase vulnerability and change trajectories, with early risk factors initiating ripple effects across domains that amplify over time.

Plutchik reported at least 23 shared risk factors for self- and other-harm.[52] Since then, research has further enhanced our understanding of the potential risk factors relevant to dual-harm.[1,56] These include early life adversity, impulsivity, sensation seeking, poor coping skills, mental health problems (e.g., substance misuse, substance use disorders, aggressive-related disorders), cruelty to animals, environmental and genetic factors, and alterations in neurochemistry,[5,38,39,57,58] such as serotonergic (5-HT) dysfunction, which has been associated with reduced cerebrospinal fluid 5-hydroxyindoleacetic acid (CSF 5-HIAA) levels.[59,60] By contrast, research on protective factors and resilience is still minimal. Differences between men and women among those engaging in dual-harm are barely explored, although it has been suggested that they may be less pronounced compared with those involved in single-harm.[39] Additionally, they might follow different transitions from the dual-harm to single-harm groups, with women more likely to transition to the self-harm group and men to the other-harm group.[7]

Findings across life course epidemiology, developmental psychopathology, and life course criminology have highlighted that childhood and adolescence are critical periods for a myriad of later outcomes, whereas antisocial, risky, and criminal behavior peak in the late teens, and early starters represent a high-risk group.[11] Enhancing the study of self-harm during this life period is crucial. Likewise, emphasizing the study of prospective longitudinal research is the only reliable path to improve our understanding dual-harm, its causes, and its trajectories. Along with the need for further theoretical development of dual-harm, models of self- and other-harm can generate hypotheses suitable for investigating risk factors and correlates of dual-harm.

PREVENTION

Special attention should be given to the prevention of dual-harm in youths from a socioecological perspective. Thus, efforts must not be limited to individual and interpersonal factors alone at the individual level. Emphasis on social and structural factors such as poverty, sexism, genderism, racism, ableism, and access to health care and education needs to be addressed[61] while deploying interventions at the community level according to the characteristics of settings such as neighborhoods or schools.[62] The aforementioned Cognitive-Emotional Model of Dual-Harm provides a good opportunity to start building prevention strategies specifically focused on individuals involved in dual-harm at the primary,

BOX 1— Issues and Gaps in Dual-Harm Research and Suggested Recommendations

Issues and Gaps	Recommendations for Future Research
Definition of self-harm	Self-harm: A nonfatal intentional self-inflicted harm covering different motives in which the intent to die is either absent or not observable. If intent to die is captured, use suicide attempt. Suicide attempt: An act in which a person harms themselves, intending to die, and survives.
Aggressive behaviors relevant to dual-harm	Focus on interpersonal aggression, specifically prioritizing moderate and severe forms of direct physical and sexual aggression. Include relational aggression in intimate relationships only if it is measured accurately.
Homicide-suicide as the most extreme form of dual-harm	Homicide-suicide is better understood as a distinct phenomenon from nonfatal dual-harm because of its uniqueness and different underlying factors rather than as part of a dual-harm continuum.
Methodological	Use validated measures of aggression and cross-informant perspectives. Level of analysis: Population health and combined individual- and population-level approaches are needed. Community and structural social determinants of health, like policy and environment, remain largely unexplored, along with intersectional approaches to age, gender, sexual orientation, and race/ethnicity. Data sources: Utilize diverse data sources beyond observational accounts and leveraging representative data sets.

secondary, and tertiary levels.[53] Primary prevention can encompass the implementation of educational programs or community outreach grounded in theory, as well as policy endeavors promoting healthy coping strategies, substance misuse awareness, and programs for educational achievement.[63,64] Secondary prevention can deploy screening programs and training for early detection, provide counseling and mental services, and offer cognitive and self-regulatory interventions to target maladaptive thoughts and behaviors.[63,64] Tertiary prevention can establish rehabilitation and support services, therapeutic approaches to reduce relapse and withdrawal—such as continuous monitoring and follow-up to detect early signs of recurrence—and intensive case management for individuals with chronic and severe aggressive behaviors.[56]

CONCLUSION

To summarize, this essay reviews the conceptual, definitional, and methodological challenges of dual-harm research, along with its theoretical basis, risk factors, and prevention strategies. Box 1 summarizes the issues and gaps, and our suggestions to advance research. We recommend following the emerging consensus on defining self-harm within the context of suicidal behaviors. We propose outlining the core aggressive behaviors relevant to the dual-harm construct before proceeding to avoid an overly inclusive or inconsistent set of behaviors that could hinder comparability and replication. Additionally, we posit that nonfatal dual-harm and homicide-suicide are distinct phenomena with different underpinnings and risk factors and should not be considered part of the same continuum. Rather, it would be beneficial to clearly distinguish homicide-suicide, an extremely rare event, from nonfatal dual-harm. However, comparative research between the two remains valuable. We also suggest the need to epidemiologically characterize the population of those who engage in nonfatal dual-harm, explore its subgroups, and shed light on the social determinants of health associated with it.[65,66]

We urge public health researchers to tackle this important topic and be mindful of existing issues and limitations. Researchers should aim for consistency in both the conceptualization and measurement. This will enable a progression from the current dichotomous view toward a more nuanced understanding, allowing comparisons of the extent and severity of behaviors within the dual-harm population. Late childhood and adolescence warrant special attention as key stages for the development of dual-harm. Future studies should contribute to developing tailored interventions and preventive measures for those engaging in or at risk for dual-harm. AJPH

ABOUT THE AUTHORS

Diego A. Díaz-Faes and Charles C. Branas are with the Mailman School of Public Health and Sonali Rajan is with Teachers College, Columbia University, New York, NY.

CORRESPONDENCE

Correspondence should be sent to Diego A. Díaz-Faes, PhD, Columbia University, Mailman School of Public Health, 722 West 168th St, New York, NY 10032 (e-mail: da3166@cumc.columbia.edu). Reprints can be ordered at https://www.ajph.org by clicking the "Reprints" link.

PUBLICATION INFORMATION

Full Citation: Díaz-Faes DA, Rajan S, Branas CC. Navigating dual-harm: integrating self- and other-harm into public health inquiry. *Am J Public Health*. 2025;115(4):596–604.

Acceptance Date: November 16, 2024.

DOI: https://doi.org/10.2105/AJPH.2024.307940

ORCID iD:

Diego A. Díaz-Faes https://orcid.org/0000-0002-0494-2260

CONTRIBUTORS

D. A. Díaz-Faes conceptualized, drafted, and reviewed the manuscript. S. Rajan and C. C. Branas edited and reviewed the manuscript.

CONFLICTS OF INTEREST

The authors declare no conflicts of interest.

HUMAN PARTICIPANT PROTECTION

This article did not involve human participants.

REFERENCES

1. O'Donnell O, House A, Waterman M. The co-occurrence of aggression and self-harm: systematic literature review. *J Affect Disord*. 2015;175:325–350. https://doi.org/10.1016/j.jad.2014.12.051
2. Shafti M, Taylor P, Forrester A, Handerer F, Pratt D. A systematic review of the co-occurrence of self-harm and aggression: is dual harm a unique behavioural construct? *Front Psychiatry*. 2023;14:1083271. https://doi.org/10.3389/fpsyt.2023.1083271
3. Gvion Y, Apter A. Aggression, impulsivity, and suicide behavior: a review of the literature. *Arch Suicide Res*. 2011;15(2):93–112. https://doi.org/10.1080/13811118.2011.565265
4. Sahlin H, Kuja-Halkola R, Bjureberg J, et al. Association between deliberate self-harm and violent criminality. *JAMA Psychiatry*. 2017;74(6):615–621. https://doi.org/10.1001/jamapsychiatry.2017.0338
5. Steeg S, Webb RT, Mok PLH, et al. Risk of dying unnaturally among people aged 15–35 years who have harmed themselves and inflicted violence on others: a national nested case–control study. *Lancet Public Health*. 2019;4(5):e220–e228. https://doi.org/10.1016/S2468-2667(19)30042-8
6. Hawton K, Saunders KE, O'Connor RC. Self-harm and suicide in adolescents. *Lancet*. 2012;379(9834):2373–2382. https://doi.org/10.1016/S0140-6736(12)60322-5
7. Steinhoff A, Ribeaud D, Eisner M, Shanahan L. Developmental trajectories of self-, other-, and dual-harm across adolescence: the role of relationships with peers and teachers. *Psychopathology*. 2023;56(1-2):138–147. https://doi.org/10.1159/000525296
8. Decker MR, Wilcox HC, Holliday CN, Webster DW. An integrated public health approach to interpersonal violence and suicide prevention and response. *Public Health Rep*. 2018;133(1 suppl):65S–79S. https://doi.org/10.1177/0033354918800019
9. Karatekin C, Gresham B, Barnes AJ, Corcoran F, Kritzik R, Mason SM. Re-politicizing the WHO's social determinants of health framework. *Health Promot Int*. 2024;39(5):daae122. https://doi.org/10.1093/heapro/daae122
10. Witt KG, Hetrick SE, Rajaram G, et al. Interventions for self-harm in children and adolescents. *Cochrane Database Syst Rev*. 2021;3(3):CD013667. https://doi.org/10.1002/14651858.CD013667.pub2
11. Moffitt TE. Male antisocial behaviour in adolescence and beyond. *Nat Hum Behav*. 2018;2(3):177–186. https://doi.org/10.1038/s41562-018-0309-4
12. Hawton K, Harriss L, Hall S, Simkin S, Bale E, Bond A. Deliberate self-harm in Oxford, 1990–2000: a time of change in patient characteristics. *Psychol Med*. 2003;33(6):987–995. https://doi.org/10.1017/S0033291703007943
13. Turecki G, Brent DA, Gunnell D, et al. Suicide and suicide risk. *Nat Rev Dis Primers*. 2019;5(1):74. https://doi.org/10.1038/s41572-019-0121-0
14. Crosby A, Ortega L, Melanson C. Self-directed violence surveillance: uniform definitions and recommended data elements. 2011. Available at: https://stacks.cdc.gov/view/cdc/11997. Accessed June 14, 2024.
15. International Society for the Study of Self-Injury. What is self-injury? 2024. Available at: https://www.itriples.org/aboutnssi. Accessed June 14, 2024.
16. De Leo D, Goodfellow B, Silverman M, et al. International study of definitions of English-language terms for suicidal behaviours: a survey exploring preferred terminology. *BMJ Open*. 2021;11(2):e043409. https://doi.org/10.1136/bmjopen-2020-043409
17. Baron R, Richardson D. *Human Aggression*. New York, NY: Plenum Press; 1994.
18. Krahé B. *The Social Psychology of Aggression*. 3rd ed. London, UK: Routledge; 2020. https://doi.org/10.4324/9780429466496
19. Voulgaridou I, Kokkinos CM. Measuring relational aggression in children and adolescents: a systematic review of the available instruments. *Aggress Violent Behav*. 2019;46:82–97. https://doi.org/10.1016/j.avb.2019.02.002
20. Zych I, Viejo C, Vila E, Farrington DP. School bullying and dating violence in adolescents: a systematic review and meta-analysis. *Trauma Violence Abuse*. 2021;22(2):397–412. https://doi.org/10.1177/1524838019854460
21. Salmivalli C. Bullying and the peer group: a review. *Aggress Violent Behav*. 2010;15(2):112–120. https://doi.org/10.1016/j.avb.2009.08.007
22. Shafti M, Steeg S, de Beurs D, et al. The interconnections between self-harm and aggressive behaviours: a general network analysis study of dual harm. *Front Psychiatry*. 2022;13:953764. https://doi.org/10.3389/fpsyt.2022.953764
23. Russo NF, Pirlott A. Gender-based violence: concepts, methods, and findings. *Ann N Y Acad Sci*. 2006;1087(1):178–205. https://doi.org/10.1196/annals.1385.024
24. Díaz-Faes DA, Pereda N. Is there such a thing as a hate crime paradigm? An integrative review of bias-motivated violent victimization and offending, its effects and underlying mechanisms. *Trauma Violence Abuse*. 2022;23(3):938–952. https://doi.org/10.1177/1524838020979694
25. Liem M. Homicide followed by suicide: a review. *Aggress Violent Behav*. 2010;15(3):153–161. https://doi.org/10.1016/j.avb.2009.10.001
26. Rouchy E, Germanaud E, Garcia M, Michel G. Characteristics of homicide-suicide offenders: a systematic review. *Aggress Violent Behav*. 2020;55:101490. https://doi.org/10.1016/j.avb.2020.101490
27. Panczak R, Geissbühler M, Zwahlen M, Killias M, Tal K, Egger M. Homicide-suicides compared to homicides and suicides: systematic review and meta-analysis. *Forensic Sci Int*. 2013;233(1-3):28–36. https://doi.org/10.1016/j.forsciint.2013.08.017
28. Slade K. Dual harm: the importance of recognising the duality of self-harm and violence in forensic populations. *Med Sci Law*. 2019;59(2):75–77. https://doi.org/10.1177/0025802419845161
29. Branas CC, Richmond TS, Schwab CW. Firearm homicide and firearm suicide: opposite but equal. *Public Health Rep*. 2004;119(2):114–124. https://doi.org/10.1177/003335490411900203
30. Loeber R, Hay D. Key issues in the development of aggression and violence from childhood to early adulthood. *Annu Rev Psychol*. 1997;48(1):371–410. https://doi.org/10.1146/annurev.psych.48.1.371
31. Taylor PJ, Jomar K, Dhingra K, Forrester R, Shahmalak U, Dickson JM. A meta-analysis of the prevalence of different functions of non-suicidal self-injury [erratum in *J Affect Disord*. 2019;259:440]. *J Affect Disord*. 2018;227:759–769. https://doi.org/10.1016/j.jad.2017.11.073
32. Cairns RB, Cairns BD. The natural history and developmental functions of aggression. In: *Handbook of Developmental Psychopathology*. Sameroff AJ, Lewis M, Miller SM, eds. New York, NY: Springer US; 2000:403–429. https://doi.org/10.1007/978-1-4615-4163-9_22
33. Slade K, Smith HP, Potter A, Baguley T. Re-examining the dual harm profile: an assessment using US prison population-level data. *Psychol Crime Law*. 2024;30(7):758–772. https://doi.org/10.1080/1068316X.2022.2127716
34. Swogger MT, Walsh Z, Homaifar BY, Caine ED, Conner KR. Predicting self- and other-directed violence among discharged psychiatric patients: the roles of anger and psychopathic traits. *Psychol Med*. 2012;42(2):371–379. https://doi.org/10.1017/S0033291711001243
35. Scocco P, Macis A, Ferrari C, et al. Self-harm behaviour and externally-directed aggression in psychiatric outpatients: a multicentre, prospective study (viormed-2 study) [erratum in *Sci Rep*. 2019;9(1):20382]. *Sci Rep*. 2019;9(1):17857. https://doi.org/10.1038/s41598-019-53993-7
36. Harford TC, Chen CM, Kerridge BT, Grant BF. Self- and other-directed forms of violence and their relationship with lifetime DSM-5 psychiatric disorders: results from the National Epidemiologic Survey on Alcohol Related Conditions–III (NESARC–III). *Psychiatry Res*. 2018;262:384–392. https://doi.org/10.1016/j.psychres.2017.09.012
37. Steeg S, Farooq B, Taylor P, et al. Childhood predictors of self-harm, externalised violence and transitioning to dual harm in a cohort of adolescents and young adults. *Psychol Med*. 2023;53(15):7116–7126. https://doi.org/10.1017/S0033291723000557
38. Richmond-Rakerd LS, Caspi A, Arseneault L, et al. Adolescents who self-harm and commit violent crime: testing early-life predictors of dual harm in a longitudinal cohort study. *Am J Psychiatry*. 2019;176(3):186–195. https://doi.org/10.1176/appi.ajp.2018.18060740
39. Steinhoff A, Bechtiger L, Ribeaud D, Eisner M, Shanahan L. Self-, other-, and dual-harm during adolescence: a prospective-longitudinal study of childhood risk factors and early adult correlates. *Psychol Med*. 2023;53(9):3995–4003. https://doi.org/10.1017/S0033291722000666
40. Spaan P, Michielsen PJS, de Neve-Enthoven NGM, et al. Dual-harm in adolescence and associated clinical and parenting factors. *Soc Psychiatry Psychiatr Epidemiol*. 2022;57(8):1615–1626. https://doi.org/10.1007/s00127-022-02258-2
41. Favril L, Rich JD, Hard J, Fazel S. Mental and physical health morbidity among people in prisons: an umbrella review. *Lancet Public Health*. 2024;9(4):e250–e260. https://doi.org/10.1016/S2468-2667(24)00023-9
42. Jaffee SR, Strait LB, Odgers CL. From correlates to causes: can quasi-experimental studies and statistical innovations bring us closer to identifying the causes of antisocial behavior? *Psychol Bull*.

2012;138(2):272–295. https://doi.org/10.1037/a0026020

43. Viding E, McCrory E, Baskin-Sommers A, De Brito S, Frick P. An "embedded brain" approach to understanding antisocial behaviour. *Trends Cogn Sci.* 2024;28(2):159–171. https://doi.org/10.1016/j.tics.2023.08.013
44. Cheng C, Messerschmidt L, Bravo I, et al. A general primer for data harmonization. *Sci Data.* 2024;11(1):152. https://doi.org/10.1038/s41597-024-02956-3
45. Beltz AM, Wright AGC, Sprague BN, Molenaar PCM. Bridging the nomothetic and idiographic approaches to the analysis of clinical data. *Assessment.* 2016;23(4):447–458. https://doi.org/10.1177/1073191116648209
46. Himmelstein G, Bates D, Zhou L. Examination of stigmatizing language in the electronic health record. *JAMA Netw Open.* 2022;5(1):e2144967. https://doi.org/10.1001/jamanetworkopen.2021.44967
47. Harrendorf S. Prospects, problems, and pitfalls in comparative analyses of criminal justice data. *Crime Justice.* 2018;47(1):159–207. https://doi.org/10.1086/696042
48. Giabbanelli PJ, Rice KL, Nataraj N, Brown MM, Harper CR. A systems science approach to identifying data gaps in national data sources on adolescent suicidal ideation and suicide attempt in the United States. *BMC Public Health.* 2023;23(1):627. https://doi.org/10.1186/s12889-023-15320-8
49. Paleczny S, Osagie N, Sethi J, Cusimano MD. Validity and reliability International Classification of Diseases-10 codes for all forms of injury: a systematic review. Simmen HP, ed. *PLoS One.* 2024;19(2):e0298411. https://doi.org/10.1371/journal.pone.0298411
50. Edmondson AJ, Brennan CA, House AO. Non-suicidal reasons for self-harm: a systematic review of self-reported accounts. *J Affect Disord.* 2016;191:109–117. https://doi.org/10.1016/j.jad.2015.11.043
51. Gomes HS, Farrington DP, Maia Â, Krohn MD. Measurement bias in self-reports of offending: a systematic review of experiments. *J Exp Criminol.* 2019;15(3):313–339. https://doi.org/10.1007/s11292-019-09379-w
52. Plutchik R. Outward and inward directed aggressiveness: the interaction between violence and suicidality. *Pharmacopsychiatry.* 1995;28(suppl 2):47–57. https://doi.org/10.1055/s-2007-979620
53. Shafti M, Taylor PJ, Forrester A, Pratt D. The co-occurrence of self-harm and aggression: a cognitive-emotional model of dual-harm. *Front Psychol.* 2021;12:586135. https://doi.org/10.3389/fpsyg.2021.586135
54. Cicchetti D, Rogosch FA. Equifinality and multifinality in developmental psychopathology. *Dev Psychopathol.* 1996;8(4):597–600. https://doi.org/10.1017/S0954579400007318
55. Masten AS, Cicchetti D. Developmental cascades. *Dev Psychopathol*. 2010;22(3):491–495. https://doi.org/10.1017/S0954579410000222
56. Lubell KM, Vetter JB. Suicide and youth violence prevention: the promise of an integrated approach. *Aggress Violent Behav.* 2006;11(2):167–175. https://doi.org/10.1016/j.avb.2005.07.006
57. Xiang C, Liu S, Fan Y, et al. Single nucleotide polymorphisms, variable number tandem repeats and allele influence on serotonergic enzyme modulators for aggressive and suicidal behaviors: a review. *Pharmacol Biochem Behav.* 2019;180:74–82. https://doi.org/10.1016/j.pbb.2019.03.008
58. Ghossoub E, Adib SM, Maalouf FT, Fuleihan GE-H, Tamim H, Nahas Z. Association between substance use disorders and self- and other-directed aggression: an integrated model approach. *Aggress Behav.* 2019;45(6):652–661. https://doi.org/10.1002/ab.21859
59. Apter A, Brown SL, Korn ML, Praag HM Van. Serotonergic parameters of aggression and suicide. In: Brown SL, Van Praag HM, eds. *Role Of Serotonin In Psychiatric Disorders.* London, UK: Routledge; 1991.
60. Hoertel N, Cipel H, Blanco C, et al. Cerebrospinal fluid levels of monoamines among suicide attempters: a systematic review and random-effects meta-analysis. *J Psychiatr Res.* 2021;136:224–235. https://doi.org/10.1016/j.jpsychires.2021.01.045
61. Nation M, Chapman DA, Edmonds T, et al. Social and structural determinants of health and youth violence: shifting the paradigm of youth violence prevention. *Am J Public Health.* 2021;111(suppl 1):S28–S31. https://doi.org/10.2105/AJPH.2021.306234
62. Kingston BE, Zimmerman MA, Wendel ML, et al. Developing and implementing community-level strategies for preventing youth violence in the United States. *Am J Public Health.* 2021;111(suppl 1):S20–S24. https://doi.org/10.2105/AJPH.2021.306281
63. Horowitz L, Tipton MV, Pao M. Primary and secondary prevention of youth suicide. *Pediatrics.* 2020;145(suppl 2):S195–S203. https://doi.org/10.1542/peds.2019-2056H
64. Jiang S, Chen Y, Wang L. Effectiveness of community-based programs on aggressive behavior among children and adolescents: a systematic review and meta-analysis. *Trauma Violence Abuse.* 2024;25(4):2845–2861. https://doi.org/10.1177/15248380241227986
65. Allen J, Balfour R, Bell R, Marmot M. Social determinants of mental health. *Int Rev Psychiatry.* 2014;26(4):392–407. https://doi.org/10.3109/09540261.2014.928270
66. Hastings PD, Guyer AE, Parra LA. Conceptualizing the influence of social and structural determinants of neurobiology and mental health: why and how biological psychiatry can do better at addressing the consequences of inequity. *Biol Psychiatry Cogn Neurosci Neuroimaging.* 2022;7(12):1215–1224. https://doi.org/10.1016/j.bpsc.2022.06.004

Outcomes of Home Isolation Care Among COVID-19 Patients During the 2021 Epidemic Crisis in the Bangkok Metropolitan Region, Thailand

Teeraboon Lertwanichwattana, MD, Supattra Srivanichakorn, MD, MPH, Sairat Noknoy, MD, MSc, Sirinapa Siriporn Na Ratchaseema, MD, MSc, Nittaya Phanuphak, MD, PhD, Kitti Wongthavarawat, PhD, Arunotai Siriussawakul, MD, Varalak Srinonprasert, MD, Pattara Leelahavarong, PhD, Parawee Chevaisrakul, MD, PhD, Putthapoom Lumjiaktase, PhD, Aree Kumpitak, BSc, Nopphan Phromsri, BSc, Yupadee Sirisinsuk, PhD, Pongtorn Kietdumrongwong, MD, Apinun Aramrattana, MD, PhD, and Ram Rangsin, MD, DrPH

Objectives. To determine the overall mortality and risk factors of COVID-19 patients who were admitted to the Home Isolation (HI) program in Bangkok, Thailand, during the epidemic crisis in 2021.

Methods. We conducted a retrospective cohort study using the data from a government telehealth application from July to December 2021. The vital status was verified from the government database on September 20, 2022. We used survival analysis to analyze the 28-day mortality and independently associated factors.

Results. Of 90 854 reported cases, the average age was 37.27 years, and half were men. Initial symptoms included being asymptomatic (51.66%), having mild symptoms (35.60%), or experiencing severe symptoms requiring nonurgent (11.27%) or urgent referral (1.47%). The 28-day mortality rate was 0.80%. Factors associated with 28-day mortality included older age, male gender, higher body mass index, severity of initial symptoms, and time to admission.

Conclusions. The Home Isolation program was able to manage a high volume of patients, including severe cases, exceeding its initial design. Thailand's COVID-19 mortality rate remained relatively low compared with other countries. Proactive bed surge planning and continuous plan improvement were crucial for future preparedness. (*Am J Public Health*. 2025;115(4):605–616. https://doi.org/10.2105/AJPH.2024.307922)

AJPH April 2025, Vol. 115, No. 4

On January 13, 2020, Thailand became the first country outside of China to report a confirmed case of COVID-19, with the infected individual being a traveler from Wuhan city.[1,2] Subsequently, on January 31, 2020, the first case of local transmission was reported.[3] Since then, the number of COVID-19 cases in Thailand steadily increased, driven by both imported cases and local transmission.[4,5] The Thai Ministry of Public Health officially declared COVID-19 a dangerous communicable disease, designating the COVID-19 epidemic as a public health emergency.[6] The initial priorities of the responses focused on preventing the entry of the virus that causes COVID-19 into Thailand and mitigating its local transmission. The implementation of a surveillance system, increased testing availability, and robust outbreak investigations and contact tracing, combined with social measures to reduce personal contacts, such as school closures, travel restrictions, and partial or complete lockdowns, contributed to a relatively limited number of COVID-19 cases between 2020 and early 2021.[7,8] Notably, Thailand policy at that time mandated an at least 14-day hospitalization even for asymptomatic individuals infected with severe acute respiratory syndrome coronavirus 2

(SARS-CoV-2), aiming to limit the community spread of infection.

However, a resurgence of COVID-19 cases occurred in April 2021, with almost 2000 patients being diagnosed per day during this wave of the epidemic.[5,9] The sharp increase in the number of COVID-19 cases was particularly observed in Bangkok, attributed to the presence of the B.1.1.7 (α) variant, followed immediately by the B.1.617.2 (Delta) variant.[10] Consequently, the Thai government then modified the treatment and care protocol by implementing the Home Isolation program, providing COVID-19 care at home for those patients who were asymptomatic or had mild symptoms.[11] This study describes the outcomes of the Home Isolation program for COVID-19 patients in the Bangkok Metropolitan Region (BMR) during the 2021 epidemic crisis from July to December 2021.

METHODS

We conducted a retrospective cohort study among COVID-19 patients in the BMR who received the Home Isolation program and were documented in the Assistive Technology and Medical Devices Research Center (AMED) Telehealth platform, developed by Thailand's National Science and Technology Development Agency. The study period covered the time from July 1 to December 31, 2021.

Study Participants

The Thai government officially implemented the Home Isolation program on July 1, 2021, starting in the BMR, the epidemic's epicenter. Eligible patients needed to meet specific criteria from the Department of Medical Services, Ministry of Public Health, including being asymptomatic or mildly symptomatic, aged younger than 60 years, in good physical condition, living alone or with 1 cohabitant, and not obese (body mass index [defined as weight in kilograms divided by the square of height in meters] ≥ 30 kg/m^2 or weight > 90 kg).[12] During the study period, all COVID-19 patients in Thailand, including foreign residents, were eligible to receive care free of charge. An at-home COVID-19 rapid antigen test was not available in Thailand during the study period. Diagnosing COVID-19 relied solely on health care professionals administering either the SARS-CoV-2 antigen rapid test or reverse transcriptase polymerase chain reaction test. Individuals testing positive could receive home treatment, supervised by their health care facilities. Hospitals or health care facilities were not required to use AMED Telehealth; they could implement their own systems, but could use AMED if lacking a telehealth platform to support or refer patients to the National Health Security Office (NHSO) system.

If the responsible health care facilities could not accommodate identified patients, they were encouraged to contact the NHSO to access the central COVID-19 care-at-home service. This could be done through 1 of 3 channels: the emergency line, online registration, or the Line messaging application. After registration, the dispatcher system promptly coordinated and matched the patient with the health care facilities for entry into the Home Isolation program.[13]

Health care providers offering care at home for COVID-19 patients under the coordination of the NHSO in the BMR during the crisis included established government hospitals, public health service centers, community private clinics partnering with the NHSO, and newly developed health care volunteer networks for crisis response, such as the Fammed-CoCare (Family Medicine Coordinated Care) and ComCOVID-19 (Community-led COVID-19 Workforce) Health Volunteer Network and the Thai Red Cross Society network.

The Fammed-CoCare and ComCOVID-19 Network, composed of more than 3000 health professionals (2249 physicians, 608 nurses, 338 pharmacists, and 33 dentists), was established in April 2021 from a network of 8 civil society organizations led by representatives of marginalized communities. These volunteers performed patient triage, delivered essential medical supplies, and codelivered health care services alongside health professionals in mobile units. Beyond symptom screening, they assessed mental health, livelihood needs, and human rights violations, and provided corresponding support.

After being matched with a health care facility, patients were monitored through the AMED Telehealth platform, which enabled remote health monitoring. This platform offered tele-medical consultations for daily assessments of symptoms, temperature, and oxygen saturation using thermometers and pulse oximeters. In addition, the platform facilitated essential medication prescriptions and provided 3 meals a day free of charge. For patients requiring a higher level of care, the Home Isolation program would refer them to the hospital for further appropriate care.[14]

In this study, a COVID-19 death was defined as the death of an individual within 28 days (inclusive) of their initial positive SARS-CoV-2 test during their most recent COVID-19 infection. This definition was adopted by public health agencies and reflected the effectiveness of policies aimed at addressing COVID-19.

Data Collection

In this study, secondary data were obtained anonymously from electronic medical records on the AMED Telehealth platform supported by the NHSO from July to December 2021. The recorded features in the platform included baseline characteristics such as gender, age, nationality, health care coverage scheme, and type of health care facility. In addition, the data encompassed clinical manifestations and the date of the first onset, daily symptoms and clinical presentations during admission to the Home Isolation program, medication prescriptions, and discharge status.

Mortality Data

To assess the mortality of the study participants, we requested the AMED Telehealth system to send the patient lists to identify the vital status of the participants by September 20, 2022 (approximately 1 year after admission into the Home Isolation program). This identification was conducted using the vital status database of the NHSO, which is linked to the Thailand National Civil Registration database, providing vital status information.

The pertinent details recorded in the death certificate related to the participants who had died during the specified time period, including the date of death, were retrieved from the national Civil Registration database by NHSO. Subsequently, this information was incorporated into the patient records from the AMED Telehealth database before being sent to the study investigator without any personal identification.

Statistical Analysis

Continuous and categorical variables were presented with the appropriate measure of central tendency and as the number and percentage, respectively. We used the Mann-Whitney U test, χ^2 test, or Fisher exact test to compare differences between COVID-19 deaths.

To estimate the time since Home Isolation program entry to death within 28 days from all causes, the primary endpoint in this analysis was death within 28 days identified from the vital status database of the NHSO and the Thailand National Civil Registration database. Those patients who were alive after 28 days were right censored on the 28 days after Home Isolation entry. We conducted a survival analysis using the Kaplan–Meier method. In addition, we employed the Cox proportional hazards model to ascertain the independent effects of various potential risk factors.

The study focused on mortality within 28 days following enrollment in the Home Isolation program as the outcome of interest. Patient demographics and risk factors associated with this mortality were assessed through both univariate and multivariate models to determine their impact on overall survival, calculated from the date of illness onset. Subsequently, a backward stepwise selection approach was applied in the Cox proportional hazard model to refine the analysis. We used a *P* value cut-off of .05 for all statistical tests. We conducted all analyses with R statistical software version 3.6.3 (R Foundation for Statistical Computing, Vienna, Austria).

RESULTS

From July 1 to December 31, 2021, a total of 90 854 COVID-19 patients were admitted to the Home Isolation program in the BMR with support from the NHSO and using data from AMED Telehealth. Nearly 70% of these participants had health insurance coverage under the NHSO Universal Coverage scheme. During this period, the Home Isolation program delivered home-based care to nearly 97% of the patients through various health care facilities, including Bangkok Metropolitan Administration Public Health Service Centers (n = 69), community private clinics partnering with the NHSO (n = 190), the Fammed-CoCare and ComCOVID-19 Network, Bangkok Metropolitan Administration–affiliated hospitals (n = 11), the Thai Red Cross Society network, and private hospitals (n = 2). Remarkably, in the initial month of the crisis (July 2021), the newly established Fammed-CoCare and ComCOVID-19 network provided home care for nearly 50% of patients, highlighting its significant contribution during this critical period. The demographics of who entered the Home Isolation program are shown in Table 1.

Home Isolation Program Outcomes

The highest daily number of new COVID-19 cases admitted to the Home Isolation program was on August 4, 2021, with a daily total of 2851 cases. In addition, the highest total admitted patients under the care of Home Isolation program in the BMR occurred on August 14, 2021, with a total number of 30 722 cases (Figure 1).

Mortality of All Cases in the Program

As of September 20, 2022 (approximately 1 year following the epidemic crisis), a total of 1339 (1.47%) COVID-19 patients died from all causes of death

TABLE 1— Demographics of COVID-19 Patients Admitted to the Home Isolation Program: Bangkok Metropolitan Region, Thailand, July–December 2021

Characteristic	Total, Mean ±SD or No. (%)
Age, y	
Mean ±SD	37.3 ±19.0
< 5	2 258 (2.7)
5–19	13 966 (16.6)
20–39	30 383 (36.1)
40–59	26 507 (31.5)
60–79	9 907 (11.8)
≥ 80	1 214 (1.4)
Gender	
Female	49 020 (54.0)
Male	41 834 (46.0)
Nationality	
Thai	85 873 (94.5)
Non-Thai	4 981 (5.5)
Body mass index,[a] kg/m^2	
Mean ±SD	24.7 ±5.1
< 18.5	5 124 (7.9)
18.5–22.9	21 152 (32.6)
23.0–24.9	12 130 (18.7)
25.0–29.9	17 325 (26.7)
30.0–34.9	6 362 (9.8)
35.0–39.9	2 015 (3.1)
≥ 40.0	759 (1.2)
Health insurance scheme	
UCS	50 587 (65.3)
SSS	21 685 (28.0)
CSMBS	4 573 (5.9)
Cash	661 (0.9)
Health care facilities	
BMA Public Health Service Centers	35 215 (38.8)
Community private clinics partnering with the NHSO	21 965 (24.2)
Fammed-CoCare and ComCOVID-19	18 950 (20.9)
BMA-affiliated hospitals	11 466 (12.6)
Thai Red Cross Society	2 489 (2.7)
Private hospitals	769 (0.8)
Initial symptoms	
Asymptomatic	38 895 (51.7)
Mild symptoms	26 803 (35.6)
Nonurgent referral needed	8 486 (11.3)
Urgent symptoms	1 110 (1.5)
Admission month	
July	16 659 (18.3)
August	57 280 (63.0)

Continued

after their admission to the Home Isolation program. This includes both deaths that occurred during the active care period and those that happened after discharge during the follow-up period. In contrast, 107 (0.12%) deaths occurred while patients were still under the direct care of the Home Isolation program, before their discharge. The approximate 1-year mortality rate after being admitted to the Home Isolation program was 1.30 per 100 person-years. The different characteristics of participants among approximately 1-year mortality outcomes is demonstrated in Table 2.

28-Day Mortality of Cases After Program Entry

Out of 90 854 patients enrolled in the Home Isolation program, 736 cases (0.80%) or 0.70 per 100 person-years resulted in death within 28 days after entering Home Isolation. Subsequently, we conducted univariate Cox proportional hazards regression to analyze potential risk factors for the mortality rate within 28 days after Home Isolation entry (Table A, available as a supplement to the online version of this article at https://ajph.org). Among the 16 variables evaluated, we retained 5 following multivariate analyses using backward stepwise selection (Table 3). The final model, determined through stepwise selection, identified the following as prognostic factors for death within 28 days after Home Isolation entry: age 40 to 49, 50 to 59, 60 to 69, and 70 years or older; being male; body mass index 30.00 to 34.99, 35.00 to 39.99, and 40.00 kg/m^2 or greater; mild symptoms; nonurgent referral needed; urgent symptoms; and time to admission (days) less than 1, 1 to 3, and 4 to 6.

TABLE 1— Continued

Characteristic	Total, Mean ±SD or No. (%)
September	11 966 (13.2)
October	3 022 (3.3)
November	1 254 (1.4)
December	672 (0.7)
Province of residence	
Bangkok	85 156 (93.7)
Samut Prakan	2 343 (2.6)
Pathum Thani	1 417 (1.6)
Nonthaburi	990 (1.1)
Nakhon Pathom	521 (0.6)
Samut Sakhon	427 (0.5)

Note. BMA = Bangkok Metropolitan Administration; ComCOVID-19 = Community-led COVID-19 Workforce operated by the Institute of HIV Research and Innovation; CSMBS = Civil Servant Benefit Scheme; Fammed-CoCare = Family Medicine Coordinated Care; NHSO = National Health Security Office; SSS = Social Security Scheme; UCS = Universal Coverage Scheme. The sample size was n = 90 854.

[a]Defined as weight in kilograms divided by the square of height in meters, in patients aged ≥ 20 years.

DISCUSSION

The outcomes of COVID-19 patients who were admitted to receiving care at home during the fourth wave of the COVID-19 epidemic in Thailand between July and December 2021 were reported in this study. This wave marked a sudden and substantial increase in number of patients after the successful implementation of public health interventions that had initially suppressed the epidemic to limited spread nationwide during the first to the third waves in 2020 and early 2021.[15–17] In addition, this wave of the epidemic hit hard in the capital city of Bangkok, which has a large and high population density and served as the epicenter of the event.[18] This made this epidemic a significant public health crisis in Thailand.

Providing the Home Isolation program for COVID-19 patients became a prevalent practice globally during the pandemic.[19–22] Since the early stages of the outbreak in March 2020, both the World Health Organization and the European Union endorsed the notion of home care for such patients. This approach, albeit implemented under varying titles across different nations,[23,24] emerged as a widely accepted strategy for managing COVID-19 cases outside traditional health care settings. Thailand's Home

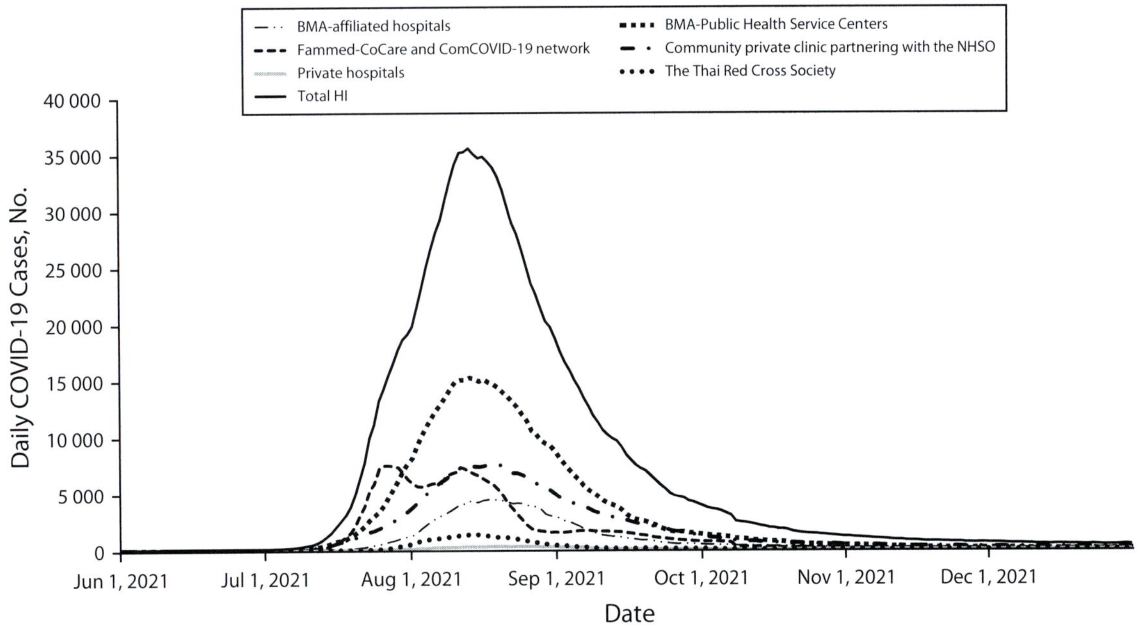

FIGURE 1— Daily Number of COVID-19 Cases Under Home Isolation Program by Type of Health Facility: Bangkok Metropolitan Region, Thailand, July–December 2021

Note. BMA = Bangkok Metropolitan Region; HI = Home Isolation program; NHSO = National Health Security Office.

TABLE 2— Overall Mortality Rate by Characteristics of the COVID-19 Patients Who Were Admitted to the Home Isolation Program: Bangkok Metropolitan Region, Thailand, July–December 2021

Characteristic	Overall Mortality, Mean ±SD or No. (%)		P^a
	No	Yes	
Overall	89 515 (98.5)	1 339 (1.5)	
Age, y			
Mean ±SD	36.9 ±18.7	67.3 ±16.3	< .001
< 40	46 537 (99.8)	70 (0.2)	< .001
40–49	14 263 (99.4)	91 (0.6)	
50–59	11 971 (98.5)	182 (1.5)	
60–69	6 759 (96.3)	262 (3.7)	
≥ 70	3 546 (86.5)	554 (13.5)	
Gender			< .001
Female	48 386 (98.7)	634 (1.3)	
Male	41 129 (98.3)	705 (1.7)	
Nationality			< .001
Thai	84 543 (98.5)	1 330 (1.5)	
Non-Thai	4 972 (99.8)	9 (0.2)	
Body mass index,[b] kg/m²			
Mean ±SD	24.7 ±5.1	24.9 ±5.7	.68
< 18.5	5 009 (97.8)	115 (2.2)	< .001
18.5–22.9	20 814 (98.4)	338 (1.6)	
23.0–24.9	11 959 (98.6)	171 (1.4)	
25.0–29.9	17 041 (98.4)	284 (1.6)	
30.0–34.9	6 258 (98.4)	104 (1.6)	
35.0–39.9	1 969 (97.7)	46 (2.3)	
≥ 40.0	738 (97.2)	21 (2.8)	
Health insurance scheme			< .001
UCS	49 759 (98.4)	828 (1.6)	
SSS	21 555 (99.4)	130 (0.6)	
CSMBS	4 447 (97.2)	126 (2.8)	
Cash	659 (99.7)	2 (0.3)	
Health care facilities			< .001
BMA Public Health Service Centers	34 692 (98.5)	523 (1.5)	
Community private clinics partnering with the NHSO	21 751 (99.0)	214 (1.0)	
Fammed-CoCare and ComCOVID-19	18 531 (97.8)	419 (2.2)	
BMA-affiliated hospitals	11 315 (98.7)	151 (1.3)	
Thai Red Cross Society	2 459 (98.8)	30 (1.2)	
Private hospitals	767 (99.7)	2 (0.3)	
Initial symptoms			< .001
Asymptomatic	38 664 (99.4)	231 (0.6)	
Mild symptoms	26 358 (98.3)	445 (1.7)	
Nonurgent referral needed	8 299 (97.8)	187 (2.2)	
Urgent symptoms	960 (86.5)	150 (13.5)	
Admission month			< .001
July	16 314 (97.9)	345 (2.1)	
August	56 438 (98.5)	842 (1.5)	

Continued

TABLE 2— Continued

Characteristic	Overall Mortality, Mean ±SD or No. (%)		P[a]
	No	Yes	
September	11 838 (98.9)	128 (1.1)	
October	3 001 (99.3)	21 (0.7)	
November	1 252 (99.8)	2 (0.2)	
December	671 (99.9)	1 (0.1)	
Province of residence			.5
Bangkok	83 892 (98.5)	1 264 (1.5)	
Samut Prakan	2 306 (98.4)	37 (1.6)	
Pathum Thani	1 399 (98.7)	18 (1.3)	
Nonthaburi	977 (98.7)	13 (1.3)	
Nakhon Pathom	517 (99.2)	4 (0.8)	
Samut Sakhon	424 (99.3)	3 (0.7)	
Prescriptions			
Favipiravir	20 485 (97.7)	490 (2.3)	< .001
Steroid	420 (86.6)	65 (13.4)	< .001
Andrographis paniculata extract	7 859 (99.4)	50 (0.6)	< .001
Body temperature upon entry, °C			
Mean ±SD	36.5 ±0.7	36.8 ±0.8	< .001
< 38	53 378 (98.9)	592 (1.1)	< .001
≥ 38	1 619 (95.9)	70 (4.1)	
Pulse rate, bpm			
Mean ±SD	86.5 ±13.6	85.7 ±15.3	.36
< 100	29 856 (98.8)	367 (1.2)	.61
≥ 100	5 875 (98.7)	77 (1.3)	
Oxygen saturation upon entry, %			
Mean ±SD	97.4 ±1.9	94.9 ±4.7	< .001
> 96	38 736 (99.2)	311 (0.8)	< .001
≤ 96	9 186 (96.6)	328 (3.4)	
Exercise-induced hypoxemia upon entry, %			.035
< 3	6 813 (98.9)	74 (1.1)	
≥ 3	455 (97.8)	10 (2.2)	
Time to admission, d			
Mean ±SD	2.4 ±3.3	1.8 ±2.6	< .001
< 1	28 621 (98.2)	525 (1.8)	< .001
1–3	38 996 (98.5)	583 (1.5)	
4–6	12 993 (98.7)	171 (1.3)	
≥ 7	8 249 (99.3)	54 (0.7)	

Note. BMA = Bangkok Metropolitan Administration; bpm = beats per minute; °C = degree Celsius; ComCOVID-19 = Community-led COVID-19 Workforce operated by the Institute of HIV Research and Innovation; CSMBS = Civil Servant Benefit Scheme; Fammed-CoCare = Family Medicine Coordinated Care; NHSO = National Health Security Office; SSS = Social Security Scheme; UCS = Universal Coverage Scheme. The sample size was n = 90 854.
[a]Wilcoxon rank sum test; Pearson χ^2 test.
[b]Defined as weight in kilograms divided by the square of height in meters, in patients aged ≥ 20 years.

TABLE 3— Univariable and Multivariable Analysis of Time to Death Within 28 Days of the COVID-19 Patients Who Were Admitted to the Home Isolation Program: Bangkok Metropolitan Region, Thailand, July–December 2021

Characteristic	Total	100 Person-Years	No. of Deaths Within 28 d[a]	Univariable Analysis, Crude HR (95% CI)	Multivariable Analysis, Adjusted HR (95% CI)
Gender					
Female	49 019	533	352	1 (Ref)	1 (Ref)
Male	41 832	452	384	1.3 (1.1, 1.5)	1.8 (1.5, 2.2)
Body mass index,[b] kg/m^2					
< 18.5	5123	55	51	1.4 (1.0, 1.9)	1.3 (0.9, 1.9)
18.5–22.9	21 150	228	152	. . .	. . .
23.0–24.9	12 130	131	83	1.0 (0.7, 1.2)	0.8 (0.6, 1.1)
25.0–29.9	17 325	187	158	1.3 (1.0, 1.6)	1.1 (0.8, 1.4)
30.0–34.9	6 362	69	72	1.6 (1.2, 2.1)	1.8 (1.3, 2.4)
35.0–39.9	2 015	22	32	2.2 (1.5, 3.2)	3.1 (2.0, 4.9)
≥ 40.0	759	8	16	3.0 (1.8, 5.0)	5.2 (2.8, 9.4)
Age, y					
< 40	46 605	509	21	1 (Ref)	1 (Ref)
40–49	14 354	157	33	5.1 (3.0, 8.8)	3.7 (1.8, 7.5)
50–59	12 152	132	78	14.0 (8.8, 23.0)	12.0 (6.3, 22.0)
60–69	7 021	75	132	42.0 (27.0, 67.0)	26.0 (14.0, 48.0)
≥ 70	4 100	40	348	197.0 (127.0, 306.0)	140.0 (78.0, 252.0)
Initial symptoms					
Asymptomatic	38 892	419	100	1 (Ref)	1 (Ref)
Mild symptoms	26 803	286	226	3.3 (2.6, 4.2)	1.6 (1.2, 2.2)
Nonurgent referral needed	8 486	91	107	4.9 (3.8, 6.5)	2.9 (2.1, 4.1)
Urgent symptoms	1 110	11	104	38.0 (29.0, 50.0)	7.0 (5.1, 9.6)
Time to admission, d					
< 1	29 143	309	302	6.2 (3.6, 11.0)	5.7 (2.7, 12.0)
1–3	39 579	427	333	5.0 (2.9, 8.5)	5.9 (2.8, 13.0)
4–6	13 164	147	83	3.7 (2.1, 6.6)	3.1 (1.4, 6.9)
≥ 7	8 303	94	14	1 (Ref)	1 (Ref)

Note. CI = confidence interval; HR = hazard ratio. The sample size was n = 90 854.
[a]Number of deaths within 28 days; the vital status as of 28 days after entry into the Home Isolation program.
[b]Defined as weight in kilograms divided by the square of height in meters, in patients aged ≥ 20 years.

Isolation program during the crisis in this study period demonstrated its ability to effectively manage a large number of patients while providing comprehensive care without discrimination. This government-led initiative, driven by community demand and readiness to co-deliver services with health professionals, granted free access to COVID-19 services for all residents, regardless of nationality or immigration status. Notably, the program's flexibility allowed for the swift admission of patients, including undocumented immigrant workers, bypassing bureaucratic hurdles. This inclusive approach ensured crucial health care access during a critical time.[23,24]

Throughout the study period, patients under the AMED Telehealth platform, serving as our study population, accounted for almost 25% of the overall COVID-19 patients in the BMR. Particularly during the peak of the epidemic in August 2021, patients under the AMED Telehealth platform constituted almost 50%.

One specific feature of the Home Isolation program in Thailand during this major event of the COVID-19 epidemic crisis in the BMR was the newly established health care networks for crisis response, namely the Fammed-CoCare and ComCOVID-19 Network and the crisis response network of the Thai Red Cross Society, which played a significant role in providing care at home, especially during the early phase of the crisis when the availability of hospital beds was very limited. These health care networks demonstrated their ability to care for severe cases and critical patients with comorbidities at home, manage patients requiring oxygen and corticosteroids, and refer to hospitals through professional networks. Using the principles of de-medicalization and differentiation, health professional volunteers and community volunteers worked with mutual respect and excelled in patient triage by symptom severity, availability of providers with various expertise and levels of clinical skills, and accessibility to clinical supply and hospital beds during the crisis.

In the first month of the study period in July 2021, the newly established health care networks for crisis response were able to provide care for almost 50% of the cases. However, starting from the second month of the epidemic onward, the health care facilities under the regular system could continue to cover the majority of the cases. This finding may be explained by the requirement that the regular health system needed more time to adapt to the crisis compared with the newly established crisis response health care networks.

Although this program was initially designed for patients with mild symptoms, aged younger than 60 years, and without underlying health conditions such as obesity or other comorbidities,[25] during this crisis event, the program had to admit patients with severe symptoms or those at risk for developing severe symptoms because of the limited availability of hospital beds, especially during the early phase in July 2021 and the peak of the epidemic in August 2021. One of the challenges regarding the scarcity of hospital beds might be, in part, attributed to the national strategy in Thailand for controlling the epidemic, which mandated the isolation of all COVID-19 cases, regardless of severity, in hospitals to limit the community spread of the virus. This strategy was lifted at the beginning of the large epidemic crisis in July 2021.

Mortality Rate Within 28 Days of Enrollment

The study population exhibited a relatively low 28-day mortality rate of 0.8%. Compared with global COVID-19 mortality rates, which range from 0.50% to 2.00%,[26] this finding suggests that Thailand's Home Isolation program, implemented during the early pandemic phase, effectively managed COVID-19 patients at a level comparable to other nations.

Our study identified sex as an independent risk factor for 28-day mortality. Males had a higher risk of death within 28 days compared with females, consistent with previous reports on COVID-19 and past respiratory virus epidemics such as the Spanish flu, severe acute respiratory syndrome coronavirus 1, and Middle East respiratory syndrome–related cornonavirus.[27–31] Possible explanations for this sex difference could be related to genetics, immune response, and the influence of varying sex hormones between males and females.

In terms of age, for each year increase, the risk of mortality within 28 days increased with the dose–response relationship. Comparing to the study in China, the case–fatality rate for COVID-19 patients increased with age. The mortality impact of COVID-19 was not limited to those aged 60 years and older but began to manifest in individuals aged as young as 40 years. This indicated the necessity for public health policies to prioritize individuals aged 40 years and older, with heightened attention to those aged 60 years and older, who face approximately twice the risk of mortality compared with younger age categories.

Obesity, as classified by the World Health Organization, emerged as a significant contributor to mortality rates during the 28-day period analyzed within the Home Isolation program. This underscores a dose–response relationship, where mortality rates increase correspondingly with higher obesity categories. Obesity can lead to metabolic syndrome, triggering chronic inflammation and disrupting immune system activation, potentially leading to a cytokine storm.[32–34] Obesity is also linked to increased risk of hypoventilation-associated pneumonia, pulmonary hypertension, and cardiac stress, all of which can worsen COVID-19 prognosis.[35]

The initial assessment of COVID-19 patients upon their admission to the Home Isolation program involved a thorough evaluation by health care providers, categorizing patients according to the severity of their symptoms ranging from asymptomatic cases to those with urgent symptoms.[36,37] Our study revealed a clear relationship between the severity of symptoms and mortality rates. However, compared with a study in South Korea reporting a transfer rate of 5.80% among patients, our Home Isolation program in Thailand exhibited fewer referrals and stricter criteria, with comprehensive evaluation protocols covering clinical presentation, vital signs, and underlying medical conditions.[38] This suggests that Thailand's

Home Isolation program implemented robust assessment measures, potentially contributing to the lower referral rate observed compared with the South Korean study.

Our analysis showed a significant correlation between time to admission and the 28-day mortality rate. Mortality rates decreased as time to admission increased, underscoring the importance of timely access to medical treatment in mitigating adverse outcomes. Prompt initiation of medical care enables timely interventions and supportive care that can prevent disease progression. Our findings emphasize the need for strategies to promote timely access to health care services, including public health campaigns to raise awareness about seeking medical care promptly upon symptom onset and initiatives to enhance accessibility to health care services. By recognizing the critical role of time to admission in determining mortality outcomes and implementing targeted interventions to facilitate prompt treatment-seeking behavior, health care systems can potentially alleviate the burden of COVID-19 and improve patient prognosis.[39,40]

Limitations

Our study had several limitations. The study population may not fully represent the spectrum of COVID-19 cases, as patients with severe conditions likely sought care in emergency departments and were thus excluded. In addition, most participants came from lower socioeconomic backgrounds, which may not reflect those of higher status who sought care at private hospitals outside our program. The non-Thai population subgroup also limits the assessment of vital status, as our method relied on national identification numbers. Finally, the lack of data on underlying conditions restricts our understanding of the impact of comorbidities on COVID-19 outcomes.

Public Health Implications

Policy recommendations should be informed by insights derived from the recent COVID-19 pandemic outbreak. During critical periods marked by a surge in case numbers and rapid community transmission, routine patient care experienced significant disruption. This disruption necessitated a transition from hospital-based care for COVID-19 patients to the establishment of a Home Isolation program. The analysis indicates that this transition had a substantial impact on the delivery of patient care and overall clinical outcomes, particularly during the initial three-month period of the outbreak. Collaborative efforts between the Family Medicine College of Thailand and the General Practitioners/Family Physicians Association aimed to address health system crises and design primary health care strategies under the Fammed-CoCare and ComCOVID-19 Network initiative. This network of medical volunteer professionals, working in partnership with civil society organizations like ComCOVID-19, quickly expanded services and ensured effective care for COVID-19 patients.

In crisis situations, specialized service units must collaborate to ensure timely care and responses. Enhancing these specialized units will enable the efficient management of crises. During noncrisis periods, a health care system that effectively leverages these specialized service units can also manage chronic conditions and provide sustained care through monitoring systems such as telemedicine, thereby decreasing the necessity for hospital visits. In conclusion, optimizing health crisis management and planning for future outbreaks of emerging diseases is crucial. Establishing responsive health care systems during the initial outbreak phase and fostering a continuous learning environment to enhance health care capability are essential. Government investment in sustaining responsive health care systems for pandemic preparedness must be prioritized. AJPH

ABOUT THE AUTHORS

Teeraboon Lertwanichwattana and Ram Rangsin are with Phramongkutklao College of Medicine, Bangkok, Thailand. Supattra Srivanichakorn, Sairat Noknoy, and Sirinapa Siriporn Na Ratchaseema are with the Royal College of Family Physicians of Thailand, Bangkok. Nittaya Phanuphak is with the Institute of HIV Research and Innovation, Bangkok. Kitti Wongthavarawat is with the National Science and Technology Development Agency, Bangkok. Arunotai Siriussawakul, Varalak Srinonprasert, and Pattara Leelahavarong are with the Faculty of Medicine Siriraj Hospital, Mahidol University, Bangkok. Parawee Chevaisrakul and Putthapoom Lumjiaktase are with the Faculty of Medicine, Ramathibodi Hospital, Mahidol University, Bangkok. Aree Kumpitak is with the Thai Network of People Living With HIV, Bangkok. Nopphan Phromsri is with the Human Settlement Foundation, Bangkok. Yupadee Sirisinsuk is with the Faculty of Pharmaceutical Sciences, Chulalongkorn University, Bangkok. Pongtorn Kietdumrongwong is with the Bangkok Dusit Medical Services, Bangkok. Apinun Aramrattana is with the Faculty of Medicine, Chiang Mai University, Chiang Mai, Thailand.

CORRESPONDENCE

Correspondence should be sent to Ram Rangsin, Phramongkutklao College of Medicine, 317 Ratchawithi Rd, Thung Phaya Thai, Ratchathewi, Bangkok, Thailand (e-mail: rrangsin@pcm.ac.th). Reprints can be ordered at https://www.ajph.org by clicking the "Reprints" link.

PUBLICATION INFORMATION

Full Citation: Lertwanichwattana T, Srivanichakorn S, Noknoy S, et al. Outcomes of home isolation care among COVID-19 patients during the 2021 epidemic crisis in the Bangkok metropolitan region, Thailand. *Am J Public Health*. 2025;115(4):605–616.

Acceptance Date: November 5, 2024.

DOI: https://doi.org/10.2105/AJPH.2024.307922

ORCID iDs:

Teeraboon Lertwanichwattana https://orcid.org/0000-0002-5960-0014

Nittaya Phanuphak https://orcid.org/0000-0002-0036-3165

Pattara Leelahavarong https://orcid.org/0000-0002-9584-0293

Ram Rangsin https://orcid.org/0000-0002-7175-0963

CONTRIBUTORS

All authors contributed to the concept and approval of the final version. T. Lertwanichwattana contributed to the design, analysis, interpretation of data, drafting, and revision of the article. S. Srivanichakorn, S. Noknoy, N. Phanuphak, and P. Chevaisrakul contributed to the revision of the article. K. Wongthavarawat contributed to the design and analysis. R. Rangsin contributed to the design, interpretation of data, drafting, and revision of the article.

ACKNOWLEDGMENTS

This study was generously funded by the Health Systems Research Institute of Thailand, whose support was critical in facilitating this research. We would like to express our sincere gratitude to all health care facilities in Bangkok and the Metropolitan Region for their invaluable support and cooperation throughout this study. Special thanks go to the medical staff, administrators, and patients who participated and provided essential data for our analysis. We also extend our appreciation to all individuals who contributed to this work but did not meet the authorship criteria; your efforts were indispensable to the success of this study.

CONFLICTS OF INTEREST

The authors declare that they have no conflicts of interest, financial or otherwise, related to this research study.

HUMAN PARTICIPANT PROTECTION

This study protocol was approved by the ethics committee of the institutional review board of the Royal Thai Army Medical Department (approval S082q/64_Exp).

REFERENCES

1. Lillie PJ, Samson A, Li A, et al. Novel coronavirus disease (COVID-19): the first two patients in the UK with person to person transmission. *J Infect.* 2020;80(5):578–606. https://doi.org/10.1016/j.jinf.2020.02.020
2. World Health Organization. Novel coronavirus—Thailand (ex-China). January 14, 2020. Available at: https://www.who.int/emergencies/disease-outbreak-news/item/2020-DON234. Accessed Accessed February 3, 2024.
3. Jindahra P, Wongboonsin K, Wongboonsin P. Demographic and initial outbreak patterns of COVID-19 in Thailand. *J Popul Res (Canberra).* 2022;39(4):567–588. https://doi.org/10.1007/s12546-021-09276-y
4. Department of Disease Control. OPENDATA Covid19 Thailand. Available at: https://covid19.ddc.moph.go.th/en. Accessed February 22, 2024.
5. World Health Organization. Novel coronavirus (2019-nCoV) situation reports. Available at: https://www.who.int/thailand/emergencies/novel-coronavirus-2019/situation-reports. Accessed February 22, 2024.
6. World Health Organization. Announcement designating COVID-19 as a dangerous communicable disease. Available at: https://www.who.int/thailand/news/detail/29-02-2020-announcement-designating-covid-19-as-a-dangerous-communicable-disease. Accessed February 22, 2024.
7. Rajatanavin N, Tuangratananon T, Suphanchaimat R, Tangcharoensathien V. Responding to the COVID-19 second wave in Thailand by diversifying and adapting lessons from the first wave. *BMJ Glob Health.* 2021;6(7):1–9. https://doi.org/10.1136/bmjgh-2021-006178
8. Wetchapanpesat, S. Strategic plan: Covid-19 strategy: managing the new wave of the Covid-19 epidemic. Ministry of Public Health. January 2021. Available at: https://ddc.moph.go.th/viralpneumonia/eng/file/main/en_Thailand%20Covid-19%20plan_MOPH_2021.pdf. Accessed January 31, 2024.
9. Department of Disease Control. Corona virus disease (COVID-19). Available at: https://ddc.moph.go.th/viralpneumonia/eng/situation.php. Accessed February 22, 2024.
10. Puenpa J, Rattanakomol P, Saengdao N, et al. Molecular characterisation and tracking of severe acute respiratory syndrome coronavirus 2 in Thailand, 2020–2022. *Arch Virol.* 2023;168(1):26. https://doi.org/10.1007/s00705-022-05666-6
11. Home isolation for asymptomatic COVID-19 patients waiting for hospital beds. Thai PBS World. Available at: https://www.thaipbsworld.com/home-isolation-for-asymptomatic-covid-19-patients-waiting-for-hospital-beds. Accessed August 12, 2023.
12. Department of Medical Services. COVID-19. Available at: https://covid19.dms.go.th/Content/Select_Landding_page?contentId=136. Accessed February 22, 2024.
13. Bangprapa M. 100K in home isolation. *Bangkok Post.* August 6, 2021. Available at: https://www.bangkokpost.com/thailand/general/2160663/100k-in-home-isolation. Accessed February 22, 2024.
14. National Science and Technology Development Agency. NSTDA develops AMED Telehealth to support COVID-19 home isolation program. September 23, 2021. Available at: https://www.nstda.or.th/en/news/news-years-2021/nstda-develops-amed-telehealth-to-support-covid-19-home-isolation-program.html. Accessed August 21, 2023.
15. Triukose S, Nitinawarat S, Satian P, et al. Effects of public health interventions on the epidemiological spread during the first wave of the COVID-19 outbreak in Thailand. *PLoS One.* 2021;16(2):e0246274. https://doi.org/10.1371/journal.pone.0246274
16. Jindahra P, Wongboonsin K, Wongboonsin P. Demographic and initial outbreak patterns of COVID-19 in Thailand. *J Popul Res (Canberra).* 2022;39(4):567–588. https://doi.org/10.1007/s12546-021-09276-y
17. Zhang W, Koetwibun C, Eng B. A comparative study of the first and second waves of the COVID-19 pandemic response in Thailand. *J Health Sci.* 2022;31(suppl 2):S234-S246.
18. Delta variant accounts for 97.6% of new COVID infections in Bangkok. Thai PBS World. Available at: https://www.thaipbsworld.com/delta-variant-accounts-for-97-6-of-new-covid-infections-in-bangkok. Accessed February 7, 2024.
19. Kumar N, Mathew G, Huchchannavar R. Home-based care programme (HBCP) for patients with COVID -19: boon or burden during pandemic management? *Biomedicine (Taipei).* 2023;43(2):649–654. https://doi.org/10.51248/.v43i02.2596
20. Dutey-Magni PF, Williams H, Jhass A, et al. COVID-19 infection and attributable mortality in UK care homes: cohort study using active surveillance and electronic records (March–June 2020). *Age Ageing.* 2021;50(4):1019–1028. https://doi.org/10.1093/ageing/afab060
21. Shaver J. The state of telehealth before and after the COVID-19 pandemic. *Prim Care.* 2022;49(4):517–530. https://doi.org/10.1016/j.pop.2022.04.002
22. FAIR Health. Monthly Telehealth Regional Tracker. Available at: https://www.fairhealth.org/fh-trackers/telehealth. Accessed February 7, 2024.
23. Home care for patients with COVID-19 presenting with mild symptoms and management of their contacts: interim guidance, 17 March 2020. Geneva, Switzerland: World Health Organization; 2020.
24. European Centre for Disease Prevention and Control. *Infection Prevention and Control in the Household Management of People With Suspected or Confirmed Coronavirus Disease (COVID-19).* 2020. Available at: https://www.ecdc.europa.eu/en/publications-data/infection-prevention-control-household-management-covid-19. Accessed February 20, 2024.
25. United Nations in Thailand. *Home Isolation Guidebook.* Available at: https://thailand.un.org/en/167490-home-isolation-guidebook. Accessed February 7, 2024.
26. Sagheb S, Gholamrezanezhad A, Pavlovic E, Karami M, Fakhrzadegan M. Country-based modelling of COVID-19 case fatality rate: a multiple regression analysis. *World J Virol.* 2024;13(1):87881. https://doi.org/10.5501/wjv.v13.i1.87881
27. Klein SL, Flanagan KL. Sex differences in immune responses. *Nat Rev Immunol.* 2016;16(10):626–638. https://doi.org/10.1038/nri.2016.90
28. Ghosh S, Klein RS. Sex drives dimorphic immune responses to viral infections. *J Immunol.* 2017;198(5):1782–1790. https://doi.org/10.4049/jimmunol.1601166
29. Matsuyama R, Nishiura H, Kutsuna S, Hayakawa K, Ohmagari N. Clinical determinants of the severity of Middle East respiratory syndrome (MERS): a systematic review and meta-analysis. *BMC Public Health.* 2016;16(1):1203. https://doi.org/10.1186/s12889-016-3881-4
30. Zumla A, Hui DS, Perlman S. Middle East respiratory syndrome. *Lancet.* 2015;386(9997):995–1007. https://doi.org/10.1016/S0140-6736(15)60454-8
31. Karlberg J, Chong DSY, Lai WYY. Do men have a higher case fatality rate of severe acute respiratory syndrome than women do? *Am J Epidemiol.* 2004;159(3):229–231. https://doi.org/10.1093/aje/kwh056
32. Um JY, Chung HS, Song MY, Shin HD, Kim HM. Association of interleukin-1β gene polymorphism with body mass index in women. Clin Chem. 2004;50(3):647–650. https://doi.org/10.1373/clinchem.2003.025858
33. Zhang C, Wu Z, Li JW, Zhao H, Wang GQ. Cytokine release syndrome in severe COVID-19: interleukin-6 receptor antagonist tocilizumab may be the key to

reduce mortality. *Int J Antimicrob Agents.* 2020;55(5):105954. https://doi.org/10.1016/j.ijantimicag.2020.105954

34. Delgado-Roche L, Mesta F. Oxidative stress as key player in severe acute respiratory syndrome coronavirus (SARS-CoV) infection. *Arch Med Res.* 2020;51(5):384–387. https://doi.org/10.1016/j.arcmed.2020.04.019
35. Stefan N, Birkenfeld AL, Schulze MB, Ludwig DS. Obesity and impaired metabolic health in patients with COVID-19. *Nat Rev Endocrinol.* 2020;16(7):341–342. https://doi.org/10.1038/s41574-020-0364-6
36. National Health Security Office. What should individuals do if they suspect they have contracted COVID-19? Available at: https://www.nhso.go.th/news/3462. Accessed February 11, 2024.
37. Phanuphak N. Home isolation, community isolation, aimed at curbing COVID-19 deaths and new infections in Thailand. National Health Security Office. July 30, 2021. Available at: https://eng.nhso.go.th/view/1/home/IN%20DEPTH/359/EN-US. Accessed February 11, 2024.
38. Park JJ, Seo YB, Lee J, Na SH, Choi YK. Original research: protocol and clinical characteristics of patients under 'at-home care' for COVID-19 in South Korea: a retrospective cohort study. *BMJ Open.* 2022;12(6):e61765. https://doi.org/10.1136/bmjopen-2022-061765
39. Thailand steps up home isolation as virus cases strain hospitals. Reuters. August 2, 2021. Available at: https://www.reuters.com/business/healthcare-pharmaceuticals/thailand-steps-up-home-isolation-virus-cases-strain-hospitals-2021-08-02. Accessed August 9, 2023.
40. Wipatayotin A. Bed shortage prompts new treatment strategy. *Bangkok Post.* June 26, 2021. Available at: https://www.bangkokpost.com/thailand/general/2138707/bed-shortage-prompts-new-treatment-strategy. Accessed August 2, 2023.

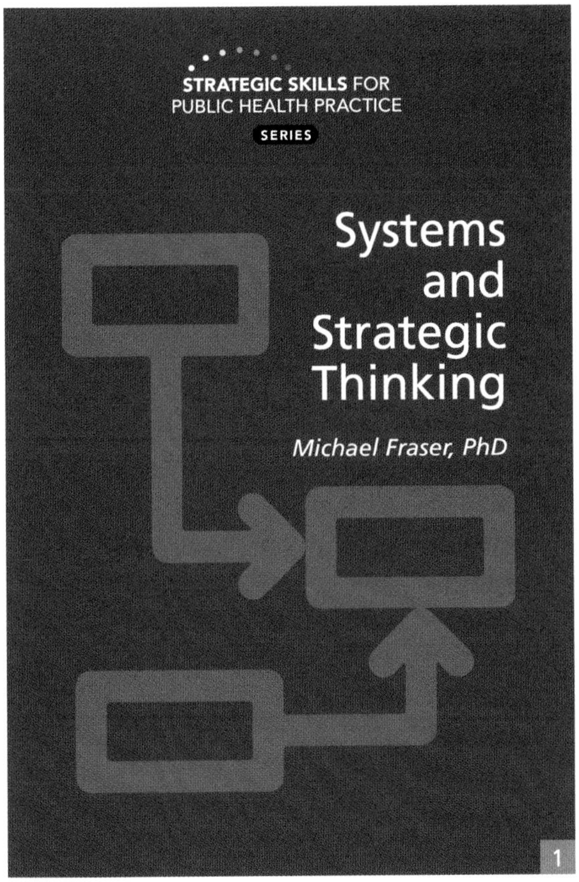

ISBN 978-0-87553-350-6, 2025, 120 PAGES,
SOFTCOVER

Strategic Skills for Public Health Practice: Systems and Strategic Thinking

By Michael Fraser

This primer defines and explains the importance of systems and strategic thinking, the essential skill for public health practitioners at the local, state, and federal levels. The book also details how systems thinking can help public health managers stimulate their teams to share different experiences, knowledge and perspectives to solve important public health challenges.

Systems and Strategic Thinking — part of the *Strategic Skills for Public Health Practice Series* — outlines a new way of approaching problems and solutions from a perspective that emphasizes interconnectedness, relationships, patterns and synergies. Systems and Strategic Thinking provides a framework practitioners can use to intervene in complex public health issues, moving their efforts from individual program silos toward approaches that take a more holistic point of view.